FIFTH EDITION

PHILOSOPHICAL *and* THEORETICAL PERSPECTIVES

for Advanced Nursing Practice

Edited by

WILLIAM K. CODY, PHD, RN, FAAN

Dean
Presbyterian School of Nursing
Queens University of Charlotte
Charlotte, North Carolina

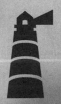

JONES & BARTLETT
LEARNING

World Headquarters
Jones & Bartlett Learning
5 Wall Street
Burlington, MA 01803
978-443-5000
info@jblearning.com
www.jblearning.com

Jones & Bartlett Learning books and products are available through most bookstores and online booksellers. To contact Jones & Bartlett Learning directly, call 800-832-0034, fax 978-443-8000, or visit our website, www.jblearning.com.

Substantial discounts on bulk quantities of Jones & Bartlett Learning publications are available to corporations, professional associations, and other qualified organizations. For details and specific discount information, contact the special sales department at Jones & Bartlett Learning via the above contact information or send an email to specialsales@jblearning.com.

Production Credits
Publisher: Kevin Sullivan
Acquisitions Editor: Amanda Harvey
Editorial Assistant: Sara Bempkins
Associate Production Editor: Sara Fowles
Marketing Manager: Elena McAnespie
V.P., Manufacturing and Inventory Control: Therese Connell
Composition: Laserwords Private Limited, Chennai, India
Cover Design: Kristin E. Parker
Cover Image: © Digoarpi/Dreamstime.com
Printing and Binding: Malloy, Inc.
Cover Printing: Malloy, Inc.

Library of Congress Cataloging-in-Publication Data
Philosophical and theoretical perspectives for advanced nursing practice--5th ed./[edited by] William K. Cody.
    p.;cm.
Includes bibliographical references and index.
ISBN 978-0-7637-6570-5 (pbk.)
I. Cody, William K.
[DNLM: 1. Nursing Theory. 2. Evidence-Based Nursing. 3. Nursing--trends. 4. Nursing Research. 5. Philosophy, Nursing. WY 86]
610.7301—dc23

2011041301

6048
Printed in the United States of America
16 15 14 13 12   10 9 8 7 6 5 4 3

Contents

Chapter 12
Healing as Appreciating Wholeness 119
W. Richard Cowling, III, RN, PhD

Chapter 13
Thinking Upstream: Nurturing a Conceptual Understanding of the Societal Context of Health Behavior 139
Patricia G. Butterfield, RN, MS

Chapter 14
Environmental Paradigms: Moving Toward an Ecocentric Perspective 149
Dorothy Kleffel, RN, MPH, DNSc

Chapter 21
Rapture and Suffering with Technology in Nursing 257
Rozzano C. Locsin, RN, PhD, FAAN and Marguerite J. Purnell, RN, PhD, AHN-BC

Chapter 22
Exploring an Alternative Metaphor for Nursing:
Relinquishing Military Images and Language 267
Gail J. Mitchell, RN, PhD, Mary Ferguson-Paré, RN, PhD, CHE,
and Joy Richards, RN, PhD

Barbara Paterson, RN, PhD

Chapter 23
Nursing Science in the Global Community 279
Shaké Ketefian, RN, EdD, FAAN and Richard W. Redman, RN, PhD

Chapter 31
The Nurse Scholar of the 21st Century 369
Sandra Schimdt Bunkers, RN, PhD, FAAN

Preface

The practice of nursing at an advanced level requires a deep understanding of theory and the ability to apply theory effectively in providing healthcare services to people. Indeed, if such understanding and ability is not found within a given nurse, in any specialty whatsoever, his or her practice cannot be considered to be advanced at all. This text, therefore, was originally edited by the late Janet Kenney and has been further revised by William Cody in this new fifth edition to meet the needs of students in graduate programs in nursing. The fifth edition establishes a reflective dialogue with a variety of contemporary perspectives of nursing practice to help students develop their own perspectives of nursing practice and to grow in their abilities to apply theories effectively.

The place of theory in nursing practice has, in reality, long been considered somewhat vague and tenuous. A situation persists today, referred to as the "theory–practice gap," in which theory and practice are perceived as interacting imperfectly, infrequently, and sometimes insignificantly. What nurses on a trajectory to enter into advanced practice must understand is that it is vital for advanced practice nurses of all stripes to possess deep understandings of knowledge that can only be learned through the formal study of nursing—which means precisely philosophical and theoretical perspectives of nursing—and to master the skills of using that knowledge in service to humankind. This value for specialized knowledge is at the core of any and every discipline.

All formalized and regulated professional practice is guided by some kind of knowledge. Such knowledge is developed, traditionally, in and between and around disciplines. Although the topographical map of disciplines across academe has shifted and morphed appreciably in the past several decades, it is still the case that disciplines exist to serve humankind through astute stewardship of knowledge within a circumscribed area. Advanced practitioners and scholars within a discipline continually push the boundaries of knowledge within that discipline and are generally the only persons sanctioned by society to do so. It would be irresponsible of any discipline to elevate persons within it to positions of authority and influence who have not demonstrated a reasonable mastery of the disciplinary knowledge.

Knowing is a process. Knowledge itself is process. It is not any one thing permanently.

The volume of information available to persons of means in the developed areas of the globe has roughly doubled every 18 months since the beginning of the information age toward the end of the previous millennium, and this process continues. Memorization of facts, data, and techniques is an entirely outmoded way of preparing professionals for practice in the new millennium. Rather, it is the process of coming to know, the values that provide the reasons for wanting to know, and the evidence that is adduced to establish a warrant for believing anything that require deep reflection, analysis, and open-ended dialogue. This book is designed to facilitate such reflective and dialogical processes.

William K. Cody, PhD, RN, FAAN

Authors

Donna L. Algase, RN, PhD, FAAN, FGSA

Othmar F. Arnold, RN, BScN

Cynthia Arslanian-Engoren, RN, PhD

Barbara E. Banfield, BSN, MSN, PhD

Anne Boykin, PhD

Anne Bruce, RN, PhD

Sandra Schmidt Bunkers, RN, PhD, FAAN

Patricia G. Butterfield, RN, MS

Barbara A. Carper, RN, EdD

William K. Cody, PhD, RN, FAAN

W. Richard Cowling, III, RN, PhD

Gweneth H. Doane, RN, PhD

Joyce J. Fitzpatrick, PhD, FAAN

Jacqueline Fawcett, RN, PhD, FAAN

Mary Ferguson-Paré, RN, PhD, CHE

Frank D. Hicks, RN, PhD

Joy L. Johnson, RN, PhD

Helga Jónsdóttir, RN, PhD

Janet W. Kenney, RN, PhD

Shaké Ketefian, RN, EdD, FAAN

Dorothy Kleffel, RN, MPH, DNSc

Merian C. Litchfield, RN, PhD

Rozzano C. Locsin, RN, PhD, FAAN

Brendan McCormack, DPhil(Oxon), BScNsg(Hons), PGCEA, RGN, RMN

Gail J. Mitchell, RN, PhD

Betty Neuman, PhD, FAAN

Rosemarie Rizzo Parse, RN, PhD, FAAN

Nola J. Pender, RN, PhD, FAAN

John R. Phillips, RN, PhD

Teri Britt Pipe, RN, PhD

Marguerite J. Purnell, RN, PhD, AHN-BC

Richard W. Redman, RN, PhD

Pamela G. Reed, RN, PhD, FAAN

Francelyn M. Reeder, RN, PhD

Joy Richards, RN, PhD

Rozella M. Schlotfeldt, RN, PhD, FAAN

Savina Schoenhofer, PhD

Colleen Varcoe, RN, PhD

Patricia Hinton Walker, PhD, FAAN

Jean Watson, PhD, FAAN

Ann L. Whall, RN, PhD, FAAN, FGSA

Judith Wuest, RN, MN

PART ONE

The Nursing Discipline and the Development of Nursing Knowledge

Florence Nightingale is hailed throughout the English-speaking world as the founder of modern nursing. Because she was a woman of action and a great advocate for improvements in health care in the 19th century British Empire, it is often forgotten that Florence Nightingale was primarily a writer.

Her great and lasting influence in health care came about through the power of her ideas laid out in prose and circulated in official reports, essays, and books.

Nightingale is sometimes thought of as the first nurse theorist (Tomey & Alligood, 2010), although it is doubtful that she would have understood what the term meant had she heard it in the 1850s. Focusing largely on hygiene, nutrition, and rest, Nightingale (1859/1969) created a system for delivering effective care to patients in the context of her time. She created schools for the training of women called to do this work, and she recorded her ideas in writing for preservation and dissemination. Formal schools modeled more or less on the Nightingale model grew up rapidly in the late 19th century. The trend spread to America, where it proliferated. Although its progenitor was unquestionably an intellectual giant of her time, nursing was not viewed by many, over the ensuing decades, as a highly intellectual pursuit. The Anglo-American tradition of nursing, from Nightingale's time until very recently, was construed largely as vocational rather than professional, as applied rather than basic science, and as a subordinate category of labor rather than a distinct and learned discipline.

Nursing history reflects a number of important events in the first century after Nightingale opened her schools, such as the emergence of formalized public health nursing and university education for nurses. The creation of new models of nursing and the dissemination of eloquent discourse about concepts and principles of nursing were hardly expected during that era, however, and developments in nursing philosophy and theory were few and far between. It was not until the publication of Hildegarde Peplau's *Interpersonal Relations in Nursing* in 1952 that a work of scholarship named as a theory of nursing by its author was published. Slowly, additions to the literature on philosophy and theory in nursing began to appear.

Considerable nursing theoretical literature in the 1950s and 1960s focused on simply naming what many nurses believed to be present in the content and context of the best nursing (e.g., Henderson, 1966). A feature of the evolving literature was the borrowing and application of theories and concepts from other disciplines, which can be detected to some extent in most of the various frameworks put forth (see Tomey & Alligood, 2010). The whole interesting project of the creation of theory to guide nursing practice became a popular topic in the scholarly nursing literature. Such endeavors came to be viewed as extremely important to nursing's future among nurse scholars who laid the groundwork for the nursing theory-based

practice movement that continues in force today.

Perhaps the most salient feature of the nursing theoretical literature that arose in the 1960s was the notion that the whole person and health in all its dimensions, taken together, comprise the proper focus of nursing care. When this idea first arose, it was taken for granted that the proper approaches for study or care planning would be to merely alternate or combine extant biological, psychological, sociological, and spiritual concepts and methods. In 1970 Martha Rogers put forward a radically different vision of nursing science as a new emergent in human history with a new and unique single focus: the unitary human being, more than and different from the sum of parts and knowable only as unitary, not through particulate approaches. Thus, a new paradigm of nursing was born.

The 1970s and 1980s were an exciting time in the evolution of nursing philosophy and theory. During those decades at least 20 significant nursing frameworks intended to guide practice were published; the notion that a nurse, a nursing unit, and a nursing school should have an explicit theoretical framework for practice was popularized; research to test and expand the extant frameworks became more common and proliferated in doctoral programs in nursing; and thus discourse about philosophy and theory in nursing became a permanent and indispensable constituent of nursing scholarship. Through the early 1990s the literature was rife with spirited dialogue and debate around issues of nursing philosophy and theory.

In the last decade much of the scholarly dialogue and debate in nursing centered around issues of practice and research in which the preceding discourses about philosophy and theory seemingly played little part. Master's programs in nursing increasingly turned into practitioner programs (and now doctor of nursing practice programs) largely teaching medical knowledge, and schools with doctoral programs in nursing increasingly focused on research that would bring in government funding, which was rarely framed in a context of nursing's disciplinary knowledge. Nevertheless, there is today a sense that a critical mass has been achieved, a corner has been turned, a milestone has been passed. Now, rooted precisely in the philosophy and theory of nursing there are very real reasons that a talented person might choose to become a nurse rather than a physician, a psychologist, or a social worker. Further, there are intriguing ideas in nursing philosophy and theory that can be explored more thoroughly through nursing scholarship than through any other means. There are also challenges to human betterment that nursing may well be the discipline best suited philosophically to meet. Whether or not nurse scholars make extensive use of nursing's extant theories or fervently embrace nursing's stated paradigms, most nurse scholars today would agree with these assertions. The distinctiveness of nursing's disciplinary knowledge base is a reality that cannot be ignored.

In Part One of this book, five scholars explore questions that are fundamental to understanding the knowledge base of the discipline. In Chapter 1, I seek to bring clarity to the evidence-based practice movement through a discussion of fundamental assumptions underlying evidence-based care and values-based practice. I propose a new way of looking at evidence and values that, hopefully, then can be used in turn to shed light and spark discussion of the remainder of the book. In Chapter 2, Schlotfeldt discusses considerations in determining what constitutes the knowledge base of the discipline of nursing, and then identifies five areas for systematic inquiry to grow the knowledge base of nursing. In Chapter 3, a much-cited article, Carper discusses fundamental patterns of knowing in nursing, which she groups into four: empirics, esthetics, personal knowledge, and moral knowledge.

In Chapter 4, Fawcett offers one view of nursing science, rooted in the value for nursing theory-guided practice and research. Fawcett finds the contemporary literature lacking in this regard and actually expresses fear for the survival of the discipline. Even a casual observer of nursing can easily discern that Fawcett's assertions are accurate regarding the dearth of nursing science in the greater portion of "nursing" research and "nursing" practice in contemporary society. What, then, does the dearth of nursing science in the activities of professional nurses mean for the future of nursing? For Fawcett, it represents an opportunity to issue a rallying cry for all nurses to become nurse scholars and for commensurate changes in our educational structures and processes. Certainly, it is clear that mastery of the complexities and subtleties inherent in values-based practice and evidence-based care requires education and scholarship that is both broad and deep. Readers are invited to picture a world in which all nurses are prepared as scholars to achieve that mastery. In Chapter 5, Phillips asks and answers the question What constitutes nursing science? In Chapter 6 (written by this author in 1994), I assert that the realization of nursing theory-guided practice is perhaps the greatest challenge that nursing as a scholarly discipline has ever faced. In light of the many challenges faced by nursing in many contexts, this is quite a claim, and it was not made lightly. I offer what I believe to be a useful definition of nursing theory. I also call for a more explicit acknowledgment of the fact that values, above all, guide practice. In Chapter 7, Litchfield and Jónsdóttir contemplate nursing as a practice discipline using a participatory model. In this section readers are invited to consider in several different ways the questions that are fundamental to generate knowledge to guide advanced practice in nursing.

References

Henderson, V. (1966). The nature of nursing: *A definition and its implications for practice, research, and education.* New York: Macmillan.

Nightingale, F. (1969). *Notes on nursing: What it is and what it is not.* New York: Dover. [Original published in 1859.]

Peplau, H. E. (1952). *Interpersonal relations in nursing.* New York: G. P. Putnam's Sons.

Rogers, M. E. (1970). *An introduction to the theoretical basis of nursing.* Philadelphia: F. A. Davis.

Tomey, A. M., & Alligood, M. R. (Eds.). (2010). *Nursg theorists and their work* (75th ed.). St. Louis, MO: Mosby.

CHAPTER 1

Values-Based Practice and Evidence-Based Care: Pursuing Fundamental Questions in Nursing Philosophy and Theory

William K. Cody, PhD, RN, FAAN

Possibly the single most important philosophical question to be posed within a practice discipline is "what guides practice?" In nursing, historically, a long list of traditions and rules from a variety of sources served to guide practice before (and since) the advent of nursing theories. In science, traditionally, the short answer to the question "what guides practice?" usually has been rendered as theory, and nursing has developed a strong body of theories; however, many powerful and subtle forces influence choices in practice. By reflecting on the manifold influences on one's choices in practice, the practitioner can construct a personal answer to the fundamental question "what guides my practice?"

A clear understanding of what guides practice helps the practitioner to pursue useful knowledge more efficiently, to represent one's disciplinary perspective more articulately, and to communicate more effectively with clients and the multidisciplinary team. This book is concerned with philosophical and theoretical perspectives to guide nursing practice. It is important to note that nursing could not take its place in the academic sun and be recognized as the distinct discipline that it is today until it could point to a domain of human knowledge specific to the discipline, knowable only through the formal study of nursing (Coyne, 1981). This domain was mapped through the creative, deliberative construction of nursing theories over the past 50 years.

Value-Laden Theory and the Fallacy of Value-Free Science

A theory's power is proportionate to the breadth of situations and events it can encompass. There are a number of frameworks in nursing that are capable of guiding nursing practice across a range of situations and events, which reflects the maturity of nursing's knowledge base. Some nurse scholars have expressed doubt that these frameworks can guide practice broadly because they are abstract or because they are humanistic in orientation or because they include nonobjective dimensions or because many have not been extensively tested under controlled conditions. Grounding of a theoretical framework in an underlying philosophy, however, strengthens the theory as a guide to practice by making explicit the assumptions and values that form its underpinnings. Many nursing frameworks have explicitly incorporated values such as caring, profound respect for all persons, and attentive presence into their conceptualizations and propositions. Learning these frameworks has profoundly changed the lives of many advanced practice nurses.

In the mid-twentieth century, a movement for "value-free" science rooted in the philosophies of science known as positivism, logical positivism, and logical empiricism wielded pervasive influence. This movement in its various guises sought essentially to purge science of all thought not arising from either empirical observation or strict rules of logic. Its influence on the sciences has lingered despite subsequent developments in philosophy of science that weakened or refuted most of its claims (Proctor, 1991). The fact that scientists are human means that science cannot be value free. Values are fundamental constituents of the human lifeworld. Indeed, there is warrant to say even that science itself is a value. That nursing's body of theory is heavily and explicitly value laden can today be seen as a strength, not a weakness, of our body of knowledge.

The hopes and expectations that grew strong in the 1980s, that nurses, nursing units, and nursing schools would adopt, use, support, and grow nursing's own theories have today been somewhat diminished by the influences of other forces converging upon the practice of nursing. These forces are multifarious and include the advent of prospective payment systems, shortened hospital lengths of stay, digitization of healthcare documentation, higher education of influential nurses in nonnursing disciplines, and the persistent need for two-year nursing programs to meet workforce demands. Along with all of these factors, the attenuated growth of the nursing theory movement can also be attributed to the failure of many members of our own discipline to recognize the uniqueness and value of our own body of knowledge and to face down criticisms from other quarters courageously.

The Clarion Call for Evidence-Based Practice

In contemporary nursing, there is a persistent clarion call to adopt evidence-based practice, implement it, teach it, study it, and standardize it (Melnyk & Fineout-Overholt, 2004). Many nurse leaders holding advanced degrees would answer the question "what guides nursing practice?" today by saying without hesitation, "Evidence." Evidence-based practice refers, in the main, to the use of rigorously derived empirical findings preferentially as the basis for intervention and nonintervention. It is not unique to nursing. The nomenclature for this movement varies, and one sees literature referring to evidence-based practice and literature referring to evidence-based care. In this chapter, a basis for differentiating the two will be proposed.

The evidence-based practice movement, although centered on the findings of empirical research and the findings of integrative reviews of empirical research, includes proponents of various different kinds of evidence, including ethical considerations and other dimensions of life (Goodman, 2003). The movement is not without its internal controversies and divergent views (e.g., Franks, 2004; Timmermans & Berg, 2003; Welsh & Lyons, 2001). Still, for the most part, the movement and the vast majority of the related literature focus on the use of rigorous and replicable research findings to inform, or even determine, questions of intervention and nonintervention in healthcare.

Standards of care can be said to approximate the state of the art in evidence-based practice. Note here the difference in terminology (standards of care), which is significant. A set of standards of care is typically based on multiple research studies accumulated over time. It is constructed by large panels of experts to provide practitioners with a well-thought out synthesis of the available evidence for intervention and nonintervention. These standards of care adhere predominantly to the medical model in their approach, but they are commonly used by nurses, health educators, and others. Some sets of standards achieve such familiarity among practitioners across disciplines that they are known chiefly by brief acronyms such as "JNC-7," which is the Seventh Report of the Joint National Committee on Prevention, Detection, Evaluation and Treatment of High Blood Pressure (U.S. Department of Health and Human Services, 2004). Equivalent sets of guidelines exist for many diseases and conditions. It would be difficult to argue against such standards of care within the parameters for which they are designed because they represent feats of combined intellectual achievement that no one person could conceivably match. They help to ensure the availability of the consensus of best reasoned options for care to millions of people.

The evidence base for many of the conventions of tradition-laden and routinized healthcare, however, the truth be told, can be rather weak. Also, for any number of possible unique acts of intervention or caregiving, there may be no research evidence at all. Does this mean, then, that we have no guide for practice in human situations in which there is insufficient research to support recommendations? Or does it mean that knowledge resources other than strongly conclusive research must be brought to bear on situations as guides to practice? Goodman (2003) proposes dealing with uncertainty (as to treatment) in medicine through "management, acknowledgement, and reduction [of the uncertainty]" (p. 131). Interestingly, Goodman does not turn to values for guidance in the absence of convincing evidence one way or another. One aim of the evidence-based practice movement is to minimize bias, and attention to the values of the practitioner can be read as an open invitation to allow bias to rule. Such an interpretation of the dynamics of personal and professional values in practice ignores the fact that many or most healthcare practitioners in fact have a value (i.e., a bias) for objective evidence of efficacy and for the use of good evidence in planning care. With or without evidence, it is the practitioner's values that drive her or his performance in providing care.

In reality, no formal guide to practice or any body of knowledge in any discipline can be both broad and specific enough to guide all actions in every situation. Practitioners are human, and life is complex, ever-changing, and unpredictable. Historically, this philosophical problem has been discussed in the discourse concerned with praxis.

Understanding Praxis

The discourse on evidence-based practice in nursing could benefit from an exploration of the literature on praxis, a concept that has been well examined from ancient times to the present. In demurring from engagement with the literature on praxis, the proponents of evidence-based practice limit discussion of considerations other than evidence that have a strong bearing on practice.

Praxis has been defined and described in several different ways. Aristotle related praxis to human situations requiring practical reasoning to inform action. Habermas (1973), Freire (1993), and Bernstein (1999), in the 20th century, have contributed to our contemporary understandings of praxis, which always unfolds embedded in human situations replete with the complications of multidimensional human interactions, the uncertain, and the unknowable. Persons pursue reasoning related to their peculiar situations based on an understanding of what is good and what contributes to human well-being. Praxis and practical reasoning always unfold in a context that is profoundly interpersonal and relatively unpredictable. The end is not predetermined, and as possible ends evolve situationally, possible means evolve as well. Thus, praxis is creative and dialogical. In political and pedagogical discourse, praxis has even been explicated as the practice of freedom.

Practice as Praxis

If practice is examined in the light of this voluminous literature of over 2,000 years, it must be viewed as driven by far more than scientific evidence alone. Even the most die-hard logical positivist would concede, at a minimum, the need for a code of ethics to provide parameters of conduct for science-based practice. Many considerations other than scientific evidence can be identified as reasons for action and as knowledge to guide practice.

The practice of nursing is intentional and deliberate action, guided by nursing science and other sources of knowledge, performed by nurses, and intended for the benefit of persons and society. In this regard, it is comparable to other professional practices. The moment-to-moment acts of nursing practice are chosen from a wide variety of options by each individual nurse in the ever-unfolding and unpredictable context of interrelationships with persons, families and communities, their meanings to the persons involved, and the values that are interwoven among the meanings. The animus underlying nursing practice is the intention to benefit people. However, the actions, behaviors, and words that provide the benefits change from moment to moment with the situation.

Each nurse is responsible for her or his own practice in a fundamental and inescapable way. The actions entailed in professional nursing practice are also the responsibility of, and occur under the stewardship of, the nursing profession itself, by way of its regulatory bodies and professional associations. These bodies determine the expectations of all the nurses within their spheres of influence, and these expectations are laid out in accord with conventions such as the nursing process and standards of ethics. In short, practice is predominantly driven by the personal and professional values of the nurse. It is owned and controlled by the individual nurse to a great extent although governed by certain bodies representing the profession and the state.

Care

Human care is a recognizable and structured interaction in human societies through which persons give and receive assistance with basic human needs, in wellness and in illness, across the lifespan, before birth, throughout life, and beyond death. Specialized care of various kinds is delivered by professionals and is largely deemed to be deliverable only by such professionals. In contemporary society, human care, hereinafter care, should be and is largely consumer driven. Care delivery is governed, at the individual level, largely by the recipient of care or the guardian or designee of the recipient, who has the right to accept or refuse whatever care is offered.

It is axiomatic across healthcare disciplines that clients have a right to be offered care based on the best evidence available. It is not for the practitioner to decide ultimately what intervention, if any, the client will receive; rather, this decision rests with the client, who has the right to be well-informed about the evidence and to make a choice. What evidence is most valued by the practitioner varies from one practitioner to the other, but all are expected to adduce evidence to justify their recommendations and offerings to clients. It is important to note that from the practitioner perspective care is offered and, within the bounds of ethics, not ordered, required, or forced, for care, in a fundamental sense, belongs to the consumer. It is the consumer's to request, accept, or reject in accord with personal values. It is the professional's responsibility to offer that for which there is best evidence. As demonstrated above, this expectation is exemplified in the standards of care that delineate the best knowledge that the health sciences have to offer at a given time.

Differentiating Practice and Care

The discourse on evidence-based practice does not differentiate clearly between practice and care. This conflation of what should be two distinct concepts is especially troubling in nursing, wherein scholars have emphasized nursing's special commitment to care and caring for generations. Upon reflection, however, one can discern a fundamental difference between the nature and structure of professional practice on the one hand and the care that is delivered by professionals on the other. In **Table 1-1**, four ways of differentiating practice and care are specified.

Practice belongs to the practitioner and is driven by values. Only the actor has the agency to initiate and cease deliberate actions. The practitioner is assumed to have control over her or his own actions and to be responsible for them. Nothing can remove the onus of individual responsibility from any professional practitioner, neither haste in service to one's charges, nor pressure from one's hierarchical superiors, nor lack of key information. This responsibility and relative autonomy is further emphasized at the societal level by assigning control and governance of the profession largely to the members of the profession itself. Professional practice is governed by the individual practitioner, her or his discipline, the governments of states and countries, laws, and societal norms. Professional practice is relatively discipline specific in that education and licensure to perform complex and sophisticated tasks to benefit others, for pay, is typically regulated in a context of disciplinary knowledge, expertise, socialization, and customary expectations.

Practice is necessarily and profoundly practitioner driven. The knowledge base and decision-making capacity of the practitioner

Table 1-1   Differentiating Practice and Care

Practice	Care
Belongs to the practitioner	Belongs to the consumer
Controlled by the practitioner, by the profession, and by society	Controlled by the consumer, by rules/laws, and by society
More discipline-specific, because it is more practitioner driven	More interdisciplinary, because it is more consumer driven
Values based	Evidence based

are among the very defining factors of professional practice. Practice, as stated before, is highly contextual and situational. Many factors impinge on moment-to-moment decision-making in practice. No external resource for decision-making can be absorbed by the practitioner thoroughly and rapidly enough to inform all action or inaction in situation to an extent equal to individual knowledge and experience. This immediacy of intention and action is in the nature of all multidimensional, deliberative interactions among human beings.

That which most fundamentally drives one's practice is one's values. Values are by definition the cherished beliefs that prompt and inspire choices and actions over time. Making similar choices repeatedly and performing similar actions repeatedly over time confirms the value as an abiding cherished belief within one's world of meaning (Parse, 1998). The way a nurse practices and the way she or he provides care to persons reflects her or his personal and professional values (Woodbridge & Fulford, 2003). Spending time with clients may reflect a value for offering attentive presence. Frequently urging clients to make changes in health maintenance routines may reflect the values of norms or problem solving. One's values are constituents of who one is and thus are reflected in all that one does.

Care is the prerogative of the consumer and is structured by evidence. Only the consumer/client (or her/his legitimate designee) has the right to accept or reject care, even though typically care is designed and prescribed or recommended by others (i.e., professionals). This assertion is an outgrowth of the ongoing paradigm shift toward person-centered care, attending to the whole person, and respect for individual and cultural differences. The professional caregiver's responsibility is to see that the consumer's choice of care is informed and that the delivery of care is carried out competently. Legal protections and social sanctions exist to ensure that the consumer's rights to be well-informed and to receive competent care are protected.

As described above, standards of care represent something close to the consensus state of the art of evidence-based care. All clients of healthcare professionals have the right to expect that care will be offered that is structured to the extent possible in accord with broadly recognized standards of care.

Values-Based Practice and Evidence-Based Care

We live our values. The strongest confirmation of a value is to act on it repeatedly, which also describes rather precisely how we construe professional practice. The practitioner chooses how to practice based on personal values. The client chooses what care to receive based on personal values. The practitioner offers care to address the client's needs and desires, care that is structured based on the best evidence available.

As the philosopher Raz (2003) has pointed out in his book The Practice of Value, "Concepts of false values cannot have instances" (p. 24). This is another way of saying essentially that we live our values. To frame this proposition more colloquially, if you don't live it, it's not your value. In contrast, there can be false evidence. Indeed, the history of science is replete with instances of evidence misinterpreted and misunderstood. Evidence is a phenomenon that emerges only as evidence of something. The answer is already halfway there when the question is posed.

Standards of care are rewritten periodically based on newly emergent evidence, and it is not unusual for standards to seesaw back and forth between yea and nay to certain procedures between one edition of guidelines and the next. Surely something more substantial, lasting, and meaningful to both nurse and client must underpin nursing practice. To this author's way of thinking, that underpinning is found in the interface of personal meanings and values with the meanings and values structured in a theoretical framework for nursing practice. Readers are invited to use this text to assist them in identifying the values and meanings that inform and inspire their practice.

Suggestions for Further Reflection

In this chapter, I have sought to inspire and facilitate reflection on the question "what guides practice?" Many of the readings throughout the rest of this book put forward ideas about philosophy and theory in nursing that will prompt further reflection, and hopefully dialogue and debate, about the question.

In Chapter 3, Carper provides a schema for organizing the knowledge necessary for nursing practice, categorized as empirics, esthetic knowing, ethical knowing, and personal knowing. How do values and evidence relate to Carper's ways of knowing? Are values and evidence equally relevant to all types of knowing, or is evidence more pertinent to one type and are values more pertinent to another?

In Chapter 15, Parse describes how adopting an explicitly values-based theoretical perspective transforms practice. In Chapter 31, Bunkers puts forward 16 tenets for framing nursing knowledge for the 21st century, all of which are explicitly value laden. Evidence is scarcely mentioned at all. Does this mean that a philosophy that is explicitly values driven does not value evidence? Or does it mean that evidence accrues when one abides with the 16 value-laden tenets? In Chapter 20, Wuest discusses the contrast between traditional values of professionalism and the values of caring and justice reflected in the feminist literature. In Chapter 23, Ketefian and Redman propose that the process of knowledge development itself is embedded in systems of cultural values and perspectives and question whether it is appropriate for Western values by their dominance in science and the professions to shape knowledge development in non-Western societies. One might well ask, "How can one accurately perceive evidence if one is using the wrong cultural lens to seek it?"

In Johnson's examination of nursing art in Chapter 16, it is easy to see that values are threaded throughout the five conceptualizations of nursing art that she puts forth, but perhaps not so easy to ferret out the role of evidence in the performance of nursing art. Cowling, in Chapter 12, explicitly connects with a values-laden ontology in describing an appreciative practice method-ology and describing an ethos of relational narrative. In Chapter 13, Butterfield points out that in many cases, the evidence one seeks in order to understand health concerns may be found not at the individual level but at the societal level. How counterproductive, and arguably inhumane, for example, to press for behavior change at the individual level to resolve a difficulty that stems fundamentally from societal neglect?

In Chapter 10, Boykin and Schoenhofer reconceptualize outcomes in a way that challenges the hegemony within the outcomes literature of strict adherence to objective and quantifiable outcomes. In the theory of nursing as caring, rather, enhancing personhood is conceptualized as the central desired outcome.

The interplay of values and evidence in determining how to practice and what kind of care to deliver occurs at the very core of healthcare decision-making. The contemporary advanced practice nurse is challenged to develop the ability to appreciate and understand a wide variety of human values in a rapidly changing multicultural society. She or he is equally challenged to develop the ability to discern strong and weak evidence and how to structure healthcare services based on the preponderance of the evidence. Both abilities are cultivated best within the context of a broad and deep appreciation of theoretical and philosophical perspectives of nursing offered in this text.

References

Bernstein, R. J. (1999). Praxis and action: Contemporary philosophies of human activity. Philadelphia: University of Pennsylvania Press.

Coyne, A. B. (1981). Prologue. In R. R. Parse, Man-living-health: A theory of nursing (pp. vii–xii). New York: John Wiley.

Franks, V. (2004). Evidence-based uncertainty in mental health nursing. Journal of Psychiatric and Mental Health Nursing, 11, 99–105.

Freire, P. (1993). Pedagogy of the oppressed (M. B. Ramos, Trans.). New York: Continuum.

Goodman, K. W. (2003). Ethics and evidence-based medicine: Fallibility and responsibility in clinical science. Cambridge, UK: Cambridge University Press.

Habermas, J. (1973). Theory and practice (J. Viertel, Trans.) Boston, MA: Beacon.

Melnyk, B. M., & Fineout-Overholt, E. (2004). Evidence-based practice in nursing and healthcare: A guide to best practice. Philadelphia: Lippincott Williams & Wilkins.

Parse, R. R. (1998). The human becoming school of thought: A perspective for nurses and other health professionals. Thousand Oaks, CA: Sage.

Proctor, R. (1991). Value-free science? Purity and power in modern knowledge. Cambridge, MA: Harvard University Press.

Raz, J. (2003). The practice of value. Oxford, UK: Oxford University Press.

Timmermans, S., & Berg, M. (2003). The gold standard: The challenge of evidence-based medicine and standardization in health care. Philadelphia: Temple University Press.

U.S. Department of Health and Human Services. (2004). Seventh Report of the Joint National Committee on Prevention, Detection, Evaluation and Treatment of High Blood Pressure. Rockville, MD: Author.

Welsh, I., & Lyons, C. M. (2001). Evidence-based care and the case for intuition and tacit knowledge in clinical assessment and decision making in mental health nursing practice: An empirical contribution to the debate. Journal of Psychiatric and Mental Health Nursing, 8, 299–305.

Woodbridge, K., & Fulford, B. (2003). Good practice? Values-based practice in mental health. Mental Health Practice, 7(2), 30–34.

CHAPTER 2

Structuring Nursing Knowledge: A Priority for Creating Nursing's Future

Rozella M. Schlotfeldt, RN, PhD, FAAN

Nursing's future will be created only as the discipline underlying nursing practices is identified, structured, and continuously updated by systematic inquiry. The kinds of knowledge contained within the discipline are identified and an approach to its structure is proposed.

There can be little doubt that one of the highest priorities for creating an appropriate future for nursing is that of identifying, structuring, and continuously advancing the knowledge that underlies the practices of professionals in the field. That statement can be made because a consensus has not yet been attained concerning the subject matter that must be mastered by those who seek to practice general and specialized nursing. Surely by the beginning of the twenty-first century, nursing's body of knowledge will be identified, selected, verified, and agreed upon by qualified professionals in the field, effectively structured, and continuously updated to reflect newly discovered knowledge. Also, knowledge judged to be erroneous, inadequate, and outdated should be deleted. This knowledge will be derived from basic and clinical scientific nursing research, both quantitative and qualitative, from philosophic and historical inquiries, and from evaluation research designed to establish valid criterion measures, devices, and approaches to establishing the efficacy and value of nursing's caring functions as they are relevant to the health, function, comfort, well-being, productivity,

Source: Schlotfeldt, R. (1989). Structuring nursing knowledge: A priority for creating nursing's future. Nursing Science Quarterly, 1(1): 35–38. Reprinted by permission of and copyright © 2002 Sage Publications, Inc.

self-fulfillment, and happiness of human beings.

The thesis of this chapter is that only qualified professionals in the field, including general and specialist practitioners, educators, administrators, investigators, historians, philosophers, and theorists, should be given responsibility by the profession (however that is defined) to identify, verify, structure, and continuously update the extant content or subject matter that, at the minimum, should be included in the intellectual armamentaria of all professional nurses. This responsibility of the profession is essential to four functions: (a) the creation of comparable programs of study at the first professional degree level; (b) control of the profession's goals, mission, and accomplishments; (c) a valid procedure for licensing (not registering) all who qualify as professionals in the field; and (d) certification of bona fide nursing specialists.

Nursing as a Profession

Two major criteria must be fulfilled by any occupational group whose members earn and achieve the status of a profession, or more appropriately for nursing, a learned helping profession. First, a profession must have an institutionalized goal or social mission. Learned professions are valued by the societies whose members give them positive sanction for two major reasons: (a) the services learned professionals render are judged to be essential and beneficial for all members of society during particular times in their lives, and (b) members of each learned profession have identified and come to a consensus about the knowledge that practitioners must master and use selectively, creatively, humanely, effectively, and ethically in providing those essential services. As a second criterion, each profession must support a cadre of investigators whose role is to advance its knowledge continuously with a view toward improving its practices.

The traditional learned professions have included the clergy, lawyers, and physicians. The clergy have been valued and supported because they are expected to be knowledgeable and skillful in providing spiritual comfort and well-being for all those who consult them. Lawyers are expected to master coded law and to apply their discipline fairly and skillfully in fulfilling the goal of preserving social harmony and justice. Physicians have been valued because knowledge of human ills and disabilities and their causes and knowledge of the means to eliminate, attenuate, or manage them and alleviate their noxious consequences are considered essential to the well-being of society. Are the caring functions and mission of nurses, namely, appraising and optimizing the health, function, comfort, independence, and potential of human beings, any less valued than spiritual comfort and well-being? Are they any less desirable than social harmony and justice? Are they any less important than finding causes for, diagnosing, and treating human ills?

Unfortunately, the caring functions typically provided by nurses were for too long considered to be mere extensions of the duties and obligations of wives and mothers, for which large amounts of professional knowledge were not considered essential (Reverby, 1987). Lay members of societies have typically not recognized and nurses themselves have been remarkably tardy in identifying and organizing the several kinds of professional knowledge that are fundamental to executing the caring functions that nurses typically provide.

The essential and often crucial nature of nurses' caring functions in promoting the health and well-being of all human beings is finally being recognized by thinking people, including scholarly nurses. There is now general agreement (at least verbal agreement) that nursing's social mission is to appraise and assist human beings in their quest to optimize their health status, health assets, and health potential (Fawcett, 1983). Furthermore, general agreement exists that there is or should be a body of structured knowledge that professionals in the field agree represents the discipline that is fundamental to general and specialty nursing practices.

Nursing scholars have discussed, described, and characterized the discipline (Donaldson & Crowley, 1978), and in the recent past, the American Association of Colleges of Nursing (1986) has reported findings from a "national effort to define the essential knowledge, practice, and values that the baccalaureate nurse should possess" (p. 1). Panel members expressed the belief that the essentials so delineated can be achieved within the traditional baccalaureate degree program in nursing and that the baccalaureate represents first-level professional preparation in nursing.

The efforts that have been made toward establishing the discipline represent significant steps toward achieving the goal of identifying, organizing, and achieving a consensus concerning the specific body of extant knowledge that underlies nursing practices. It must be noted, however, that there has not yet been a concerted effort to identify and obtain agreement about the currently available knowledge that is fundamental to nursing's growing number of declared specialties or even to obtain a consensus about the requisite knowledge and skills that define what nursing's specialties are. It must be recognized also that the subject matter that constitutes the discipline has not yet been identified and structured, and agreement has not been reached concerning appropriate and needed inclusions from qualified professionals in the field. This paper presents an approach to organizing the several kinds of knowledge contained within the discipline, a possible next step toward having qualified professionals select and structure the specific extant subject matter of the discipline about which agreement is needed.

Knowledge of the Discipline

Figure 2-1 shows the kinds of professional knowledge contained within the discipline, which is depicted as a large sphere having a permeable and expandable membrane (represented by the second sphere) to permit the continuous addition of newly discovered knowledge and the deletion of

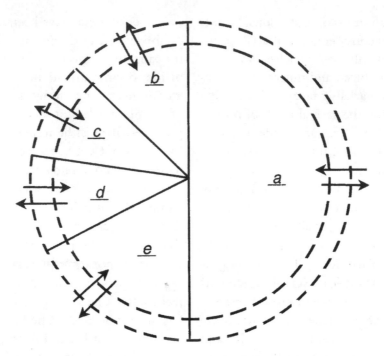

FIGURE 2-1 The Nursing Discipline

Source: Schlotfeldt, R. (1989). Structuring nursing knowledge: A priority for creating nursing's future. Nursing Science Quarterly, 1(1): 35–38. Reprinted by permission of and copyright © 2002 Sage Publications, Inc.

that found through systematic inquiry to be erroneous, inadequate, or irrelevant.

The largest segment of the sphere (**Figure 2-1a**) represents nursing's scientific subject matter. Therein belongs all of nursing science (i.e., the verified facts, principles, and laws that have been discovered through scientific inquiry to be valid, relevant, and useful for nursing practice); included also are extant scientific theories that guide scientific investigations in nursing and those that have been proposed by scholarly nurses as promising explanations of phenomena that are of particular concern to nurses.

To date, much of nursing science has been discovered by basic scientists and subsequently found through empirical evidence and systematic study to be relevant. Nurse investigators have also been adding to nursing's scientific knowledge by testing the relevance and utility of theories generated by basic scientists in clinical nursing situations (Chinn, 1984). Few investigations have yet been reported that test scientific theories regarding human phenomena that are of particular concern to nurses but not to basic scientists (Silva, 1986). A plausible reason is that there is little agreement among nurses concerning the human phenomena that are of concern to nurses and how they should be characterized and classified and how knowledge of them should be advanced.

In general, nurses accept the notion that human beings are biopsychosocial beings (Engel, 1977). It is proposed here that the subjects that nurses serve also exemplify assets of the human spirit of which relevant knowledge is inadequate. Those assets surely include human spirituality and other qualities of the human spirit, such as determination, verve, courage, beliefs, hope, and aspiration. Nurses surely hold responsibility for advancing knowledge of those health-seeking assets. In sum, human beings' health-seeking mechanisms and behaviors, beliefs, and propensities can be classified as biological, psychological (both emotional and cognitive), and sociocultural and as assets of the human spirit; all of them are directly relevant to the natural efforts by humans to seek and attain optimal health. Because so much scientific nursing knowledge remains to be discovered, it is safe to predict that nursing science will likely always represent the largest and most rapidly changing aspect of the discipline. Furthermore, nurses are increasingly recognizing the relevance of scientific knowledge from disciplines not traditionally judged to be relevant for nursing. Included, for example, are concepts, principles, and theories from economics, political science, administration and management, and computer science. The science fundamental to education has long been incorporated as an integral part of the discipline of nursing.

A second important segment of the sphere representing the nursing discipline is historical knowledge (**Figure 2-1b**). Included is knowledge of the heritage of the occupation and the developing profession of nursing, including knowledge of people, circumstances, and events that have shaped that development. Included also is the history of nursing knowledge as it has been transmitted to generations of practitioners.

The third section of the sphere (**Figure 2-1c**) represents philosophic nursing knowledge. Included are the profession's accepted values and codes of professional behavior. Included also should be the several philosophic theories that have been tested, found useful and relevant to nurses' work, and accepted as philosophic guides to practice. Illustrative are selected theories of value, justice and morality, and ethical theories. Because nurses are encountering increasing numbers of moral and ethical dilemmas and because nurses are increasingly manifesting interest in becoming scholars in the discipline of philosophy, it is predicted that nursing knowledge henceforth will include increasing amounts of tested and relevant philosophic knowledge that will be incorporated into the discipline.

The fourth section of the sphere (**Figure 2-1d**) represents knowledge of nursing strategies, approaches, and technologies along with the scientific and artistic principles essential to their execution. Included also is knowledge of the prevailing health care system. Relationships between the goals and caring functions of nurses and the goals and practice functions of other health professionals in the existing health care systems represent another important segment of the discipline.

Another significant segment of nursing's body of knowledge has always been knowledge of factors that influence the health status, health assets, and health potential of human beings, both favorably and unfavorably (**Figure 2-1e**). Included is knowledge of biological, physical, and cognitive abilities with which people are naturally endowed and knowledge of environmental factors, economic and social circumstances, and changes associated with normal development, including the aging process. In the nursing perspective presented here, pathologies and medical diagnoses and treatments are factors that affect the health of human beings. Nurses must have adequate knowledge of these factors: such knowledge is an integral part of the discipline that must be mastered by nurse practitioners.

There is yet another kind of knowledge that is directly relevant to and essential for nursing practice. It is the knowledge that professionals must gain from relevant data concerning each person being served and that obtained through astute and perceptive observations. Personal knowledge of individuals and groups of persons is needed for nurses to respect the uniqueness of those for whom they provide exemplary services. For that reason, there can be no prescriptive nursing practice theories or professional approaches to nursing care that are universally generalizable.

In summary, conceptualizing the discipline of nursing as an expandable and permeable sphere made up of segments of varying size provides an approach to classifying and organizing the several kinds of knowledge that constitute the nursing discipline. Such

an approach demonstrates the vast and growing amounts of knowledge that professionals in the field must master and be able to use selectively, creatively, artistically, humanely, and skillfully to provide exemplary care.

Nursing should be recognized as a learned helping profession and a respected academic discipline. Surely nursing scholars will ensure the attainment of those goals by the beginning of the twenty-first century. Crucial to their attainment is identifying and attaining agreement about the human phenomena that are of particular concern to nurses, enhancing scholarly clinicians' involvement in generating promising relevant theories, and testing those theories as the means to discover knowledge through which to continuously improve nursing practices. Such an approach will ensure the availability of valid nursing knowledge in the twenty-first century and its currency during all centuries to come.

References

American Association of Colleges of Nursing. (1986). *Essentials of college and university education for professional nursing*. Washington, DC: Author.

Chinn, P. (1984). From the editor. *Advances in Nursing Science, 6*(2), ix.

Donaldson, S., & Crowley, D. (1978). The discipline of nursing. *Nursing Outlook, 26*, 113–120.

Engel, G. (1977). The need for a new medical model: A challenge for biomedicine. Science, 196, 129–136.

Fawcett, J. (1983). Hallmarks of success in nursing theory development. In P. Chinn (Ed.), Advances in nursing theory development (pp. 3–17). Rockville, MD: Aspen.

Reverby, S. (1987). A caring dilemma: Womanhood and nursing in historical perspective. Nursing Research, 36, 5–11.

Silva, M. (1986). Research testing nursing theory: State of the art. Advances in Nursing Science, 9(1), 1–11.

CHAPTER 3

Fundamental Patterns of Knowing in Nursing

Barbara A. Carper, RN, EdD

It is the general conception of any field of inquiry that ultimately determines the kind of knowledge the field aims to develop as well as the manner in which that knowledge is to be organized, tested, and applied. The body of knowledge that serves as the rationale for nursing practice has patterns, forms, and structure that serve as horizons of expectations and exemplify characteristic ways of thinking about phenomena. Understanding these patterns is essential for the teaching and learning of nursing. Such an understanding does not extend the range of knowledge, but rather involves critical attention to the question of what it means to know and what kinds of knowledge are held to be of most value in the discipline of nursing.

Identifying Patterns of Knowing

Four fundamental patterns of knowing have been identified from an analysis of the conceptual and syntactical structure of nursing knowledge.[1] The four patterns are distinguished according to logical type of meaning and designated as (1) empirics, the science of nursing; (2) esthetics, the art of nursing; (3) the component of a personal knowledge in nursing; and (4) ethics, the component of moral knowledge in nursing.

Empirics: The Science of Nursing

The term nursing science was rarely used in the literature until the late 1950s. However,

---

Source: Carper, B. A. (1978). Fundamental patterns of knowing in nursing. ANS, 1 (1): 13–24.

since that time, there has been an increasing emphasis, one might even say a sense of urgency, regarding the development of a body of empirical knowledge specific to nursing. There seems to be general agreement that there is a critical need for knowledge about the empirical world, knowledge that is systematically organized into general laws and theories for the purpose of describing, explaining, and predicting phenomena of special concern to the discipline of nursing. Most theory development and research efforts are primarily engaged in seeking and generating explanations that are systematic and controllable by factual evidence and that can be used in the organization and classification of knowledge.

The pattern of knowing that is generally designated as "nursing science" does not presently exhibit the same degree of highly integrated abstract and systematic explanations characteristic of the more mature sciences, although nursing literature reflects this as an ideal form. Clearly, there are a number of coexisting, and in a few instances competing, conceptual structures—none of which has achieved the status of what Kuhn calls a scientific paradigm. That is, no single conceptual structure is as yet generally accepted as an example of actual scientific practice "which include[s] law, theory, application, and instrumentation together . . . [and] . . . provide[s] models from which spring particular coherent traditions of scientific research."[2(p10)] It could be argued that some of these conceptual structures seem to have greater potential than others for providing explanations that systematically account for observed phenomena and may ultimately permit more accurate prediction and control of them. However, this is a matter to be determined by research designed to test the validity of such explanatory concepts in the context of relevant empirical reality.

New Perspectives What seems to be of paramount importance, at least at this stage in the development of nursing science, is that these preparadigm conceptual structures and theoretical models present new perspectives for considering the familiar phenomena of health and illness in relation to the human life process; as such, they can and should be legitimately counted as discoveries in the discipline. The representation of health as more than the absence of disease is a crucial change; it permits health to be thought of as a dynamic state or process that changes over a given period of time and varies according to circumstances rather than a static either/or entity. The conceptual change in turn makes it possible to raise questions that previously would have been literally unintelligible.

The discovery that one can usefully conceptualize health as something that normally ranges along a continuum has led to attempts to observe, describe, and classify variations in health, or levels of wellness, as expressions of a human being's relationship to the internal and external environments. Related research has sought to identify behavioral responses, both physiological and psychological, that may serve as cues by which one can infer the range of normal variations of health. It has also attempted to identify and categorize significant etiological factors that serve to promote or inhibit changes in health status.

Current Stages The science of nursing at present exhibits aspects of both the "natural history stage of inquiry" and the "stage of deductively formulated theory." The task of the natural history stage is primarily the description and classification of phenomena that are, generally speaking, ascertainable by direct observation and inspection,[3] but current nursing literature clearly reflects a shift from this descriptive and classification form to increasingly theoretical analysis, which is directed toward seeking, or inventing, explanations to account for observed and classified empirical facts. This shift is reflected in the change from a largely observational vocabulary to a new, more theoretical vocabulary whose terms have a distinct meaning and definition only in the context of the corresponding explanatory theory.

Explanations in the several open-system conceptual models tend to take the form commonly labeled functional or teleological.[4] For example, the system models explain a person's level of wellness at any particular point in time as a function of current and accumulated effects of interactions with his or her internal and external environments. The concept of adaptation is central to this type of explanation. Adaptation is seen as crucial in the process of responding to environmental demands (usually classified as stressors) and enables an individual to maintain or reestablish the steady state, which is designated as the goal of the system. The developmental models often exhibit a more genetic type of explanation in that certain events, the developmental tasks, are believed to be causally relevant or necessary conditions for the normal development of an individual.

Thus, the first fundamental pattern of knowing in nursing is empirical, factual, descriptive, and ultimately aimed at developing abstract and theoretical explanations. It is exemplary, discursively formulated, and publicly verifiable.

Esthetics: The Art of Nursing

Few, if indeed any, familiar with the professional literature would deny that primary emphasis is placed on the development of the science of nursing. One is almost led to believe that the only valid and reliable knowledge is that which is empirical, factual, objectively descriptive, and generalizable. There seems to be a self-conscious reluctance to extend the term knowledge to include those aspects of knowing in nursing that are not the result of empirical investigation. There is, nonetheless, what might be described as a tacit admission that nursing is, at least in part, an art. Not much effort is made to elaborate or to make explicit this esthetic pattern of knowing in nursing—other than to associate vaguely the "art" with the general category of manual and/or technical skills involved in nursing practice.

Perhaps this reluctance to acknowledge the esthetic component as a fundamental pattern of knowing in nursing originates in the vigorous efforts made in the not-so-distant past to exorcise the image of the apprentice-type educational system. Within the apprentice system, the art of nursing was closely associated with an imitative learning style and the acquisition of knowledge by accumulation of unrationalized experiences. Another likely source of reluctance is that the definition of the term art has been excessively and inappropriately restricted.

Weitz suggests that art is too complex and variable to be reduced to a single definition.[5] To conceive the task of esthetic theory as definition, he says, is logically doomed to failure in that what is called art has no common properties—only recognizable similarities. This fluid and open approach to the understanding and application of the concept of art and esthetic meaning makes possible a wider consideration of conditions, situations, and experiences in nursing that may properly be called esthetic, including the creative process of discovery in the empirical pattern of knowing.

Esthetics Versus Scientific Meaning Despite this open texture of the concept of art, esthetic meanings can be distinguished from those in science in several important aspects. The recognition "that art is expressive rather than merely formal or descriptive," according to Rader, "is about as well established as any fact in the whole field of esthetics."[6(p xvi)] An esthetic experience involves the creation and/or appreciation of a singular, particular, subjective expression of imagined possibilities or equivalent realities that "resists projection into the discursive form of language."[7] Knowledge gained by empirical description is discursively formulated and publicly verifiable. The knowledge gained by subjective acquaintance, the direct feeling of experience, defines discursive formulation. Although an esthetic expression required abstraction, it remains specific and unique rather than

exemplary and leads us to acknowledge that "knowledge—genuine knowledge, understanding—is considerably wider than our discourse."[7(p23)]

For Wiedenbach, the art of nursing is made visible through the action taken to provide whatever the patient requires to restore or extend his [sic] ability to cope with the demands of his [sic] situation,[8] but the action taken, to have an esthetic quality, requires the active transformation of the immediate object—the patient's behavior—into a direct, nonmediated perception of what is significant in it—that is, what need is actually being expressed by the behavior. This perception of the need expressed is not only responsible for the action taken by the nurse but reflected in it.

The esthetic process described by Wiedenbach resembles what Dewey refers to as the difference between recognition and perception.[9] According to Dewey, recognition serves the purpose of identification and is satisfied when a name tag or label is attached according to some stereotype or previously formed scheme of classification. Perception, however, goes beyond recognition in that it includes an active gathering together of details and scattered particulars into an experienced whole for the purpose of seeing what is there. It is perception rather than mere recognition that results in a unity of ends and means that gives the action taken an esthetic quality.

Orem speaks of the art of nursing as being "expressed by the individual nurse through her creativity and style in designing and providing nursing that is effective and satisfying."[10(p155)] The art of nursing is creative in that it requires development of the ability to "envision valid modes of helping in relation to 'results' which are appropriate."[10(p69)] This again invokes Dewey's sense of a perceived unity between an action taken and its result—a perception of the means of the end as an organic whole.[9] The experience of helping must be perceived and designed as an integral component of its desired result rather than conceived separately as an independent action imposed on an independent subject. Perhaps this is what is meant by the concept of nursing the whole patient or total patient care. If so, what are the qualities that enable the creation of a design for nursing care that eliminate or would minimize the fragmentation of means and ends?

Esthetic Pattern of Knowing

Empathy—that is, the capacity for participating in or vicariously experiencing another's feelings—is an important mode in the esthetic pattern of knowing. One gains knowledge of another person's singular, particular, felt experience through empathic acquaintance.[11,12] Empathy is controlled or moderated by psychic distance or detachment in order to apprehend and abstract what we are attending to and in this sense is objective. The more skilled the nurse becomes in perceiving and empathizing with the lives of others, the more knowledge or understanding will be gained of alternate modes of perceiving reality. The nurse will thereby have available a larger repertoire of choices in designing and providing nursing care that is effective and satisfying. At the same time, increased awareness of the variety of subjective experiences will heighten the complexity and difficulty of the decision making involved.

The design of nursing care must be accompanied by what Langer refers to as sense of form, the sense of "structure, articulation, a whole resulting from the relation of mutually dependent factors, or more precisely, the way the whole is put together."[7(p16)] The design, if it is to be esthetic, must be controlled by the perception of the balance, rhythm, proportion, and unity of what is done in relation to the dynamic integration and articulation of the whole. "The doing may be energetic, and the undergoing may be acute and intense," Dewey says, but "unless they are related to each other to form a whole," what is done becomes merely a matter of mechanical routine or of caprice.[9]

The esthetic pattern of knowing in nursing involves the perception of abstracted particulars as distinguished from the recognition of abstracted universals. It is the knowing of a unique particular rather than an exemplary class.

The Component of Personal Knowledge

Personal knowledge as a fundamental pattern of knowing in nursing is the most problematic, the most difficult to master and to teach. At the same time, it is perhaps the pattern most essential to understanding the meaning of health in terms of individual well-being. Nursing considered as an interpersonal process involves interactions, relationships, and transactions between the nurse and the patient-client. Mitchell points out that "there is growing evidence that the quality of interpersonal contacts has an influence on a person's becoming ill, coping with illness and becoming well."[13(p4950)] Certainly the phrase "therapeutic use of self," which has become increasingly prominent in the literature, implies that the way in which nurses view their own selves and the client is of primary concern in any therapeutic relationship.

Personal knowledge is concerned with the knowing, encountering, and actualizing of the concrete, individual self. One does not know about the self; one strives simply to know the self. This knowing is a standing in relation to another human being and confronting that human being as a person. This "I-Thou" encounter is unmediated by conceptual categories or particulars abstracted from complex organic wholes.[14] The relation is one of reciprocity, a state of being that cannot be described or even experienced—it can only be actualized. Such personal knowing extends not only to other selves but also to relations with one's own self.

It requires what Buber refers to as the sacrifice of form, that is, categories or classifications, for a knowing of infinite possibilities, as well as the risk of total commitment.

> Even as a melody is not composed of tones, nor a verse of words, nor a statue of lines—one must pull and tear to turn a unity into a multiplicity—so it is with the human being to whom I say You. . . . I have to do this again and again; but immediately he is no longer You.[14(p59)]

Maslow refers to this sacrifice of form as embodying a more efficient perception of reality in that reality is not generalized nor predetermined by a complex of concepts, expectations, beliefs, and stereotypes.[15] This results in a greater willingness to accept ambiguity, vagueness, and discrepancy of oneself and others. The risk of commitment involved in personal knowledge is what Polanyi calls the "passionate participation in the act of knowing."[16(p17)]

The nurse in the therapeutic use of self rejects approaching the patient-client as an object and strives instead to actualize an authentic personal relationship between two persons. The individual is considered as an integrated, open system incorporating movement toward growth and fulfillment of human potential. An authentic personal relation requires the acceptance of others in their freedom to create themselves and the recognition that each person is not a fixed entity, but constantly engaged in the process of becoming. How then should the nurse reconcile this with the social and/or professional responsibility to control and manipulate the environmental variables and even the behavior of the person who is a patient in order to maintain or restore a steady state? If a human being is assumed to be free to choose and chooses behavior outside of accepted norms, how will this affect the action taken in the therapeutic use of self by the nurse? What choices must the nurse make in order to know another self in an authentic relation apart from the category of patient, even when categorizing for the purpose of treatment is essential to the process of nursing?

Assumptions regarding human nature, McKay observes, "Range from the existentialist to the cybernetic, from the idea of an information processing machine to one of a many splendored being."[17(p399)] Many of these assumptions incorporate in one form or another the notion that there is, for all individuals, a characteristic state which they, by virtue of membership in the species, must strive to assume or achieve. Empirical descriptions and classifications reflect the assumption that being human allows for prediction of basic biological, psychological, and social behaviors that will be encountered in any given individual.

Certainly empirical knowledge is essential to the purposes of nursing, but nursing also requires that we be alert to the fact that models of human nature and their abstract and generalized categories refer to and describe behaviors and traits that groups have in common. However, none of these categories can ever encompass or express the uniqueness of the individual encountered as a person, as a "self." These and many other similar considerations are involved in the realm of personal knowledge, which can be broadly characterized as subjective, concrete, and existential. It is concerned with the kind of knowing that promotes wholeness and integrity in the personal encounter, the achievement of engagement rather than detachment, and it denies the manipulative, impersonal orientation.

Ethics: The Moral Component

Teachers and individual practitioners are becoming increasingly sensitive to the difficult personal choices that must be made within the complex context of modern health care. These choices raise fundamental questions about morally right and wrong action in connection with the care and treatment of illness and the promotion of health. Moral dilemmas arise in situations of ambiguity and uncertainty, when the consequences of one's actions are difficult to predict and traditional principles and ethical codes offer no help or seem to result in contradiction. The moral code that guides the ethical conduct of nurses is based on the primary principle of obligation embodied in the concepts of service to people and respect for human life. The discipline of nursing is held to be a valuable and essential social service responsible for conserving life, alleviating suffering, and promoting health, but appeal to the ethical "rule book" fails to provide answers in terms of difficult individual moral choices, which must be made in the teaching and practice of nursing.

The fundamental pattern of knowing identified here as the ethical component of nursing is focused on matters of obligation or what ought to be done. Knowledge of morality goes beyond simply knowing the norms or ethical codes of the discipline. It includes all voluntary actions that are deliberate and subject to the judgment of right and wrong—including judgments of moral value in relation to motives, intentions, and traits of character. Nursing is deliberate action, or a series of actions, planned and implemented to accomplish defined goals. Both goals and actions involve choices made, in part, on the basis of normative judgments, both particular and general. On occasion, the principles and norms by which such choices are made may be in conflict.

According to Berthold, "Goals are, of course, value judgments not amenable to scientific inquiry and validation."[18(p196)] Dickoff, James, and Wiedenbach also call attention to the need to be aware that the specification of goals serves as "a norm or standard by which to evaluate activity . . . [and] . . . entails taking them as values— that is, signifies conceiving these goal contents as situations worthy to be brought about."[19(p422)]

For example, a common goal of nursing care in relation to the maintenance or restoration of health is to assist patients to achieve a state in which they are independent. Much of the current practice reflects an attitude of value attached to the goal of independence and indicates nursing actions to assist patients in assuming full responsibility for themselves at the earliest possible moment or to enable them to retain responsibility to the last possible moment. However, valuing independence and attempting to maintain it may be at the expense of the patient's learning how to live with physical or social dependence when necessary—for example, in instances when prognosis indicates that independence cannot be regained.

Differences in normative judgments may have more to do with disagreements as to what constitutes a "healthy" state of being than lack of empirical evidence or ambiguity in the application of the term. Slote suggests that the persistence of disputes, or lack of uniformity in the application of cluster terms, such as health, is due to "the difficulty of decisively resolving certain sorts of value questions about what is and is not important." This leads him to conclude, "That value judgment is far more involved in the making of what are commonly thought to be factual statements than has been imagined."[20(p220)]

The ethical pattern of knowing in nursing requires an understanding of different philosophical positions regarding what is good, what ought to be desired, what is right; of different ethical frameworks devised for dealing with the complexities of moral judgments; and of various orientations to the notion of obligation. Moral choices to be made must then be considered in terms of specific actions to be taken in specific, concrete situations. The examination of the standards, codes, and values by which we decide what is morally right should result in a greater awareness of what is involved in making moral choices and being responsible for the choices made. The knowledge of ethical codes will not provide answers to the moral questions involved in nursing, nor will it eliminate the necessity for having to make moral choices, but it can be hoped that

The more sensitive teachers and practitioners are to the demands of the process of justification, the more explicit they are about the norms that govern their actions, the more personally engaged they are in assessing surrounding circumstances and potential consequences, the more "ethical" they will be; and we cannot ask much more.[21(p221)]

Using Patterns of Knowing

A philosophical discussion of patterns of knowing may appear to some as a somewhat idle, if not arbitrary and artificial, undertaking having little or no connection with the practical concerns and difficulties encountered in the day-to-day doing and teaching of nursing, but it represents a personal conviction that there is a need to examine the kinds of knowing that provide the discipline with its particular perspectives and significance. Understanding four fundamental patterns of knowing makes possible an increased awareness of the complexity and diversity of nursing knowledge.

Each pattern may be conceived as necessary for achieving mastery in the discipline, but none of them alone should be considered sufficient. Neither are they mutually exclusive. The teaching and learning of one pattern do not require the rejection or neglect of any of the others. Caring for another requires the achievements of nursing science, that is, the knowledge of empirical facts systematically organized into theoretical explanations regarding the phenomena of health and illness, but creative imagination also plays its part in the syntax of discovery in science, as well as in developing the ability to imagine the consequences of alternative moral choices.

Personal knowledge is essential for ethical choices in that moral action presupposes personal maturity and freedom. If the goals of nursing are to be more than conformance to unexamined norms, if the "ought" is not to be determined simply on the basis of what

is possible, then the obligation to care for another human being involves becoming a certain kind of person—and not merely doing certain kinds of things. If the design of nursing care is to be more than habitual or mechanical, the capacity to perceive and interpret the subjective experiences of others and to imaginatively project the effects of nursing actions on their lives becomes a necessary skill.

Nursing thus depends on the scientific knowledge of human behavior in health and in illness, the esthetic perception of significant human experiences, a personal understanding of the unique individuality of the self, and the capacity to make choices within concrete situations involving particular moral judgments. Each of these separate but interrelated and interdependent fundamental patterns of knowing should be taught and understood according to its distinctive logic, the restricted circumstances in which it is valid, the kinds of data it subsumes, and the methods by which each particular kind of truth is distinguished and warranted.

The major significances to the discipline of nursing in distinguishing patterns of knowing are summarized as (1) the conclusions of the discipline conceived as subject matter cannot be taught or learned without reference to the structure of the discipline—the representative concepts and methods of inquiry that determine the kind of knowledge gained and limit its meaning, scope, and validity; (2) each of the fundamental patterns of knowing represents a necessary but not complete approach to the problems and questions in the discipline; and (3) all knowledge is subject to change and revision. Every solution of an existing problem raises new and unsolved questions. These new and as yet unsolved problems require, at times, new methods of inquiry and different conceptual structures; they change the shape and patterns of knowing. With each change in the shape of knowledge, teaching and learning require looking for different points of contact and connection among ideas and things. This clarifies the effect of each new thing known on other things known and the discovery of new patterns by which each connection modifies the whole.

References

1. Carper, B. A. "Fundamental Patterns of Knowing in Nursing." PhD dissertation, Teachers College, Columbia University, 1975.
2. Kuhn, T. The Structure of Scientific Revolutions (Chicago: University of Chicago Press, 1962).
3. Northrop, F. S. C. The Logic of the Sciences and the Humanities (New York: The World Publishing Co., 1959).
4. Nagel, E. The Structure of Science (New York: Harcourt, Brace and World, Inc., 1961).
5. Weitz, M. "The Role of Theory in Aesthetics" in Rader, M., ed. A Modern Book of Esthetics, 3rd ed. (New York: Holt, Rinehart and Winston, 1960).
6. Rader, M. "Introduction: The Meaning of Art" in Rader, M., ed. A Modern Book of Esthetics, 3rd ed. (New York: Holt, Rinehart and Winston, 1960).
7. Langer, S. K. Problems of Art (New York: Charles Scribner and Sons, 1957).
8. Wiedenbach, E. Clinical Nursing: A Helping Art (New York: Springer Publishing Co., Inc., 1964).
9. Dewey, J. Art as Experience (New York: Capricorn Books, 1958).
10. Orem, D. E. Nursing: Concepts of Practice (New York: McGraw-Hill Book Co., 1971).
11. Lee, V. "Empathy" in Rader, M., ed. A Modern Book of Esthetics, 3rd ed. (New York: Holt, Rinehart and Winston, 1960).
12. Lippo, T. "Empathy, Inner Imitation and Sense-Feeling" in Rader, M., ed. A Modern Book of Esthetics, 3rd ed. (New York: Holt, Rinehart and Winston, 1960).
13. Mitchell, P. H. Concepts Basic to Nursing (New York: McGraw-Hill Book Co., 1973).
14. Buber, M. I and Thou. Translated by Walter Kaufman (New York: Charles Scribner and Sons, 1970).
15. Maslow, A. H. "Self-Actualizing People: A Study of Psychological Health" in Moustakas, C. E., ed. The Self (New York: Harper and Row, 1956).
16. Polanyi, M. Personal Knowledge (New York: Harper and Row, 1964).

17. McKay, R. "Theories, Models and Systems for Nursing." Nurs Res 18:5 (September–October, 1969).

18. Berthold, J. S. "Symposium on Theory Development in Nursing: Prologue." Nurs Res 17:3 (May–June, 1968).

19. Dickoff, J., James, P., and Wiedenbach, E. "Theory in a Practice Discipline: Part I." Nurs Res 17 (September–October, 1968).

20. Slote, M. A. "The Theory of Important Criteria." J Philosophy 63 (April 14, 1966).

21. Greene, M. Teacher as Stronger (Belmont, CA: Wadsworth Publishing Co., Inc., 1973).

CHAPTER 4

The State of Nursing Science: Hallmarks of the 20th and 21st Centuries

Jacqueline Fawcett, RN, PhD, FAAN

Science generally is regarded as the systematic, controlled, empirical, and critical activities undertaken to generate and test theories. Nursing science, therefore, comprises those systematic, controlled, empirical, and critical activities undertaken to generate and test nursing theories. This column focuses on my view of the state of nursing science circa 1999. My comments reflect countless hours of solitary thought, as well as 35 years of dialogue with colleagues and students in classrooms and at local, regional, national, and international workshops and conferences. I have become increasingly troubled by the state of our science but have retained sufficient optimism to accept the invitation to write this column and share my vision of what we can do if we want to save our discipline and advance our science.

Hallmarks of 20th-Century Nursing

During the 1980s, I published a trilogy of articles that reflected my excitement with the state of nursing science and my optimism for the future of the discipline of nursing. In the first article, I identified four hallmarks of success in nursing theory development (Fawcett, 1983). In the second article, I identified three hallmarks of success in nursing research (Fawcett, 1984). In the third article, a colleague and I identified four hallmarks

Source: Fawcett, J. (1999). The state of nursing science: Hallmarks of the 20th and 21st Centuries. Nursing Science Quarterly, 12(4): 311–315. Reprinted by permission of and copyright © 1999 Sage Publications, Inc.

of success in nursing practice (Fawcett & Carino, 1989).

The four hallmarks of success in nursing theory development that I identified were specification of a metaparadigm for nursing, explication of conceptual models of nursing, explication of unique nursing theories, and theories shared with other disciplines. The meaning and content of the nursing metaparadigm, conceptual models, and unique nursing theories most likely are well known to readers. Shared theories may require some explanation. Simply put, a shared theory is one that has been borrowed from another discipline and then tested to determine its empirical adequacy in nursing situations. If the theory is found to be empirically adequate in legitimate nursing situations, it may be considered to be a shared theory.

The three hallmarks of success in nursing research that I identified were specification of the boundaries of nursing research, explication of the types of research needed by the professional discipline of nursing, and delineation of research activities appropriate for nurses according to educational preparation. The boundaries of nursing research were, I maintained, set by the metaparadigm of nursing and by the rules of research that are inherent in each conceptual model of nursing. The metaparadigm sets the global boundary for research as examination of nursing's efforts to facilitate person–environment interactions having to do with health. Each conceptual model of nursing provides an interpretation of that boundary and presents more circumscribed boundaries in the form of a set of conceptual and methodologic rules for research.

Drawing from the notion that nursing is a professional rather than an academic discipline, I maintained that basic, applied, and clinical types of research are required. An academic discipline has as its mission only the development and dissemination of knowledge. A professional discipline, in contrast, has as its mission the development, dissemination, and utilization of knowledge. Basic research focuses only on development of knowledge, without regard to its later use; this type of research is conducted by the members of both academic and professional disciplines. Applied research focuses on determination of the practical limits of knowledge, that is, determination of the range of practical situations in which each theory is empirically adequate. Applied research also is conducted by members of both academic and professional disciplines. Clinical research focuses on the effects of actual implementation of theories in clinical practice situations; this type of research is conducted only by members of professional disciplines.

For the third hallmark of success in nursing research, delineation of research activities appropriate for nurses according to educational preparation, I drew from the American Nurses' Association Commission on Nursing Research 1981 statement of guidelines for the investigative functions of nurses. The commission issued guidelines for participation in a wide range of research-related activities that took into account distinct differences in research capabilities between the graduates of associate degree nursing programs, baccalaureate nursing programs, master's degree nursing programs, practice-oriented doctoral programs (DNSc), and research-oriented programs (PhD).

The four hallmarks of success in nursing practice that Carino and I identified were the use of conceptual models of nursing to guide nursing practice, development of classification systems, establishment of formal linkages between nursing education and nursing service, and recognition of clinical scholars and clinical scholarship. The first three hallmarks are self-explanatory. The fourth hallmark characterizes clinical scholarship as a professional imperative and the consequent emergence of nurse clinicians as clinical scholars. Clinical scholarship takes many forms, including the development and testing of assessment formats and intervention protocols and the application of clinical nursing research findings in daily clinical practice. Clinical scholars are nurse clinicians who practice nursing in an increasingly thoughtful manner. "They continually contemplate situations and stretch their minds toward insights into nursing practice and helping people to improve their health. Nurses who are true clinical scholars are noted for their ability to make novel connections between things or ideas—mental leaps and intuitive lunges that improve nursing practice and, therefore, enhance the well-being of their patients" (Fawcett & Carino, 1989, p. 6).

Current Trends in Nursing Science

Throughout the 1990s, my excitement about the advances in nursing science that led to the trilogy of hallmark articles has been progressively dampened. I have been particularly discouraged because I have seen little that might indicate a need for updates in those hallmark works. That is, although I do not see any evidence of a loss of ground for the existing hallmarks, I do not see any progress either. Even more to the point, I have seen nothing that might qualify as a new hallmark of success in nursing theory development, nursing research, or nursing practice. Moreover, my early optimism has turned to pessimism, reflecting a very real concern for the continued existence of the discipline of nursing.

Research conducted by nurses has increased in quantity and, some might argue, in quality in recent years, but I can no longer support the maxim that research conducted by nurses is, by definition, nursing research. That is because the current trend in research by nurses signals a major threat to the very survival of our discipline. More specifically, much of the research conducted by contemporary nurse researchers (i.e., those nurses who are academically qualified to advance science through research) has not been nursing research and has done nothing to advance nursing science. Instead, much of the research has employed nonnursing methodologies to generate new theories guided by nonnursing conceptual frameworks and to test theories developed by members of other disciplines. Note, for example, that just 6 of the 73 studies (8%) reported in Nursing Research and Research in Nursing and Health in 1998 involved the generation or testing of nursing theories using nursing methodologies. However, 2 of the 6 studies were designed to test ad hoc theories that combined concepts from nursing and some other discipline, and another 2 of the 6 tested ad hoc nursing theories developed from an interdisciplinary literature exclusive of nursing. Thus, just 2 of the 73 studies (3%) were guided by widely recognized nursing theories, namely, Leininger's theory of culture care diversity and universality and Pender's theory of health promotion. Clearly, much science was produced in 1998, but very little nursing science.

The argument could be advanced that the studies that were guided by nonnursing conceptual frameworks and theories were focused on the development of shared nursing theories, which I previously identified as a hallmark of success in nursing theory development (Fawcett, 1983). However, the investigators who reported those studies did not identify the development of shared theory as a goal, nor did they explicitly discuss any modifications in the original theories that might be required for their use in legitimate nursing situations.

Turning to practice, services offered by nurses have become seemingly more comprehensive and sophisticated, but I can no longer support the maxim that practice by nurses is, by definition, nursing practice. That is because the current trend in practice by nurses, especially by so-called advanced practice nurses, signals another major threat to the survival of our discipline. More specifically, many of the services offered by contemporary nurse practitioners (i.e., those nurses academically and professionally qualified to utilize science through practice) have not been based on nursing science and have done nothing to inform nursing science. Instead, nurse practitioners increasingly base their

practice on medical science and perform tasks "traditionally within the domain of medical practice" (Orem, 1995, p. 41). Note, for example, that nurse practitioners are said to resemble physicians' assistants (Martha Rogers, cited in Huch, 1995), junior doctors (Meleis, 1993), or pseudodoctors (Kendrick, 1997) engaged in nursing qua medicine (Watson, 1996).

The reasons for the current trends in research and practice most likely are many and complex. With regard to research, perhaps editors and peer reviewers think that the use and testing of nonnursing conceptual frameworks and theories will increase the visibility of research conducted by nurses among members of other disciplines and the public. Perhaps researchers who base their studies on conceptual models of nursing and nursing theories do not submit their reports to the two journals cited here because they think that such studies are not published in those journals. I would be remiss, then, if I did not mention that almost every report of research based on an explicit conceptual model of nursing that I have submitted to either journal has been published. Thus, it is unlikely that systematic bias against nursing science is operating. However, in contrast to Nursing Science Quarterly and Visions: The Journal of Rogerian Nursing Science, neither of the other two journals cited requires research to reflect advances in nursing science through the testing of a conceptual model of nursing or a nursing theory.

With regard to practice, perhaps practitioners think that if they emulate medical practice, their services will be more highly valued by the public and other health professionals, or perhaps many nurses feel so oppressed by physicians that they, like virtually all oppressed persons, have a disdain for the science of their own discipline and identify with the science of the perceived oppressor, medicine.

The Hallmark of 21st-Century Nursing: A Prediction

While in the depths of pessimism, I began to think of a way to save our discipline. It has become increasingly clear to me that the discipline of nursing can survive if, and only if, we end our romance with medical science and the conceptual frameworks, theories, and methodologies of nonnursing disciplines. We see evidence of that romance every day in the reports of studies conducted by nurses but guided by nonnursing conceptual frameworks, theories, and methodologies. We also see evidence of that romance in advertisements for either a nurse practitioner or a physician's assistant—as if they were interchangeable professions. And, perhaps most disturbing, we see evidence of that romance every time that nurse practitioners are featured in the news media, including the nursing media, and talk about how they provide the same services as primary care physicians and receive—or hope to soon receive—the same reimbursement as physicians for those services from third-party payers. No wonder, then, that physicians claim that nurses are infringing on medical turf. No wonder, then, that we tolerate and even support Nurse Practice Acts that require supervision of nurse practitioners by a licensed physician.

If we do not end the romance with nonnursing disciplines. I predict that we will not survive as a distinct discipline. If, however, we do end the romance, we have a chance at survival but only under certain conditions. Those conditions, I believe, involve embracing nursing science through the integration of research and practice, which will require a change in the educational preparation of all nurses and will mandate a change in the employment conditions of nurses. More specifically, I believe that our discipline will not only survive but flourish through rapid advances in nursing science if all nurses become nurse scholars. I envision nurse scholars as nurses who integrate nursing science versions of the roles of nurse researcher and nurse practitioner. Today's separate roles of nurse researcher and nurse practitioner will no longer exist. Rather, all nurses will perform a single role—that of nurse scholar. The immediate and obvious advantage of a single role is the elimination of the so-called research-practice gap. If actualized, I predict that the single role of nurse scholar will become the one hallmark of the success of 21st-century nursing.

I envision nurse scholars as academically and professionally qualified to develop and utilize nursing science. More specifically, I envision nurse scholars as qualified to conduct nursing discipline-specific research and to practice from a nursing discipline-specific perspective. Nurses will focus on discipline-specific research and practice and employ nursing methodologies to generate, test, and apply nursing theories within the context of conceptual models of nursing. Only when that occurs can the research and practice activities of nurses be said to advance nursing science, and only then can research and practice be said to contribute to the discipline of nursing.

All nurse scholars will actively engage in integrated research-practice activities, using nursing methodologies to test and apply conceptual models of nursing and nursing theories in the provision of nursing services to people. Clearly, nurse scholars are not the nurse researchers or nurse practitioners of today but, rather, are nursing practitioners (Orem, 1995) or senior nurses (Meleis, 1993) who are engaged in nursing qua nursing (Watson, 1997). Inasmuch as nurse scholars constantly conduct nursing discipline-specific research and engage in nursing discipline-specific practice, they advance nursing science continuously.

Nurse scholars are initially prepared for their integrated role responsibilities in post-baccalaureate doctorate of nursing (ND) programs. I believe that today's diversity in entry levels cannot continue to exist if our discipline is to survive. Thus, I envision the ND as the entry level for all nursing. Moreover, given the holistic, comprehensive nature of nursing discipline-specific practice, I envision no need for unlicensed assistive nursing personnel. ND-prepared nurse scholars want to be at the patient's side, which is the only place where they can perform integrated research and practice role activities.

ND-prepared nurse scholars use nursing methodologies, which are derived from explicit conceptual models of nursing and nursing theories, to guide their integrated research and practice activities. The integration of research and practice is evident as ND-prepared nurse scholars use the data obtained from every encounter with a patient for nursing research purposes. Every nurse-patient encounter, then, becomes a case study, with an individual patient serving as his or her own control (Wood, 1978). Thus, each case study is an experiment that tests the efficacy of the conceptual model and theories used to guide the nurse-patient encounter. In other words, ND-prepared nurse scholars use the clinical data available to them in every patient situation to determine the credibility of existing conceptual models of nursing and the empirical adequacy of existing nursing theories, thereby contributing constantly to nursing science.

Rather, their area of expertise or specialization is in a particular conceptual model of nursing or nursing theory. These scholars carry out their role responsibilities with the individuals, families, and/or communities regarded as legitimate patients within the context of that particular conceptual model of nursing or nursing theory. In addition, they apply the relevant nursing methodology to the full range of conditions and situations encompassed by the conceptual model or theory.

ND-prepared nurse scholars receive advanced preparation in doctor of philosophy (PhD) programs. The focus of PhD programs in nursing science is on the use of nursing methodologies, derived from conceptual models of nursing and nursing theories, with groups of patients rather than with individual patients. More specifically, PhD-prepared nurse scholars use aggregate data obtained from multiple encounters with patients to determine the credibility of various existing conceptual models of nursing and the empirical adequacy of various existing nursing theories. They also use those data to develop new conceptual models of nursing, nursing theories, and nursing methodologies. In other words, they combine single case studies to advance nursing science.

Rather than specialize in a particular conceptual model of nursing or nursing theory, PhD-prepared nurse scholars are generalists who examine the differential efficacy of two or more conceptual models of nursing or nursing theories with diverse patients with diverse conditions in diverse situations. The results of such examinations ultimately will lead to a better understanding of the "fit" of a particular intellectual perspective with a particular patient and, therefore, a substantial advance in nursing science.

ND- and PhD-prepared nurse scholars function as "attending nurses," that is, nurses who are with patients continuously wherever they are "in and outside of institutions, schools, homes, clinics, and community settings" (Watson, 1996, p. 163). Thus, each patient always has his or her own nurse scholar, who collaborates with other health professionals when the patient requires services from others. Attending nurses, of course, carry out integrated research and practice role responsibilities. As attending nurses, ND- and PhD-prepared nurse scholars may work in nurse corporations, which

are made up of nurse scholars in equal partnership with one another, or they may elect to be self-employed. Nurse corporations contract with individuals, families, communities, medical centers, community and specialty hospitals, home care agencies, hospices, and other agencies and organizations for the provision of distinctively nursing services guided by conceptual models of nursing, nursing theories, and nursing methods. The idea of nurse corporations was proposed by Sills (1983), who explained this:

> The conceptual key to the corporation proposal is that it changes the fundamental nature of the social contract. The professional nurse would no longer be an employee of the hospital or agency, but rather a member of a professional corporation that provides nursing services to patients and clients on a fee-for-service basis. ... Such a change in the nature of the social contract is, it seems to me, fundamentally necessary for the survival of nursing as a profession rather than an occupational group of workers employed by other organizations. (p. 573)

Sills viewed nurse corporations as a solution to the problem of collective bargaining by nurses and an organizational way to address the economics of nursing practice.

I envision nurse corporations as extending beyond the provision of nursing services to the provision of programs of nursing education. In this case, nurse corporations contract with universities to design and implement

ND and PhD programs. Universities, of course, have the right and responsibility to appoint only those partners in the nurse corporation who meet the university's criteria for faculty. Furthermore, universities, as well as clinical agencies, might elect to contract with more than one nurse corporation. Self-employed nurse scholars are entrepreneurs who contract directly with universities for appointment to the faculty and with clinical agencies for practice and research privileges. Alternatively, they engage in private practice, contracting directly with patients for certain nursing services, with students for such educational services as tutoring and mentoring, and with nurse corporations for the continuing education of the partners.

Conclusion

Achievement of the proposed hallmark of 21st-century nursing depends on our individual and collective willingness to take potentially enormous risks and "have the courage to take a position about why people need nursing and about what nursing can and should be" (Orem, 1995, p. 414). Clearly, if we want to ensure the survival of our discipline, all of us must fall in love with nursing science now and develop a passion for the destiny of the discipline of nursing.

References

Fawcett, J. (1983). Hallmarks of success in nursing theory development. In P. L. Chinn (Ed.), Advances in nursing theory development (pp. 3–17). Rockville, MD: Aspen.

Fawcett, J. (1984). Hallmarks of success in nursing research. Advances in Nursing Science, 7(1), 1–11.

Fawcett, J., & Carino, C. (1989). Hallmarks of success in nursing practice. Advances in Nursing Science, 11(4), 1–8.

Huch, M. H. (1995). Nursing and the next millennium. Nursing Science Quarterly, 8, 38–44.

Kendrick, K. (1997). What is advanced nursing? Professional Nurse, 12(10), 689.

Meleis, A. I. (1993, April). Nursing research and the Neuman model: Directions for the future. Panel discussion at the Fourth Biennial International Neuman Systems Model Symposium, Rochester, NY.

Orem, D. E. (1995). Nursing: Concepts of practice (5th ed.). St. Louis: C. V. Mosby.

Sills, G. M. (1983). The role and function of the clinical nurse specialist. In N. L. Chaska (Ed.), The nursing profession: A time to speak (pp. 563–579). New York: McGraw-Hill.

Watson, J. (1997). The theory of human caring: Retrospective and prospective. Nursing Science Quarterly, 10, 49–52.

Watson, M. J. (1996). Watson's theory of transpersonal caring. In P. H. Walker & B. Neuman (Eds.), Blueprint for use of nursing models: Education, research, practice, and administration (pp. 141–184). New York: NLN Press.

Wood, K. W. (1978). Casework effectiveness: A new look at the research evidence. Social Work, 23, 437–458.

CHAPTER 5

What Constitutes Nursing Science?

John R. Phillips, RN, PhD

Science is an organized body of knowledge concerning human beings and their worlds; it encompasses "the attitudes and methods through which this body of knowledge is formed" (Chernow & Vallasi, 1993, p. 2452). Chernow and Vallasi (1993) also state that since scientific methods do not always guarantee scientific discovery, other factors such as intuition, experience, and good judgment "contribute to new developments in science" (p. 2452). In addition, a survey of the evolution of knowledge shows that abstract thinking is integral to the advancement of science. This broad view of science is essential in understanding the development of any particular science and its phenomena of concern.

This is especially true for nursing science with its unique body of knowledge. Controversy arises, however, when attempts are made to identify this body of knowledge, where some nurses make little distinction between nursing knowledge and the knowledge of other sciences, such as medicine. Too, some nursing models and theories still include knowledge from other sciences that has not been transposed into a nursing perspective. Furthermore, it must be determined how or if these nursing models and theories can be used to generate nursing knowledge that constitutes nursing science.

Some nurses may say this is a moot point and probably not worthy of further pursuit. However, one needs to realize that it

Source: Phillips, J. R. (1996). What constitutes nursing science? Nursing Science Quarterly, 9(2): 48–49. Reprinted by permission of and copyright © 2002 Sage Publications, Inc.

is nursing science that gives direction to the further generation of nursing knowledge, and it is nursing science that provides the knowledge for all aspects of nursing. Moreover, it is through the art of nursing, "the imaginative and creative use of knowledge" (Rogers, 1988, p. 100), that nurses can know and understand the health care needs of people. How adequately can this be achieved if nursing science is not constituted with nursing knowledge?

Fawcett (1993, 1995) in her metaparadigm of nursing has helped to provide an understanding of what constitutes nursing science. Her analysis and evaluation of nursing models and theories make it clear that there is a particular perspective of the metaparadigm concepts for each of the nursing models and theories. For example, the definitions of person, environment, health, and nursing are different for each model and theory. Since each nursing model and theory has a different philosophical and theoretical foundation, nurses who use them have different realities of nursing. How are these differences related to what constitutes nursing science?

Parse (1987) and Newman (1992) in their paradigms of nursing and Fawcett (1993) in her worldviews of nursing address these differences and provide for further understanding of what constitutes nursing science. The use of these paradigms and worldviews reveals that some nursing models and theories are composed of conflicting philosophical and theoretical foundations. Too, some nursing models and theories overlap more than one paradigm or worldview. If a nursing

model or theory lacks coherence within its philosophical and theoretical foundation and overlaps more than one paradigm or worldview, then a close examination of it is needed to determine whether it constitutes nursing science. Will a time come when particular nursing models or theories will no longer be appropriate to constitute nursing science?

Nursing models and theories provide multiple diverse and divergent nursing realities. These realities foster creative ideas and insights that are essential to the methods that are used to discover knowledge. It is time, however, to evaluate how the various scientific methods contribute to the development of nursing science. Realizing, for example, that statistics is only one language of science, nurses can no longer be satisfied with only the traditional scientific methods that often give a cloudy vision of what nursing science is. Nurses must emerge from the womb of other sciences so as to give birth to scientific methods that give a clear vision of what nursing is and can be, knowing that today there is only an inkling of the future of nursing science.

Nurses can design these new methods through a creative synthesis of the various aspects of science and the human processes such as intuition and lived experiences. Some of our current nursing scientific methods already provide for imaginative, abstract, and logical reasoning processes that are required to discover knowledge to develop nursing science. Such scientific methods will give unity to nursing science through the diversity of nursing models and theories. This assumption is acceptable when Moody (1990) quote of Bronowski is considered: "Science is nothing else than the search to discover unity in the wild variety of nature or . . . in the variety of our experiences" (p. 18).

A cumulative body of knowledge that is flexible and open to change flows from the unitary nature of nursing science. The wholeness of this knowledge provides further understanding of the ambiguity and uncertainty found in the multiple realities of nursing models and theories. This understanding will reveal the rigid and static nature of knowledge from other sciences, which in many instances is outdated and not from a nursing perspective. However, as nurses develop knowledge through the use of nursing models and theories, they must remain in doubt and be open to changes in it (Wilson, 1985). This is essential if nurses are to advance a nursing science that provides the knowledge for the changing art of nursing, where there is concern for the wholeness of people.

Questions of what constitutes nursing science have revealed an evolving phenomenon in nursing. The revelation is that facts alone do not constitute nursing science, however important they may be; it is the pattern of knowledge that gives unity to nursing science. As the pattern is revealed, nurses are being challenged to relook at what constitutes nursing science. Needless to say, the focus on the pattern of knowledge brings a profound provocation to create a new vision of nursing science, a vision that will eventually sever the umbilical cord of subjugation to the knowledge of other sciences. This new vision may save some of the nursing models and theories from becoming obsolete, even extinct.

The recognition and use of the pattern of knowledge is moving nursing science to the forefront of science in general. This new, prominent position enables nurses to respond to the public's desire for quality health care, where the concern is the healing of the whole person. In such an arena of health care, nurses will not compete with other health care providers since they will be using nursing knowledge for the practice of nursing, rather than knowledge from other sciences, particularly medicine. Can we say that the "gap" between theory and practice will disappear as nurses continue to use nursing models and theories that constitute the nursing science for their practice?

Yes, nursing models and theories do constitute nursing science. Nurses must not accept the perennial denigration of nursing models and theories and the call to abandon them for the knowledge from other sciences. If nurses do, nursing will become a wasteland filled with "illiterate nurses" where all of humanity will suffer in immeasurable ways.

Nursing models and theories are the savior of nursing science, and nurses' ravenous use of them will bring redemption from a wasteland composed of knowledge from other sciences. This is the power that nursing models and theories give nurses in determining what constitutes nursing science, its knowledge, and its scientific methods. As nurses continue to use nursing models and theories, nursing science will no longer be invisible in the world of science.

References

Chernow, B. A., & Vallasi, G. A. (1993). The Columbia encyclopedia (5th ed.). New York: Columbia University Press.

Fawcett, J. (1993). Analysis and evaluation of nursing theories. Philadelphia: Davis.

Fawcett, J. (1995). Analysis and evaluation of conceptual models of nursing (3rd ed.). Philadelphia: Davis.

Moody, L. E. (1990). Advancing nursing science through research, Vol. 1. Newbury Park, CA: Sage.

Newman, M. A. (1992). Prevailing paradigms in nursing. Nursing Outlook, 40, 10–13, 32.

Parse, R. R. (1987). Nursing science: Major paradigms, theories, and critiques. Philadelphia: Saunders.

Rogers, M. E. (1988). Nursing science and art: A prospective. Nursing Science Quarterly, 1, 99–102.

Wilson, H. S. (1985). Research in nursing. Menlo Park, CA: Addison-Wesley.

CHAPTER 6

Nursing Theory-Guided Practice: What It Is and What It Is Not

William K. Cody, PhD, RN, FAAN

The full realization of nursing theory-guided practice is perhaps the greatest challenge that nursing as a scholarly discipline has ever faced. There may be multiple theories guiding practice within the discipline, but it is imperative that these be nursing theories. There is not space here to explicate the many benefits to humanity that emanate from true nursing theory-guided practice. Rather it is the intention of this column to elucidate the proposition that it is essential to the advancement of nursing science and the future of the discipline to seek greater clarity as to what constitutes nursing theory-guided practice. This phrase is often heard in the halls and classrooms of schools of nursing, but not everyone using the term "nursing theory" means the same thing.

Sometimes the term "theory" is used in nursing to refer to any knowledge that is useful in general health care or the care of a particular population—as in the content of most undergraduate courses, for example. For many nurses, including some advanced practitioners and faculty, all of this knowledge may be called "nursing theory." For others, the term "nursing theory" is used to refer only to the particular knowledge that has to do directly with planning and implementing conventional nursing care, as in the steps of the generic "nursing process." Nurses using the term in this way are more selective

---

Source: Cody, W. K. (1994). Nursing theory-guided practice: What it is and what it is not. Nursing Science Quarterly, 7(4):144–145.

as to what they admit as "nursing theory," yet they do not see the necessity of using a specific nursing framework to guide practice. Another assertion often heard is that "most nursing theories haven't been tested yet." Such a use of the term "theory" is closely related to the legacy of positivism, in which a "theory" must be empirically verifiable on the basis of objective measurement. This belief system also gives rise to the term "research-based practice," which reflects the belief that it is appropriate to take empirical findings directly into practice.

A distinct use of the term "nursing theory" and one with which readers of Nursing Science Quarterly are, no doubt, familiar, refers specifically to a distinct and well-articulated system of concepts and propositions rooted explicitly in a philosophy of nursing and intended solely to guide nursing practice and research. These attributes are the minimal criteria for any conceptual system to be called a nursing theory. Merely to have been written by a nurse or used by nurses does not and cannot turn knowledge into nursing theory. This use of the term is not original with the author, it is simply commensurate with the use of the term "theory" in all other academic disciplines. Of course, all knowledge is open to anyone to learn and use, but members of a discipline have the obligation to concern themselves specifically with the knowledge base of their discipline, to participate in its development, to guide its use, and to evaluate the work of their colleagues on the basis of the work's relation to the extant theory base of that discipline.

In Nightingale's time, and for years thereafter, nurses were the nutritionists, the sanitarians, the physical therapists, and the respiratory therapists in Wald's time, they were the social workers and health educators. All of these roles have evolved into distinct professions, and nowhere is the nurse considered the chief expert in any of these fields today. To expect contemporary nurses to have extensive knowledge in such non-nursing areas is unfair and impractical. To call such knowledge nursing knowledge is plainly retrogressive and antithetical to the advancement of nursing science. The same is true of medical knowledge, but medicine still dominates nursing politically, and many nurses actually value having the medical tasks delegated to them. The resulting inter-disciplinary dynamic creates the impression among many nurses that mastery of much of the medical canon is the chief requisite to practice nursing. It is important for contemporary nurses to understand that what is merely delegated from another (more powerful) discipline can also be taken away. As more and more nurses recognize the distinction between the knowledge base and goals of medicine and nursing, nursing will be free to progress more rapidly toward full standing as an autonomous discipline.

The notion that research findings do or should guide practice is quite prevalent in contemporary nursing. This idea, as mentioned previously, is associated with the interpretation of the term "theory," which holds that any theory must be testable in a quantitative manner. Thus, the idea that research findings guide practice is linked to the objectivistic, reductionistic legacy of logical positivism, but even under logical positivism, it was not the empirical findings that were said to provide direction for future practice but rather the theory as supported through empirical testing. Theory was believed to guide research and practice. The research findings were to feed back into the theory, which would then (continue to) guide research and practice. This was the dominant model of the theory-research-practice triad throughout the much-heralded yet largely disastrous era of "value-free science" (Jacox & Webster, 1986).

More recently, it has been widely acknowledged that all scientific endeavors are value laden. Especially in the social or human sciences, it has become increasingly clear that values, above all, guide practice. Theory must be rethought for the postmodern age to explicitly address the question of values—not only what values but whose. For example, if any discipline within the human sciences is to be norm based, then who determines those norms and why should they be valued by others? In nursing science, if human health is conceptualized within a framework of norms, then what value is demonstrated for persons whose health is judged to be outside the norm—for what purpose, and with what consequences?

A nursing theory that explicitly posits a value for the human, regardless of societal norms and expectations, guides the nurse to practice in a wholly respectful way that precludes labeling and trying to change the person (Parse, 1992). It is true, as Habermas (1974) and others have charged, that the theories of a bygone era, falsely purged of values, are now and always were incapable of meaningfully guiding practice in human affairs, but theories that incorporate and explicate their proponents' values certainly have the capacity to guide practice. It is always, essentially, values that guide practice of any kind.

There is a kind of investigation frequently published in nursing literature that has to do with problem solving in the practice arena. These investigations address practical problems of hands-on health care practice, such as dressings, positioning, and pulmonary toilet, sometimes comparing two techniques. Surely the time has come for nursing as a scholarly discipline to realize that these investigations constitute practical problem solving and do not constitute scholarly research undertaken to advance the knowledge of the discipline. Scholarly research is guided by and develops, expands, or tests theory. This is one of its defining characteristics. Much of the nursing problem-solving literature is like testing two methods of slicing onions: you will favor the method that makes your eyes tear less. Certainly it can be said that if a nurse tested two ways of promoting decubitus healing and the decubiti treated one way healed faster, without untoward consequences, then that way could be tentatively recommended for future use. This is not nursing research per se it is problem solving. Neither does such a procedure really guide practice. What guides practice here is the value for promoting healing and the desire to do so while avoiding harm to the person.

Nursing theory-guided practice is based on theory that is specific to the discipline of nursing, explicitly rooted in a philosophy of nursing, and intended solely to guide nursing practice and research. True theory-guided practice is far more comprehensive and complex than mere application of the results of problem-solving investigations. Only when nurses everywhere are guided in their practice by a theory base specific to nursing will nursing have achieved parity with other scholarly disciplines. As a discipline coming of age in the late 20th-century dawning of the postmodern era, nursing is poised to make a remarkable contribution to 21st-century human science and practice. Nursing as a scholarly discipline comprises not only what it is and has been, but also what it can become. History tells us plainly that nursing not guided by nursing theory becomes something else!

References

Habermas, J. (1974). Theory and practice (J. Viertel, Trans.). Boston: Beacon. (Original work, 4th ed., published in German in 1971).

Jacox, A., & Webster, G. (1986). Competing theories of science. In L. Nicoll (Ed.), Perspectives on nursing theory (pp. 333–341). Boston: Little, Brown.

Parse, R. R. (1992). Human becoming: Parse's theory of nursing. Nursing Science Quarterly, 5, 35–42.

CHAPTER 7

A Practice Discipline That's Here and Now

Merian C. Litchfield, RN, PhD

Helga Jónsdóttir, RN, PhD

A practice discipline of nursing would enable nurses to articulate the significance of what they do as an essential thread of contemporary healthcare provision, but as yet one does not exist. The purpose of this article is to develop the meaning and possibilities of a practice discipline for nursing. Tuning into the general shift in thought about our human condition across disciplines and nations, we consider features of a participatory paradigm, which, when refocused on the humanness of the health circumstance, informs our approach to a practice discipline. Knowledge is personal and participatory, evolving in the here and now of health systems. Research integral to practice and service innovation illustrates the way of looking at and talking about a new phase in discipline development. The discipline is relational and creative in practice, evolving in the forums for dialogue. Each one of us as nurses has responsibility in participation.

Key words: *dialogue, health circumstance, health experience, humanness, nursing knowledge, nursing practice, participatory paradigm, practice discipline, relational.*

> *We cannot solve our problems with the same thinking that created them.*
>
> —*Albert Einstein*

The escalating problems of providing health care in all nations call for new thinking. The shortage of nurses now, as part of the general workforce predicament, is indication of our unsustainable systems. Workplace pressures are constraining the nursing that we as nurses know is needed. As has been so throughout our history, we seek the freedom

Source: Litchfield, M., Jonsdottir, H. A practice discipline that's here and now. Advances in Nursing Science, 31 (1): 79-91. Reprinted by permission of and copyright © 2008 Lippincott Williams & Wilkins, Inc.

appropriate forums what is essential about nursing that contributes directly to health and society and what conditions are necessary for these given scarce resources. The decades of scholarship in nursing have given us a range of theories, yet the vision—and promise—of a distinct discipline of nursing is not reflected in the strategizing that gives direction to health system reform.

In this discipline vacuum, extensive lists of nurse competencies have only served to portray nursing as a set of activities given meaning as the nurse's work in the health system already defined by the social relevance of medical science. The service mission is rooted in the prevailing health paradigm of prevention, diagnosis, and treatment of disease, its signs, symptoms, and dangers. This obfuscates what nursing knowledge is and how we could be contributing to health in the lives of all people and the nation. The nursing needed as a professional practice is obscure in health policy and system development, whereas the health missions of service providers/funders define the nature of the work of nurses as employees to be managed as part of their pool of resources.

Health systems are increasingly shaped by the drive to cost-effectiveness in our world of expanding and extravagant possibilities for the cure and control of disease and disability. The challenge is intensifying to articulate our discipline in a way that influences the roles and positions for nurses in the service configuration providing essential health care. Our respective research projects have brought us to the realization that we should be vigorously pursuing the articulation of

the discipline of nursing with the scope of research broadened to the health system context—the policies, strategies, service design, and delivery—in which nursing care is inextricably woven. We do not want to just slot practitioners into the workforce; we do want to see them positioned to contribute to changes and to say what needs to happen for health care to be socially relevant as well as economically sustainable.

We write this article to energize dialogue around nursing as a practice discipline, across nations, not with the idea of reaching consensus of what nursing is, which theory is right or best, or what should be achieved. Rather, it is to enliven nursing practice, research, and education in our different ways in different places in the interests of all peoples. We have developed our thesis by taking account of the historical evolution of the discipline and locate it now within contemporary thought about the human condition to articulate the significance of nursing in its context of healthcare and service delivery. It is intended to contribute among the efforts of many nurses to make sense of our predicament and as a form of response to the call to "conscience and action" of the Nursing Manifesto project inspired in the United States at the turn of the millenium.[1]

Call of the Discipline

The nursing academy is divided into distinct camps of scholarship. In general, the efforts to develop nursing as a discipline have been separated from the pragmatics of nurses' employment as the mainstay of health service delivery—the workforce and allotted work. This division seems inevitable in hindsight. In their seminal 1978 article on "The Discipline of Nursing," Donaldson and Crowley[2] urged the differentiation of the discipline (development of the body of knowledge) from the activities of practitioners (the profession) to liberate nursing from its vocational status and to enable us to claim its social relevance. Clinical practice, they said, is concerned with here-and-now activities, whereas a discipline gives knowledge of its important expansive scope through past, present, and future for use in any place. They recommended "lessening our preoccupation with the process of nursing and pedagogy and placing emphasis on content as substance."[2] (p. 251)

This distinction must have been a confirmation, perhaps a relief, to the cadre of scholars constructing and evaluating theories. We can now see it as a necessary phase of laying claim to a distinctly nursing knowledge. But, as the often cited theory–practice gap, it created a vacuum for the kind of knowledge that could give identity and value to nursing—as a practice, in practice—that is integral to everyday health care, service delivery, and sector development. We see the consequence continuing in the age-old confusion of education and training for nurses. Paradoxically, the division is accentuated in the current drive to *integration* of health care when, by default, the disciplinary perspective brought to health assumes medical science as foundational knowledge, privileging the practice of medicine. Medical knowledge has become a generic pool of health knowledge, practiced

by physicians and selectively *applied* as the work of nurses.

The division was addressed directly—and most helpfully—in a recent debate published in *Nursing Science Quarterly* between Mitchell and Bournes[3] on one side, arguing that an extant theory is foundational for nurses to even start practicing, and Reed[4,5] and Rolfe[5,6] on the other side, arguing that theorizing is rooted responsively in the pragmatics of everyday activities. We could both agree and disagree with each side. Neither satisfies the vacuum for a contemporary practice discipline.

We are concerned about the collapse of the vision of professional nursing into the schism between efforts to create a discipline (to date) and the pragmatics of work and workforce. We believe it is timely to juxtapose these seemingly irreconcilable points of view and camps of scholarship and consider anew what is meant by a practice discipline, looking to a future of globalizing yet locally attentive health care.

The vacuum for a nursing practice discipline has been recognized from outside nursing. Weinberg,[7] a sociologist in the United States, set out to respond to the question "what do nurses do?" She observed the impotence of nurses to claim their share of scarce resources in a tight economic climate. She urged the articulation of nursing in context: "If nurses want to protect themselves and patient care, they cannot wait for interested observers to figure out what is going on. . . . The first step is to articulate what nurses as professionals do and why the little things are really big things."[7] (p. 43)

Joining the effort toward a nursing discipline, our questions are about the coherence of what nursing is about, looking to contemporary wise thinking about the human condition, life, society, and health to give relevance. In the effort to reconcile knowledge and activities in the complex context of health services and workforce, we see that nurses framing nursing as a practice—practice wisdom—is the task of discipline development for this era.

An Era of Practice

The political rhetoric is about changing the culture of health systems from a curative/reactive to a preventive/responsive orientation. Attention has turned to the workforce to achieve it, assuming division of labor according to the generic health–disease outcomes. Yet, we know people need "nursing" not usefully represented in either orientation. For nursing to be recognized in the drive to integration through multidisciplinary projects, the challenge is to be articulate about our own discipline as *practice* in situ: what nurses achieve in relation to other health-care workers and under what conditions. We see this challenge illustrated in a Canadian Health Services Research Foundation report written by nurses working on policy and mindful of the talk of multitasking and interchangeability of healthcare workers: "The question that must be asked is not 'who *can* do this set of tasks or activities?' but rather 'who *should* and why?' given the context and population."[8(p. iv)] The question is complex, arising in the discipline vacuum.

Methodologies for developing nursing knowledge have derived, often adopted, from other disciplines. They have been useful but found wanting in satisfying the vacuum for a distinct practice discipline. Thorne and colleagues, among many others, explained the inadequacies of both traditional quantitative science and the qualitative tradition for providing the scope and depth of the study needed for the "general knowledge of the sort that enhances particularization in practice."[9(p. 171)] Swinging to the pragmatic side, they argued that "interpretive description" of health and illness experiences would be more appropriate to bring nursing knowledge into its practice context. The interpretive turn was further reflected in writing about praxis from the 1990s. Connor[10] proposed a time of praxiology entering the new millennium. Doane and Varcoe[11] explained the usefulness of pragmatic enquiry to attend to experience and "ultimately reshape "'reality.'" Methodology is left implicit in whatever the nurse does.

Leaving aside the efforts to develop nursing as a discipline, and with a pragmatic orientation, Liaschenko and Peter found that the current statements of ethics of nursing are outdated in assuming it can be a profession with autonomy in controlling its own work: the statements are "no longer adequate to address the social realities and moral challenges of healthcare work."[12(p. 488)] Alternatively, they argued that considering nursing—and medicine too—as "work" would more appropriately accord value in the workplaces of contemporary health care; it could achieve the collective ethical responsibility of all healthcare providers to work collaboratively and interdependently. We see this stance as important in our efforts to acknowledge the value of everyday activities of nurses in context, but we are concerned the social relevance of nursing would continue to be obscured within the hegemony of the current service delivery culture.

Thus, attention has been turning to who the nurse is and moral agency: praxiology has continued to echo in procedures for reflective practice to recognize moral agency. However, reflection on practice remains an ad hoc academic procedure if nurses (as practitioners and educators) do not have the capability of articulating the nature of nursing knowledge in relation to health that signifies the process of a practice as part of the whole provision of health care. Nursing knowledge is tacit, research framed within the methodologies of other disciplines, nurse employment exploited, and outcomes of health care skewed and depleted of essential nursing care.

We acknowledge the pragmatic stance of many nurse scholars. It turns attention to the action of nursing as relational, dynamic, and responsive. But it is the vacuum for a discipline we continue to address, focusing on practice as we look for coherence between the pragmatics of nurses as workforce and the evolution of thinking about the nature of nursing knowledge: a *practice* discipline that conveys our ethical foundation.

In the mid-1970s, from their study of the theoretical frameworks for nursing curricula, Torres and Yura[13] identified four major concepts: person, society, health, and nursing. With some variations these have been recognized as the key elements of the discipline.[14]

As a member of the theorist group writing at the later end of that era, Margaret Newman[15] took a retrospective look at the trajectory of their emergence. She traced them as a sequential refocusing of theory development to maintain the social relevance of nursing scholarship: "What the theorist chose to examine reflected the needs of that particular time."[15(p.29)] She construed the trajectory as environment, nursing (nurse–client process), person (the human being) and, for the 1980s, "health," which she saw was cumulative, giving meaning to all the concepts.

Now we pick up on this historical trajectory to add *practice* as the contemporary integrative theme. We believe this opens scholarship to exploration of the pragmatic vis-à-vis discipline threads. It has turned us to the nurse-person-environment-health interrelationship as fundamental and therefore to the process of nursing in relation to content and its social relevance. Our challenge to find coherence that will accord us a practice discipline has brought us to a paradigm that is participatory.

A Participatory Paradigm

We refer to a participatory paradigm we see as an expression of the widespread shift in Western thought about how we understand our human condition now emerging across nations and disciplines. The word "participatory" orients us to practice as relational; we are prompted to turn our attention to the action of nursing, elaborating beyond just the presence of the nurse with patients/clients, applied knowledge, and a set of activities she or he performs. It is about the self-in-relation, complementary in our sense of community. This calls for a fresh look at temporality beyond causality, at responsibility and ethics. We see the efforts to develop a nursing discipline resonating within the movement. In this section we refer to a selective range of authors to point to some features of a participatory paradigm we believe are important for the articulation of nursing as a practice discipline.

World View in Nursing

In retrospect, we can see the emergence of a participatory paradigm in the nursing academy unfolding through the last half century. The theorists looked to the great philosophers, sages, and popularizers of contemporary thought about our human world to articulate an ontology of contemporary relevance for nursing, albeit mostly viewed through the lens of other disciplines. It was inevitable that, for a time, methodologies of the respective disciplines and their schools of thought framed the knowledge such that knowledge was abstract to be applied by nurses. The theories were used and tested, mostly confirmed as guides for nurses.

The ontologies published as grand theories each brought coherence to knowledge in their own frameworks. But the theorists and the practitioners inhabited different worlds of scholarship. Each theory, named to emphasize difference, had its own language for nursing knowledge, its own premises to frame research process and findings, and thus each attracted its own community of scholars. A fragmented discipline has been

no match for the coherence of medicine to inform health sector change.

As a second generation from Martha Rogers' articulation of a unique discipline in her "nursing science of unitary human beings," some theories have—separately—intensified an orientation to the engagement of the nurse with patients/clients. They give it significance according to the particular theory. For example, knowledge is represented by Parse[16] as cocreated and presented in the language of "human becoming" and by Newman[17] as life patterns recognized through the intersubjectivity of nurse and patient/client and depicted as the expansion of consciousness of each. Newman framed her theory as praxis where "the form that nursing research takes is the form of practice"[18(p. 100)] to point to knowledge as—and of—a process through which a transformative change in all participating activities can be achieved. Hence, nurses have been viewed as increasingly knowledgeable as engaged practitioners, even if their methods and "health" ends have been differently construed by each theory.

The theories importantly drew attention to the nurse–patient function, making a difference to the experience of people when they are patients/clients, as well as nurses, impacting on their lives.[19] However, what this means for health in relation to service design and delivery has had little attention. Moreover, as forms of knowledge the nurse brings to "what she ought to do," the theories remain as tentative paradigms, coexisting, if not competing, in pockets. Their significance for the employing organization's mission is subtle and fragile. As the workforce, nurses are employed to work in a causal paradigm where knowledge is product—the evidence for discrete interventions. Activities expected of nurses are rooted in the mission of the organization. They continue to be subject to the service boundaries, resources, and conditions that support health care within the hegemonic medical cure and control paradigm. The vacuum for the practice discipline of nursing seeks a further turn in a participatory paradigm to move further into the relational nature of nursing—beyond packages of interventions—to bring the coherence of a practice.

Meanwhile, others have been taking an epistemological approach. Benner[20] held her focus on the activities of nurses in their workplaces. She emphasized the embodied moral agency of nurses in caring—socially embedded—and its expression in their expanding capability to practice knowledgeably. The participatory nature of a practice is clear in the depiction of "embodied interdependence" of nurse with patients/clients as well as in practitioner communities. Doane and Varcoe emphasized the inventiveness of nurses "to create and recreate their knowing in each moment of practice."[11(p. 89)]

The detour of nursing scholarship through other disciplines and the separate theoretical and pragmatist approaches emerging from it have been important in our consciousness of different paradigms of knowledge in nursing. But although all the leaders of the factions emphasize the importance of communities of scholars, trying to move between them to question and articulate the nature of nursing

practice is fraught with misunderstanding. The ontological and epistemological efforts to date call forth new thinking for an inclusive nursing community.

We have been searching alongside many others for ways of developing the discipline of nursing both for and in practice, such as Boyd,[21] Connor,[22] Doane and Varcoe,[11] Picard and Jones,[19] Reed,[4] and Roy and Jones.[23] Now, as part of this movement, we take our stand in a participative paradigm to look beyond the divisions, while still preserving diversity in how practitioners contribute to "health" in the various places and times of healthcare provision.

A Shifting World View

A broad scan of literature reveals a general shift well underway in Western societies in the way we understand our human condition. We refer to some authors to point to features of a participatory paradigm that we believe are of greatest significance for the dialogue in nursing. In particular, we see the significance lies in how we situate ourselves in the world we seek to understand. We are exploring the meaning this lens brings to nursing as a "discipline."

Theological scholars[24–26] have written about a period of transition in human culture over the past centuries from the transethnic world of the great religions to this point of emergence of a global secular world in which we understand ourselves as coparticipants in the creation of lives in our shared places and time, with responsibility for it. Geering writes, "We humans are slowly coming to realise that what each of us inhabits is a world of meaning, which we ourselves have put together."[26(p. 5)] Cupitt[25] writes about "be-ing" to refer to our here-and-now evolving communal world. All these authors use the term "secular" to mean attention to this world of diverse beliefs and values of the sacred.

Insights from discoveries in the physical sciences have led scientists—and many popularizers—to write about a shift to a paradigm in which observer and observed, knower and known, merge. Schrodinger's cat story of the 1930s has been cited repeatedly to popularize the revelations from quantum physicists: the interrelationship of observer, tools, and observation determine our reality. David Bohm, U.S./British physicist-turned-philosopher, said, "World views—it's really a self-world-view because it includes yourself."[27(p. 25)]

In biology, Chilean biologists Maturana and Varela[28] pioneered a "science of cognition," coining the term "autopoiesis" to convey their observations of a dynamic interrelationship of part and whole in cellular systems. They write their insight as follows: "We live our field of vision . . . we cannot separate our history of actions" biological and social "from how this world appears to us."[28(p. 23)] Furthermore, it is relational: "We have only the world that we bring forth with others, and only love helps us bring it forth."[28(p. 248)] Lynn Margulis, an evolutionary biologist from Massachusetts, writing with Dorian Sagan,[29] argued the inadequacy of the hegemonic reductionism of evolutionary theory after Darwin, where knowledge is framed as linear and competitive. From another world view, she reinterpreted observations and drew on recent genome studies to depict evolution as integrative. Conveyed in the term "symbiogenesis," the origins of species, humans included, are explained as ecological interrelationships at the cellular level; complexity increases through cooperation and new forms of community emerge. This realization led the duo to address the big human question "What is life?" to which they answer (in part) "a question the *universe poses to itself* in the form of a human being. . . . we are only a single theme of the orchestrated lifeform . . . *our life is embedded* . . . in the rest of Earth's sentient symphony" (emphasis added).[30(p. 199)]

M. C. Escher, living and working in western Europe, creatively depicted the participatory thinking in 1956. Choosing to call himself an artisan—"a graphic artist 'with heart and soul',"[31(p. 8)] he explored the human capability of representing three-dimensional reality in two-dimensional drawings. A drawing called Print Gallery shows a man in a gallery looking at a picture in which his "looking at the picture" is an integral part. He described it as follows: ". . . we come to the logical conclusion that the young man himself also must be part of the print he is looking at. He actually sees himself as a detail of the picture; reality and image are one and the same."[31(p. 67)]

Historically, tracing ideas of science, theology, and philosophies, Skolimowski, of Polish origin, addressed directly the "new order of reality" as "the participatory mind": "We are woven into the universe we explore."[32(p. 88)] The world we experience as complex continuously evokes our efforts to simplify: "The patterns and configurations of the world are not there independently of mind, but are the patterns of our knowledge through which our minds work."[32](p. 88) Furthermore, "the power of creation is the power of articulation."[32](p. 14) A participatory world view is a new understanding of ontology and epistemology. The meanings of these terms require us to consider them together: "they elicit from each other what they assume in each other."[32](p. 76) Knowledge is in process as comprehension, and "to know is to *constitute* the world."[32](p. 81)

A proactive ecological philosopher born and based in the United States, Abram[33] also draws on great philosophical writing along with varied depictions of the worlds of indigenous oral peoples and his own experience as a sleight-of-hand magician performing as part of everyday life in many countries. He conveys the participatory thinking inherent in the interrelatedness of human cognition and the natural world. Always, he says, there is an active interplay between the perceiving body and that which it perceives: "We always retain the ability to alter or suspend any particular instance of participation. Yet we can never suspend the flux of participation itself."[33](p. 59) We are immersed in a sensuous world. We make sense of this world humanly through our language: "The human mind is not some otherworldly essence that comes to house itself inside our physiology. Rather, it is instilled and provoked by the sensorial field itself, induced by the tensions and participations between the human body and the animate earth."[33](p. 262) "The common

field of our lives and the other lives with which ours are entwined . . . our experience of this field is always relative to our situation in it."[33](p. 40)

The participatory thinking has also been emerging in the writing about the general organization of societies and workplaces. The participatory theme has been integral to the women's movement. It shows in Wheeler and Chinn's[34] reframing of group process as community represented by the acronym PEACE: Praxis, Empowerment, Awareness, Consensus, Evolvement. It is also found in Margaret Wheatley's[35] explanation of transformational leadership for the management of organizations, linking directly to "the participative nature of the universe" emerging from quantum physics. Danah Zohar's experience in childbirth led her to become a popularizer of the new physics revelations with a participatory interpretation. With psychiatrist/psychotherapist Ian Marshall, she is now reaching into the business worlds and corporate culture, elaborating the relational theme of "changing ourselves to change the world."[36]

In these selected but wide-ranging writings, we can see a participatory shift. All authors noted the inadequacy now of our former views of knowledge of past eras. These views have increasingly obscured the humanness of living our lives—experience, spirituality, sentience, and mystery. But this participatory view does not negate previous ways of thinking, nor even transcend them. Everything just looks different. Cupitt[25] uses the terms "contingency," "immanence," and "outsidelessness" to refer to our humanness.

All authors bring coherence to their reasoning with reference to community and love. We are participants in a creative world in the moment, constantly evolving as participants in it and together making sense of it in our own particular ways. Our spirituality is our interrelationship, as participants, in the sensuousness and communion of our living universe. We seek to understand, see patterns, find order, and theorize, knowing we are ourselves inside what we write about. Temporality moves beyond the linear; we live and act in the here and now: "always in the middle of things," Cupitt says.[25(p. 64)] The meaning of the past–future is unfolding and enfolding in the moment of "holomovement," Bohm[27] says. Hence we are brought to the realization of our vulnerability and our responsibility in action.

Expressing these features, a participatory world view has language at its core. Geering explains language as evolving meaning: "Language is the collective product of the powers of human imagination and creativity," where words to syntax to stories construe our cultural heritage, such that "by means of stories we create the world we live in."[26(pp. 18, 41)] Abram views language as evolving from and expressing the participatory nature of the universe: "The sensuous, perceptual life-world, whose wild, participatory logic ramifies and elaborates itself in language . . . a vast, living fabric continually being woven by those who speak."[33(pp. 83–84)] Bohm's[27] physics led him to focus his thinking about language on the dialogical nature of our human world of unfolding, meaning where "meaning is active," making sense of things; culture construes language, and dialogue is a form of "social meditation" unfolding among us in what we attend to.

In the academy of social sciences, John Heron and Peter Reason[37] have been elaborating their earlier work on cooperative enquiry and action research and now articulate their methods as expression of a participatory paradigm. They describe a participative paradigm: "the mind's conceptual articulation of the world is grounded in its experiential participation in what is present, in what there is."[37(p. 277)] Critical subjectivity extends to critical intersubjectivity. To elaborate the participatory nature of knowledge, they added axiology to ontology, epistemology, and methodology. Axiology makes explicit the ethics of knowledge development in the question: "What sort of knowledge is intrinsically valuable in human life?"[37(p. 277)] Ethics is now inherent in the whole process.

Reason and Bradbury present their edited book on "participatory inquiry and practice" as part of what they describe as the revolutionary transition in world view "emerging at this historical moment."[38(p. 1)] In their introduction they too trace the roots historically—from the reinvention of humanism in the 1950s through the cognitive and linguistic turns of the postmodern era that alerted us to the relationship between power and language, and so to the participatory world view of today that draws on and takes us into a socially constructed world. They connect to Bohm, Abram, and Skolimowski among many other contemporary sages to elaborate an action science that "continually enquires into the meaning and purpose of our practice,"[38(p. 7)] relational and concerned with the betterment of the world and life in it. We attend to what we have come to know through an instrumental paradigm "to draw on techniques and knowledge of positivist science and to frame these within a human context."[38(p. 7)] They too emphasize the linguistic nature of things: "As soon as we attempt to articulate ('real' reality) we enter a world of human language and cultural expression."[38(p. 7)] They talk of knowledge as a verb rather than a noun in dialogue, evoking attention to the ethical and political. Knowledge is "a living, evolving process of coming to know rooted in everyday experience."[38(p. 2)] In their view, inquiry is about the healing of the splits and alienation in contemporary experience.

Our consciousness of the trend in thought about the nature of human knowledge has given us a new lens on the discipline to see how the once-separated discipline and activities of nurses are one as process. After Reason and Bradbury[38] and Geering,[26] let us consider the discipline of nursing as a verb inviting the syntax to express culture and stories that convey nuances; it is the process of practice in context and informed in dialogue. Dialogue brings nursing theoretical insights and the schools of knowledge into the complexity of healthcare provision.[11] In nursing communities our attention is drawn to the language, texts, and discourses that have confused and divided us and alienated many. Our professional responsibility is to participate in open, inclusive dialogue.

But this meaning of discipline begs a focus that orients practice to the social relevance of nursing: a nursing take on "the common good" to draw us into dialogue. Reason and Bradbury stated their moral purpose for inquiry, using terms appropriated from the literature through the ages: "The flourishing of life, the life of human persons, of human communities, and increasingly of the more-than-human world of which we are a part."[38(p. 10)] We can agree with this too but want a focus that enables us to participate in a *nursing* community about nursing practice. For this, we have looked to our discipline's history.

Focus of the Discipline

Each theorist proposed a focus for nursing—the theory—as she or he had conceptualized it. For other scholars it has been implicit. Also, there have been many threads of nurses' work and roles developing worldwide, in health systems without a specifically nursing purpose. We see the elaboration of advanced practice nursing happening within specialty fields and practices, the focus closely aligned with medical science concerning assessment–diagnosis–prescription or defined by the mission of employing organizations. As educators, we have observed students searching for a nursing purpose to anchor their theses, often reaching into other disciplines for ideas of social relevance.

Newman, with Sime and Corcoran-Perry,[39] in describing their framework of three research paradigms, recognized the need for a focus statement to convey the social mandate of nursing. Noting the predominance of caring and health as integrative concepts in the nursing literature, they proposed the phrase "caring in the human health experience." Newman explained: "Caring designates the nature of the nursing practice participation . . . the experiential dimension characterizes the phenomenon (of human health) as something beyond the traditional objective-subjective perspective."[40(p. 48)] The phrase as a whole was the focus of the discipline. This statement has been important in drawing attention to the social relevance of our research efforts. In a phrase, the concepts of caring and health had more meaning for nursing than when considered separately; there is deeper meaning in expression of culture and history.

As students, our beginning research was underway at this time. We explored what the focus statement might mean as we studied the nature of practice. This led to the explication of a research-as-if-practice process.[41–44] But separateness still bothered us; a researcher is not a practitioner in the sense of having a work role and status within the health service organization. We must be able to state the social relevance of our practice, given our paradigm of a participatory, always-evolving-in-the-moment idea of knowledge. It must have meaning for the practice of all other nurses and for health service and policy trends.

In retrospect, we can see the 1991 focus statement representing its era and cultural context. The relational caring/experiential aspect of nursing was growing as a counterbalance to the expanding challenges of technological advances and fiscally driven health service reforms. We can see the strong influence of phenomenology, grounded theory, and hermeneutics on nurses' studies of "the lived experience" of people as patients and clients. Hence, the focus on experience privileges these methodologies and their parent disciplines—primary attention to individuals. Although it acknowledges the moral relational core, the phrase separates "what is important" to be attended to from the action that addresses it. It is difficult to see how it focuses knowledge development for much of the work of nurses in established roles and career pathways.

Through our research projects in our respective countries and writing together to explore the nature of nursing practice in context, we have sought a broader statement: a cohesive statement that is more inclusive of the different forms of knowledge and that resolves the current splitting of the relational and the technical. For this, we have turned our attention now to *humanness*.

This tunes us into the 1991 focus statement[39] and recent writing such as the *Consensus Statement on Emerging Nursing Knowledge* orchestrated by the Boston Group.[24] But, in replacing the action concept (caring) we are opening to all paradigms of action, whatever the nature of change and whatever part the nurse plays in change. Furthermore, although we agree that attention to people's experience is vital in nursing, we are now lifting our sights to more broadly attend to the *health circumstance*. For us, the discipline focus is *the humanness of the health circumstance*.

With this focus we look beyond the separateness of human beings as nurse and patient in engagements to being human whatever the health predicament, whoever is implicated in it, and however located in time and place. It contrasts with, but is essentially complementary to, the medical discipline focus on the incidence of disease, differential diagnosis, and treatment to date framed within a deterministic paradigm.

The phrase expresses social relevance. The public looks to nurses for a human face in the technically and fiscally oriented world; our understanding of health circumstance is what enables us to advocate the humanness of people's experience in the strategizing for service development and in community development. It gives a common focus to research framed within the extant theoretical orientations, research addressing the practicalities of specific activities expected of nurses, and research on issues of workforce and service management. It calls forth the examination of the ethics of nursing.

In Action

The lens of a participatory paradigm makes everything look different: practice, research, management, education, service design, and policy development. Our understanding of the paradigm has evolved through our research endeavors, as we sought to address the vacuum for a contextualized practice discipline. It has opened our thinking not only to an alternative form of nursing practice but also to the form of leadership through which policy, service development, and management can be constructed to support the health care provided by all nurses, whatever the paradigms for their activities. We can think now of an integrative people-pivotal paradigm for healthcare provision.[45] The following is a glimpse of our growing consciousness of the significance of nursing practice for health care and possibilities for action. In this we are not "proving" or "demonstrating" our thesis, we just want to illustrate a way of seeing and talking about nursing in context.

Importantly, our research starting point was the process of practice. We knew that to explore the relational nature of nursing we had to be practicing. We awoke to a general trend in thinking about our humanness and connected into the discourses referring to a "participatory paradigm."[41–44] Initially undertaken according to academic requirements, the research was not integral to the sanctioned, pressured yet seductive health service design, workforce, and professional structures. But it was *as if* practice; it was as close to the reality of practice as possible without being swallowed into the system.

The process we described was of partnership with people as patients/client (considered as collective) such that, through our conversations extending in time (multiple meetings), we made sense of what was happening for them. Holding the humanness of the circumstance as our orientation, *everything* happening and talked about, place and time, had relevance, as far as our minds allowed us: outsideless.[25] There was insight into how the predicament had come about and what it meant in life ahead for family, work, and play; meaning was actualized in the statements of action that each could, and would, take in the moment. In action, people as families and groups with really complex health circumstances managed tangled difficult times,[44] accessed services discerningly, made the best of health care available conscious of scarce resources, and addressed health matters that would have implications for later years or for following generations.[45] The insights alerted us in our practitioner role to our responsibilities around the personal predicament as well as community life, collaboration among healthcare workers to orchestrate health care, health service management, and policy development. Hence, action was more than a set of activities; it was coherence in action around whatever was needed for everyone to get on with life as patients/clients, family and community members, citizens, and as nurses in their professional world. It included—but not necessarily—the *conventions* of health care. Knowledge was participatory in process for all; it was practice wisdom. As researchers we developed narratives that presented the humanness of the health circumstance, and these were used for influence in the various forums where policy and funding decisions are made.

Our interest turned to nurse roles, new and traditional, and how they might be complementary in contributing to the expected "health outcomes" of contracted services and the organization's mission. Projects were funded as practice and service innovation.[44,45] Education looked different; roles of

teacher and learner had changed. As educators-researchers we took one step back from the practitioner role—to mentorship with practitioners. Learning was integral to the dialogue of practice; roundtable forums were the medium.

As mentors-researchers we came with our novice experience. We could see in our participation the expression of our own respective culturally and historically grounded education and wise mentorship from our earlier professional lives that had shaped our values, viewpoints, and hang-ups. The practitioners took their own lead in developing their practice in relation to each other. Together, we challenged our different languages, constantly reexamining viewpoints as a process of theorizing, each with our own take on the task to articulate practice, what it achieves, and the service model to support it. There was work to be done to create a practice, personally and culturally expressive and responsive within health service environments. It was intense work, but it evoked new vitality in its creativity and was deeply appreciated by all participants. One nurse said she had "come home to nursing."[46]

Research, practice, service development, management, and education began to collapse into the dialogical process, with the patient/client and nurse partnership being pivotal.[45] Health care can become a dynamic collaborative endeavor. Now the new practice role is influencing reconfiguration in service delivery, integrative in the traditional silo structure of primary, secondary, and tertiary sectors and specialist divisions. In a participatory paradigm nursing practice is collective. Nurses work in different paradigms, their activities given coherence in the core dialogue centered on and reaching out from partnerships with patients/clients. Professional forums are essential where the ethics of practice can take form for each nurse and standards continually examined. There is more work to be done.

Hence, with this eversion in healthcare provision, discipline development is in practice, leadership comes from practice, and attention primarily focused on the humanness of the health circumstance. Service models are shaped by and around practice. The roundtable forums expand and contract to dynamically address the current issues and challenges. They take account of the diversity of community life, other healthcare workers, service and policy developers, funders, health economists, and politicians. It is not all easy and smooth, but the possibilities are open. There is even more work to be done.

Conclusion

This discussion is intended as a contribution to the dialogue around the discipline, not a proposal of "how to" or theory. The separation of knowledge development in the academy from the activities of nurses-as-workforce has created a vacuum for a practice discipline that would enable nurses to articulate the significance of nursing, so essential in contemporary healthcare provision. We have tuned into the trend in thought around the human condition represented in the emergence of a participatory paradigm

and explored its meaning for nursing in the context of health service delivery to have social relevance today. Turning our focus to the humanness of the health circumstance, our research has brought us to an understanding of the discipline as relational and evolving in the process of nursing practice in context. The discipline is here and now, alive and creative in forums for dialogue. Each one of us has responsibility in participation.

References

1. Cowling R, Chinn PL, Hagedorn S. *A Nursing Manifesto: A Call to Conscience and Action.* http://www.nursemanifest.com/manifesto.htm. Published 2000. Accessed July 29, 2007.
2. Donaldson S, Crowley D. The discipline of nursing. In: Nicoll L, ed. *Perspectives on Nursing Theory.* Boston. Little Brown & Co; 1986:241–251.
3. Mitchell GJ, Bournes DA. Challenging the athoretical production of nursing knowledge: a response to Reed and Rolfe's column. *Nurs Sci Q.* 2006;19(2):116–119.
4. Reed PG. The practice turn in nursing epistemology. *Nurs Sci Q.* 2006;19(1): 36–38.
5. Reed PG, Rolfe G. Nursing knowledge and nurses' knowledge: a reply to Mitchell and Bournes. *Nurs Sci Q.* 2006;19(2):120–122.
6. Rolfe G. Nursing praxis and the science of the unique. *Nurs Sci Q.* 2006;19(1): 39–43.

7. Weinberg DB. When little things are big things. In: Nelson S, Gordon S, eds. *The Complexities of Care: Nursing Reconsidered.* Ithaca, NY: ILR/Cornell University Press; 2006:30–43.

8. Besner J, Doran D, Hall LM, et al. *A Systematic Approach to Maximizing Nursing Scopes of Practice.* Canadian Health Services Research Foundation. http://www.chsrf.ca/final_research/ogc/besner_e.php. Published September 2005. Accessed July 29, 2007.

9. Thorne S, Kirkham SR, MacDonald-Emes J. Interpretive description: a non-categorical qualitative alternative for developing nursing knowledge. *Res Nurs Health.* 1997;20:169–177.

10. Connor MJ. The practical discourse in philosophy and nursing: an exploration of linkages and shifts in the evolution of praxis. *Nurs Philos.* 2004;5:54–66.

11. Doane GH, Varcoe C. Toward compassionate action: pragmatism and the inseparability of theory/practice. *Adv Nurs Sci.* 2005;28(1):81–90.

12. Liaschenko J, Peter E. Nursing ethics and conceptualizations of nursing: profession, practice and work. *J Adv Nurs.* 2004;46(5):488–495.

13. Torres G, Yura H. *Today's Conceptual Framework: Its Relationship to the Curriculum Development Process.* New York: National League for Nursing; 1974.

14. Meleis AI. *Theoretical Nursing: Development and Progress.* 3rd ed. Philadelphia: Lippincott; 1997.

15. Newman MA. The continuing revolution: a history of nursing science. In: Chaska NL, ed. *The Nursing Profession: A Time to Speak.* New York: McGraw-Hill; 1983:385–393.

16. Parse RR. *The Human Becoming School of Thought: A Perspective for Nurses and Other Health Professionals.* Thousand Oaks, CA: Sage; 1998.

17. Newman MA. *Health as Expanding Consciousness.* 2nd ed. New York: National League for Nursing; 1994.

18. Newman MA. The research-practice relationship. *Nurs Sci Q.* 1991;4(3):100–101.

19. Picard C, Jones D, eds. *Giving Voice to What We Know: Margaret Newman's Theory of Health as Expanding Consciousness in Nursing Practice, Research and Education.* Sudbury, MA: Jones & Bartlett; 2005.

20. Benner P. The roles of embodiment, emotion and lifeworld for rationality and agency in nursing practice. *Nurs Philos.* 2000;1:5–19.

21. Boyd CO. Toward a nursing practice research method. *Adv Nurs Sci.* 1993:16(2):9–25.

22. Connor MJ. *Courage and Complexity in Chronic Illness: Reflective Practice in Nursing.* Wellington, NZ: Daphne Brasell Press/Whitireia Publishing; 2004.

23. Roy C, Jones DA, eds. *Nursing Knowledge Development and Clinical Practice.* New York: Springer; 2007.

24. Armstrong K. *A History of God.* London: William Heinemann; 1993.

25. Cupitt D. *The Revelation of Being.* London: SCM Press; 1998.

26. Geering L. *Tomorrow's God: How We Create Our Worlds.* Wellington, NZ: Bridget Williams Books; 1994.

27. Bohm D. *Unfolding Meaning: A Weekend of Dialogue with David Bohm.* London: Routledge; 1985.

28. Maturana HR, Varela FJ. *The Tree of Knowledge: The Biological Roots of Human Understanding.* Revised ed. Boston: Shambhala; 1992.

29. Margulis L, Sagan D. *Acquiring Genomes: A Theory of the Origins of the Species.* New York: Basic Books; 2002.

30. Margulis L, Sagan D. *What Is Life?* New York: Simon & Schuster; 1995.

31. Escher MC. *Exploring the Infinite: Escher on Escher.* van Hoorn WJ, Wierda F, compiler; Oneindige H, trans. New York: Harry N Abrams; 1989.

32. Skolimowski H. *The Participatory Mind. A New Theory of Knowledge and of the Universe.* London: Penguin Books; 1994.

33. Abram D. *The Spell of the Sensuous: Perception and Language in a More-Than-Human World.* New York: Vintage Books; 1996.

34. Wheeler CE, Chinn PL. *Peace and Power: A Handbook of Feminist Process.* 3rd ed. New York: National League for Nursing; 1991.

35. Wheatley MJ. *Leadership and the New Science: Learning About Organization From an Orderly Universe.* San Francisco: Berrett-Koehler; 1992.

36. Zohar D, Marshall IN. *Spiritual Capital: Wealth We Can Live By.* San Francisco: Berrett-Koehler; 2004.

37. Heron J, Reason P. A participatory inquiry paradigm. *Qual Inq.* 1997;3(3): 274–294.

38. Reason P, Bradbury H. Introduction: inquiry and participation in search of a world worthy of human aspiration. In: Reason P, Bradbury H, eds. *Handbook of Action Research: Participative Inquiry and Practice.* London: Sage; 2001:1–14.

39. Newman MA, Sime AM, Corcoran-Perry SA. The focus of the discipline of nursing. In: Newman MA, ed. *A Developing Discipline: Selected Works of Margaret Newman.* New York: National League for Nursing; 1995:33–42.

40. Newman MA. Prevailing paradigms in nursing. In: Newman MA, ed. *A Developing Discipline: Selected Works of Margaret Newman.* New York: National League for Nursing; 1995:43–54.

41. Litchfield MC. Practice wisdom. *Adv Nurs Sci.* 1999;22(2):62–73.

42. Pharris MD. Coming to know ourselves as community through a nursing partnership with adolescents convicted of murder. *Adv Nurs Sci.* 2002;24(3): 21–42.

43. Jónsdóttir H, Litchfield MC, Pharris MD. The relational core of nursing: practice as it unfolds. *J Adv Nurs.* 2004;47(3): 241–250.

44. Jónsdóttir H. Research-as-if-practice: a study of family nursing partnership with couples experiencing severe breathing

difficulties. *J Fam Nurs*. 2007;13(4): 443–460.

45. Litchfield MC. *Towards a People-Pivotal Paradigm for Healthcare: Report of the Turangi Primary Health Care Nursing Innovation 2003–2006*. New Zealand Ministry of Health. Accessed September 6, 2011, from http://www.moh.govt.nz/ publicationpending.

46. Litchfield M, Laws M. Achieving family health and cost containment outcomes: innovation in the New Zealand health sector reforms. In: Cohen E, De Back V, eds. *The Outcomes Mandate: Case Management in Health Care Today*. St. Louis, MO: Mosby; 1999: 306–316.

Conceptualizations of Human Beings, Health, Environment, and Nursing Practice

In Part Two of this text, scholars offer the opportunity to reflect on the role of people and experiences in advanced nursing practice. In Chapter 8, Reed explicates the ontology of the discipline of nursing in a unique way in which nursing is "an inherent human process of well-being." This construct can be related to the notion of nursing as a basic human science. Reed speaks of nursing as a way of knowing, a way of doing, and a way of being. In Chapter 9, Bansfield develops a philosophical method to examine the fundamentals of Orem's self-care deficit nursing theory.

In Chapter 10, Boykin and Schoenhofer, whose framework of nursing as caring posits enhancing personhood as a goal of nursing, discuss how enhancing personhood can be viewed as an outcome of nursing practice. Personhood is here defined as "a process of living grounded in caring." Although "outcomes" represents a buzzword and a necessity in today's healthcare universe, it has rarely been defined qualitatively. This chapter challenges us to "suppose that nursing is not a quantity but a quality."

In Chapter 11, Pender explicates old and new views of health along with nursing's contribution to nurturing new conceptualizations. Although nursing's contributions to paradigmatic shifts in views of health in society have gone largely unrecognized, nurse scholars can certainly point to works in our literature from 1970 onward that offered a vision of health as experiential and unitary and patterned rather than normed. These views from the nursing literature largely predated similar paradigmatic shifts now occurring at the cultural and societal levels.

In Chapter 12, continuing the theme of emerging views of health, Cowling describes a reconceptualization of healing in a new paradigm as the process of appreciating wholeness. Cowling links this theory-based practice explicitly to transformational praxis and describes in detail how one can practice fundamentally from a theoretical perspective and from one's values in moment-to-moment relating with a client. In Chapter 13, Butterfield explains why nurses and other health professionals must look beyond individuals' immediate behaviors, when considering health behaviors, to the societal contexts in which these occur. In many cases in which population health is negatively impacted, improvement stems not from actions at the individual level to change behaviors among those affected but rather from social actions aimed at significant changes in socioeconomic structures and processes that may affect thousands or millions. Butterfield's conceptualization of environment captures all of the dimensions that Fawcett outlined.

In Chapter 14, Kleffel further expands the concept of environment by explicating an ecocentric paradigm in contrast to an egocentric paradigm and a homocentric paradigm. The ecocentric approach is "grounded in the cosmos" and represents a view of environment as whole, living, interconnected, and one with humanity. Clearly, environmental perspectives offer many opportunities for both values-based practice with populations and evidence-based care for populations but in ways that are qualitatively different from practice with individuals. In Chapter 15, Parse explores the transformation of nursing practice when it is guided by the human becoming school of thought. Nursing practice from this frame of reference is explicitly based on values and beliefs. Parse writes, "The form of nursing in the transformational practice guided by the human becoming principles is true presence: a non-routinized way of being with others that honours the others' views and choices on changing health patterns and quality of life." Parse asserts that nurses as professionals have an ethical responsibility to practice from an explicitly nursing frame of reference. She cites literature that documents changes in quality of life when care is delivered from the human becoming framework. Readers are invited to reflect on how their adoption of a nursing framework impacts (or would impact) the values on which their practice is based and their use of evidence as the basis for care.

In Chapter 16, Johnson, in a philosophical study, examines nursing practice as an art. Johnson makes several provocative claims, such as her assertion that the capacity of the nurse to grasp meaning in patient situations is not affected by the intellect and not based in reflection or reasoning. Ironically, there follows a lengthy section on the nurse's ability to determine rationally an appropriate course of action in which the meaning of the situation for the patient is not mentioned. Could the introduction of the overarching constructs of values-based practice and evidence-based care offer a coherent logical and humane alternative interpretation?

Articles about the "graying of America" and related themes frequently report on the prevalence of various chronic diseases, the necessity of more forms of gerontological care, and a myriad of concerns. In Chapter 17, McCormack introduces a conceptual framework for person-centered practice with older people. The central idea of person-centered practice is respect for persons and their right to self-determination, which McCormack links to the concept of autonomy as authentic consciousness, an explicitly value-laden view. In Chapter 18, Doane and Varcoe consider nursing relationships, values, and goals in today's terms, understanding recent developments in health care have increased the challenging nature of these components. Influences on nursing relationships are examined and the authors explain the use of relational inquiry as a tool to navigate through contemporary nursing practice.

Collectively, these chapters represent the need for advanced practice nurses to place persons and their experiences at the center of the caring process while maintaining a broad perspective of their environments, communities, and societies. This all-at-once seemingly contradictory stance is actually core to nursing as a scholarly discipline, and it must be understood for the advanced practice nursing to have a scholarly understanding of the discipline. These chapters offer ample opportunities for reflection.

CHAPTER 8

Nursing: The Ontology of the Discipline

Pamela G. Reed, RN, PhD, FAAN

The purpose of this article is to contribute to clarifying the ontology of the discipline by extending existing meanings of the term nursing to propose a substantive definition. In this definition, nursing is viewed as an inherent human process of well-being, manifested by complexity and integration in human systems. The nature of this process and theoretical implications of the new nursing are presented. Nurses are invited to continue the dialogue about the meaning of the term and explore the implications of nursing, substantively defined, for their practice and science.

Key words: *deconstruction, knowledge development, metaparadigm, ontology, postmodernism.*

Distinguishing the term nursing as a noun from its use as a verb was put forth most profoundly by Rogers (1970), whose vision extended the scholarship of earlier nursing theorists to thrust nursing forward to be recognized as both a scientific discipline as well as a professional practice. It is time, however, to push back the frontier once again, beyond these two important understandings of nursing, by proposing a new meaning of nursing. With this new meaning, the term itself represents the nature and substance of the discipline. In other words, nursing is the ontology of the discipline.

The ideas put forth here are done so in the spirit of accepting Watson's (1995) "postmodern challenge" to exploit the climate of deconstruction of nursing (see Rampragus, 1995; Reed, 1995) to extend and, by some

Source: Reed, P. (1997). Nursing: The ontology of the discipline. Nursing Science Quarterly. 10(2):76–79.
Reprinted by permission of and copyright © 2002 Sage Publications, Inc.

degree, reconstruct current understandings of nursing. Smith's (1988a) article outlined the ongoing dialogue about two meanings of nursing, as a verb and a noun. This dialogue is revisited here for the purpose of further clarifying what is the ontology of the discipline, long considered a crucial question by seminal thinkers in nursing (Ellis, 1982; Rogers, 1970; Roy, 1995).

Continuing the Dialogue: Nursing as a Process of Well-Being

It is proposed here that there exists a third and perhaps most basic definition of nursing in which nursing represents the substantive focus of the discipline. Disciplines are characterized by their substantive focus: archaeology is the study of the archaeo, or what is ancient and primitive. Astronomy is the study of the astro, astronomical phenomena such as the motion and constitution of celestial bodies. Biology is a branch of knowledge about biol, or living matter. Chemistry deals with the processes and properties of chemical substances. Physics is the study of physical properties and processes. Psychology is the study of the psyche, referring to mental processes and activities associated with human behavior, and nursing, the discipline, is proposed here to be the study of nursing processes of well-being, inherent among human systems.

This meaning of nursing, as an inherent process of well-being, derives in part from the root word, nurse, defined as a process of nourishing, of promoting the development or progress of something. The meaning also derives from synonyms of nurse meaning to heal, to foster, to sustain (Laird, 1971; Webster's New Collegiate Dictionary, 1979). These descriptions signify that nursing involves a process that is developmental, progressive, and sustaining, and by which well-being occurs.

The Inherent Nursing Process

The theme of human beings' inherent nursing processes as the substantive focus of the discipline is supported in nursing theorists' works from Nightingale in 1859, to the mid-20th century writings of Henderson, to the contemporary turn-of-the-century ideas of Schlotfeldt. Nightingale (1859/1969) wrote about the person's "innate power" and the inner "reparative process." Henderson (1964) eloquently symbolized the power of the nurse within, describing nursing as "the consciousness of the unconscious, the love of life of the suicidal . . . the eyes of the newly blind, a means of locomotion for the infant . . . the voice for those too weak or withdrawn to speak" (p. 63). Watson (1985) referred to "self-healing processes," and Schlotfeldt (1994) stressed human beings' "inherent ability and propensity to seek and attain health." In addition, this nursing process is not necessarily based upon a reversal of a disease process, but more upon a moving forward, to gain a sense of well-being in the absence or presence of disease.

The discipline's understanding of how a nursing process is manifested is shifting away from the mid-20th century mechanistic conception of nursing as a process external to patients and conducted by the nurse, that is, the old nursing process. The process of nursing is viewed now more from a relational perspective, congruent with contextual and transformative conceptions of the world (see Newman, 1992; Pepper, 1942). Nursing is a participatory process that transcends the boundary between patient and nurse and derives from a valuing of what Rogers (1980, 1992) described as human systems' inherent propensity for "innovation and creative change."

"Human systems" refers to an individual or a group of human beings (Rogers, 1992, p. 30). As such, human systems, whether in the form of individuals, dyads, groups, or communities, emanate and participate in nursing processes. Nursing processes may be manifested, for example, in the grieving that an individual experiences, in the caring that occurs among people and their families and nurses, in the healing practices shared by a culture, or in many other as yet undiscovered patterns of nursing. Today, these patterns may be described as intentional or unconscious, automatic or contemplative, relational or chemical, or simply unknown. Nevertheless, with continued nursing research, education, and practice, nursing processes can be learned and knowingly deployed to facilitate well-being. Murphy's (1992) visionary book, for example, addresses some of these possibilities. He proposes a future wherein people are more aware of their innate healing potential and employ it to more purposefully enhance health.

Nightingale did not invent nursing, described here in terms of an inherent propensity for well-being. Just as earthquakes existed before geologists and photosynthesis before botanists, nursing processes existed in human beings, ultimately described by Nightingale (1859/1969) as that which nurses were to facilitate by placing the patient in the best situation possible. It follows, then, that nursing does not belong exclusively to certain groups of people, such as "well" persons or professional nurses, it belongs to human nature.

Defining the substance of the discipline of nursing in terms of a well-being process inherent among human beings does not negate the importance of knowledge of factors that interface with nursing to influence well-being and healing. Examples of these factors, often the focus of study in ancillary professions and disciplines, include the environmental, financial, cultural, surgical, and pharmacological. However, any sense of well-being involves, most basically, a nursing process. The quest for nursing is to understand the nature of and to facilitate nursing processes in diverse contexts of health experiences.

The Nature of Nursing Processes

What is the nature of nursing processes that distinguishes them from other human processes? It is proposed that the intersection of at least three characteristics—complexity, integration, well-being—distinguishes human processes as nursing specifically, nursing processes are manifested by changes in complexity and integration that generate well-being. Importantly, other distinguishing characteristics of nursing processes may be identified as the dialogue continues beyond this article.

This new understanding of the nature of nursing processes derived from various theorists' work, such as von Bertalanffy's (1981) systems view of human beings, Rogers' (1970, 1992) science of unitary human beings, Lerner's (1986) developmental contextualism and complexity theory (see Kauffman, 1995; Waldrop, 1992). Although the translation of these theorists' ideas may not be entirely congruent with those presented here, their ideas nonetheless can help inform development of a new nursing ontology.

Human beings are viewed as open, living systems and not as passive but intrinsically active and innovative. As an open system, human systems are capable of self-organizing, where self refers to the system as a whole. Self-organization is an inherent capacity for generating qualitative change out of ongoing events in the life of a system and its environment.

In his seminal work on development, Werner (1957) explained this process of qualitative change as his "orthogenetic principle," which posits that living organisms change over time from lower to higher levels of differentiation and integration. Werner (1957) called this change "development," in contrast to mechanistic processes of change, which are not developmental.

Similarly, Rogers' (1980) principles of homeodynamics describe the inherent innovative patterning of change that occurs in open systems, both environmental and human. Her three principles of helicy, resonancy, and integrality together depict the nature of qualitative change in human beings in terms of ongoing movement from lower to higher levels of diversity.

Complexity theorists (e.g., Kauffman, 1995; Waldrop, 1992) and developmentalists (e.g., Lerner, 1986; Werner, 1957) in particular have clarified a distinction between quantitative and qualitative change, both of which are necessary for development contrasting terms such as complexity and order and differentiation and organization depict this distinction. Similarly, two distinct forms of change can be identified in Rogers' (1980, 1992) works, namely diversity and innovation (Reed, 1997).

Because of the articulation between quantitative and qualitative change, human systems are not simply complex systems (SCS) but rather are complex innovative systems (CIS) (see Stites, 1994). In the context of nursing, then, nursing processes entail at least two forms of change, complexity and integration.

Complexity Complexity refers to the number of different types of variables that can be identified in a given situation. A variable is simply something that varies (Webster's, 1979). Complexity occurs when human systems experience or express variables (e.g., life events, physiologic events) as parts, separated from the whole, rather than as patterns of the whole. Thus, for example, complexity is evident when loss of a loved one or chronic illness introduces many new and seemingly disconnected variables into an individual's life, on various levels of awareness. Increasing complexity means change in quantity (size or number) not change in quality of the whole this would become chaotic were it not accompanied by corresponding changes in integration.

Integration Integration refers to a synthesizing and organizing of variables such that there is a change in form, not just change in size or number of events. A certain level of complexity is needed for integration to occur. Integration is evident, for example, when people construct meaning or identify a pattern in the variables or events experienced. Integration may also occur on levels of awareness that are not yet so readily apparent. Integration is transformative, involving qualitative change in form.

Well-Being

While changes in complexity and integration may be used to explain many facets of human development and systems' changes, this process may also be used to understand health, healing, and well-being. The rhythm between complexity and integration is proposed here to be a means by which innovative change occurs, as a manifestation of the underlying process called nursing. Thus, well-being may be explained in part by changes in complexity that are tempered by changes in integration. Complexity provides life with diversity, specialization, and depth in experiences, whereas integration provides organization, coherence, and breadth.

Examples of nursing processes are abundant. For example, groups incorporate new attachments or children into an organization called family. Persons with spinal cord injuries develop different pathways that link together shattered parts of life and bodily functions. Premature infants' behaviors become more innovative as they organize the complexity of their environment. Adults reminisce to integrate past life events and inevitable death. Healing after the loss of a loved one or the occurrence of chronic illness requires an integration of what seem like disjointed events and experiences, including memories of the past, future dreams, altered rhythms and routines, physical pain and other bodily symptoms, sadness, anguish, and self-doubt. Further, Sachs (1995) depicted what can be called nursing processes through his stories about people with various maladies, such as a colorblind painter and a surgeon with Tourette's syndrome. These people were able to create a new organization that fit with their altered needs and world. These health events, in all their initial complexity and heartbreak, gave way to metamorphoses and innovation. Regardless of whether there is a "cure" that can reverse a particular ailment, well-being occurs when the particulars of a life experience are brought together and synthesized in a coherent way. Any less, and people risk feeling dis-integrated, dis-associated, dis-organized.

While the centrality of well-being as a focus in nursing has been established, other disciplines also may be concerned with well-being and its correlates. However, promoting well-being based on a perspective of the inherent process of complexity and integration is distinctly nursing.

Challenging the Status Quo: Nursing Reconstructed

The definition of nursing proposed here is that of an inherent process of well-being, characterized by manifestations of complexity and integration in human systems. The substantive focus of the discipline, then, is not how nurses per se facilitate well-being but, rather, how nursing processes function in human systems to facilitate well-being. The focus is, in a very basic sense, how nurses can facilitate nursing.

Refocusing the Lens

This new construction of nursing provides another lens of focus for nursing researchers and practitioners. Smith (1988b) wrote metaphorically about three different camera lenses used to view human wholeness. One in particular, the motion lens, focuses on process and rhythmic flow and requires a "creative leap" to identify this process. Nurses typically encounter people in motion, in dynamic flow with their environment, whether in life-threatening experiences or perceived memory loss, chronic illness or acute pain.

The creative leap necessary for formulating the motion lens of nursing inquiry may be to address the rhythmic processes of complexity and integration that enhance well-being across these health experiences. From premature infants to dying adults and their families and communities, it is proposed that human systems have nursing processes, that is, inherent resources for well-being based on a capacity to integrate their complexities.

Debates on holism and on what represents the critical focus of nursing may be enlivened by including a new ontology of nursing—an ontology that transcends debates about part versus whole, person versus environment. Nursing processes are not necessarily bound by dimensions such as biologic, environmental, or social. Instead, the lens is focused on any human process that manifests complexity and integration related to well-being. Looking through this new lens, researchers and practitioners may identify a myriad of human manifestations of wholeness, whether they be labeled physiologic, phylogenic, or philosophic, that are integral to well-being.

Nursing as a Metaparadigm Concept

Given this reconstructed view of nursing, as a substantive focus of the discipline, the term nursing should be a central concept in the nursing metaparadigm. In the past, for good reason, some have suggested the elimination of the term nursing from the metaparadigm (Conway, 1985). However, rather than remove the term nursing from the metaparadigm, this fin-de-siècle may be the time in nursing history to consider renaming the discipline to something other than a verb, to better distinguish the disciplinary label from the substantive focus of the science and practice.

To help clarify this distinction, a term such as Paterson and Zderad's (1976) "nursology," or another disciplinary label with the "nurs" prefix could be developed, while reserving the term nursing as the process word and verb that it is, for the metaparadigm. By identifying nursing as a substantive, metaparadigm concept, nurses can better claim their unique focus and clarify the ontology of their discipline.

Approaching the Frontier

Rogers (1992) explained that one could not push back the frontier of knowledge until one approached it. This article has not been about maintaining the status quo but about approaching a frontier so that others might join in a dialogue that pushes back the frontier a bit more. In this era of healthcare reform, the discipline must define nursing as nurses truly envision it and not necessarily as others would have it be defined. Nurses may decide against renaming the discipline as was suggested here. Nevertheless, within a broadened and partially reconstructed view of the discipline that embraces nursing at its most fundamental meaning, new understandings that blend with the old can emerge to present a fuller picture of the discipline.

Nursing (as practice and praxis) is a way of doing that creates good actions that facilitate well-being. Nursing (as syntax and science) is a way of knowing that creates goods in the form of knowledge, and nursing (the substance and ontology) is a way of being that creates patterns of changing complexity and integration experienced as well-being in human systems.

Nurses are invited to try on the substantive definition of nursing to see how it fits within the context of their practice and science. Ongoing philosophic dialogue about the ontology of the discipline will help ensure that nurse theorists are theorists of nursing in its fullest sense and, likewise, that nurse researchers are researchers of nursing and that nurse practitioners are practitioners of nursing.

References

Conway, M. E. (1985). Toward greater specificity in defining nursing's metaparadigm. Advances in Nursing Science, 7(4), 73–81.

Ellis, R. (1982). Conceptual issues in nursing. Nursing Outlook, 30(7), 406–410.

Henderson, V. (1964). The nature of nursing. American Journal of Nursing, 64(8), 62–68.

Kauffman, S. (1995). At home in the universe: The search for laws of self-organization and complexity. New York: Oxford University Press.

Laird, C. (1971). Webster's new world thesaurus (rev. ed.). New York: Simon and Schuster.

Lerner, R. M. (1986). Concepts and theories of human development (2nd ed.). New York: Random House.

Murphy, M. (1992). The future of the body: Explorations into the further evolution of human nature. New York: J.P. Tarcher.

Newman, M. (1992). Prevailing paradigms in nursing. Nursing Outlook, 40, 10–13.

Nightingale, F. (1969). Notes on nursing: What it is and what it is not. New York: Dover (Original work published 1859).

Paterson, J. G., & Zderad, L. T. (1976). Humanistic nursing. New York: Wiley.

Pepper, S. P. (1942). World hypotheses: A study in evidence. Berkeley: University of California Press.

Rampragus, V. (1995). The deconstruction of nursing. Brookfield, VT: Ashgate.

Reed, P. G. (1995). A treatise on nursing knowledge development for the 21st century: Beyond postmodernism. Advances in Nursing Science, 17(3), 70–84.

Reed, P. G. (1997). The place of transcendence in nursing's science of unitary human beings. In M. Madrid (Ed.), Patterns of Rogerian knowing (pp. 187–196). New York: National League for Nursing Press.

Rogers, M. E. (1970). Introduction to the theoretical basis of nursing. Philadelphia: F. A. Davis.

Rogers, M. E. (1980). A science of unitary man. In J. P. Riehl & C. Roy (Eds.), Conceptual models for nursing practice (2nd ed., pp. 329–337). New York: Appleton-Century-Crofts.

Rogers, M. E. (1992). Nursing science and the space age. Nursing Science Quarterly, 5, 27–34.

Roy, C. L. (1995). Developing nursing knowledge: Practice issues raised from four philosophical perspectives. Nursing Science Quarterly, 8, 79–85.

Sachs, O. (1995). An anthropologist on Mars: Seven paradoxical tales. New York: A. Knopf.

Schlotfeldt, R. (1994). Resolving opposing viewpoints: Is it desirable? Is it practicable? In J. F. Kikuchi & H. Simmons (Eds.), Developing a philosophy of nursing (pp. 67–74). Thousand Oaks, CA: Sage.

Smith, M. J. (1988a). Nursing: What's in a name? Nursing Science Quarterly, 1, 142–143.

Smith, M. J. (1988b). Perspectives of wholeness: The lens makes a difference. Nursing Science Quarterly, 1, 94–95.

Stites, J. (1994). Complexity research on complex systems and complex adaptive systems. Omni, 16(8), 42–50.

von Bertalanffy, L. (1981). A systems view of man (P. A. La Violette, Ed.). Boulder, CO: Westview Press.

Waldrop, M. M. (1992). Complexity: The emerging science at the edge of order and chaos. New York: Simon and Schuster.

Watson, J. (1985). Nursing: Human science and human care. Norwalk, CT: Appleton-Century-Crofts.

Watson, J. (1995). Postmodernism and knowledge development in nursing. Nursing Science Quarterly, 8, 60–64.

Webster's New Collegiate Dictionary. (1979). Springfield, MA: G. & C. Merriam Co.

Werner, H. (1957). The concept of development from a comparative and organismic point of view. In D. B. Harris (Ed.), The concept of development (pp. 125–148). Minneapolis: University of Minnesota Press.

CHAPTER 9

Philosophical Position on Nature of Human Beings Foundational to Orem's Self-Care Deficit Nursing Theory

Barbara E. Banfield, BSN, MSN, PhD

Through a process of philosophical inquiry, the philosophical assumptions and beliefs foundational to Orem's self-care deficit nursing theory (SCDNT) were explicated. This chapter describes the position on the nature of human beings that underlies the SCDNT. Based on the philosophy of moderate realism, Orem's view of the nature of human beings is that of dynamic unitary beings engaged in an ongoing process of development, striving for their self-ideal, and possessing uniquely human qualities such as free will. Orem's position on nursing-specific views of human beings is also discussed.

Key words: *moderate realism, nature of human beings, Orem's self-care deficit nursing theory, philosophical inquiry.*

Ambiguity and misunderstanding of a nursing theory are more likely to occur when the philosophical foundations of the theory are not clearly stated. Sarter (1988b) claims that the extant nursing theories are "laden with philosophical assumptions which are not always explicitly acknowledged" (p. 52). To ensure an accurate, comprehensive understanding of a nursing theory, the philosophical foundations of the theory need to be identified.

Sarter's (1988b) point regarding the philosophical foundations of extant nursing theories applies to the self-care deficit nursing theory (SCDNT). Orem (2001) identifies the SCDNT as a general theory, one that is descriptively explanatory of nursing. Her work pertaining to the SCDNT focuses on the human requirements of persons for nursing and the processes for the production of nursing. Although not specifically addressed, the SCDNT does rest on certain beliefs and assumptions regarding the nature of reality and of human beings. Rather than being clearly identified, these philosophical assumptions and beliefs are implicit. Uys (1987) and Smith (1987) both criticized Orem's work because the philosophical foundations have not been clearly articulated.

The lack of explicitness with regard to the philosophical foundations of the SCDNT has contributed to misinterpretations of Orem's work. For example, Parse (1987) claims that Orem describes human beings as organisms with self-care capabilities. Instead of accurately representing Orem's position regarding the nature of human beings, this statement has been taken out of context. In contrast to Parse's position, Sarter (1988c) states that "although it is not as readily apparent, Orem's self-care theory of nursing expresses a view of human beings and health that also finds philosophical support from evolutionary idealism" (p. 102). Orem's general theory is not based on evolutionary idealism; it is based on the philosophical system of moderate realism.

The positions of both Parse and Sarter represent inaccurate interpretations of Orem's work. In this chapter the philosophical position of the nature of human beings that is foundational to the SCDNT is presented and discussed. The method of philosophical inquiry used for this analysis is also described.

Philosophical Inquiry Process

A philosophical inquiry of Orem's nursing theory was carried out using a six-phase inquiry process (Banfield, 1997). One of the inquiry questions was "What is the view regarding the nature of human beings that underlies Orem's SCDNT?" Because this question is a philosophical one, the appropriate way to address it is through the use of a philosophical approach. Kikuchi (1992) makes the point that "what is of concern is that nurses are erroneously subjecting to scientific study nursing questions that are nonscientific, beyond the scope of science to answer" (p. 26). As a systematic method of inquiry, philosophical inquiry involves the use of reason to critically examine, clarify, and interpret meanings and positions.

The six phases of the inquiry process are (1) critical reading and examination of Orem's work with the identification of statements pertaining to the inquiry question, (2) examination and analysis of these statements, (3) examination and analysis of the work of authors cited by Orem, (4) comparison between Orem's work and the work of the cited authors, (5) construction of the answer to the inquiry questions, and (6) evaluation of the findings. This discussion focuses on the process used to identify and clarify the philosophical position on the nature of human beings that is foundational to the SCDNT.

First Phase

The first phase involved the critical reading and examination of Orem's work to identify statements pertaining to the nature of human beings. The work of Orem that was examined included five editions of *Nursing Concepts of Practice* (1971, 1980, 1985, 1991, 1995), two editions of *Concept Formalization in Nursing* (1979), an article on views of human beings specific to nursing (Orem, 1997), and an article about positive mental health (Orem & Vardiman, 1995). The sixth edition of *Nursing Concepts of Practice* was published after this inquiry was completed. (All references to *Nursing Concepts of Practice* have been updated for the 2001 edition.) During this initial phase the aim was to identify statements and phrases pertaining to the nature of human beings rather than to analyze the meaning of these statements and phases. To ensure that the examination was comprehensive and complete, each of these works was read in its entirety a minimum of two times.

Second Phase

The second phase involved the analysis of the identified statements and phrases. These statements and phrases were grouped according to the topic or areas to which they pertained. For example, statements that pertained to human development were grouped together, statements that pertained to human freedom were grouped together, and so on. These statements were then critically examined to clarify meaning and to identify unstated or implicit assumptions. The process involved an analysis of the statements as well as the examination of the sections of the text from which the statements and phrases had been extracted. The aim of this phase of the inquiry was to gain an initial understanding of Orem's position on the nature of human beings.

Third Phase

After the analysis of Orem's work was completed, the work of authors cited by Orem was read and examined. The work read included the work of philosophers such as Harre (1970), Lonergan (1958), Macmurray (1957,1961), and Wallace (1979); psychologists such as Allport (1955), Arnold (1960a, 1960b), and Fromm (1956/1989); sociologists such as Parsons (1949, 1951) and Plattel (1965); and the work of Catholic theologians such as de Montcheuil (1954), Gannon (1956), Gilby (1970, 1974), and Rahner (McCool, 1975). (It is important to keep in mind that the choice of words used by these authors is a reflection of the language used at the time of publication.) During this phase of the inquiry the goal was to understand the positions put forth by the authors whom Orem cited.

Fourth Phase

The fourth phase involved further analysis of the identified statements. The consistency or compatibility between Orem's statements regarding human beings and the work of the cited authors was examined and analyzed. The cited work often provided a more comprehensive treatment of the topic being addressed. This served to clarify the points made or alluded to by Orem. The aim of this phase of the inquiry was to achieve a comprehensive understanding of Orem's position regarding the nature of human beings and to identify and resolve any apparent discrepancies or ambiguities.

Fifth Phase

The fifth phase of the inquiry focused on formulating an answer to the inquiry question. The answer was constructed in light of the work of Orem and others. Through this process Orem's views were synthesized into a coherent, comprehensive description on the nature of human beings.

Sixth Phase

The final phase of the inquiry was the evaluation. Unlike quantitative studies in which numerical scores reflect the reliability of the instruments and the significance of the findings, the evaluation of philosophical inquiries is a matter of judgment. Criteria identified for the evaluation of such inquiries include rigorous, clear, and precise thinking (Soltis, 1978); significance of the inquiry questions and the meaningfulness of the inquiry for enlightenment and for ordering understandings and meanings in nursing (Ellis, 1983, p. 225), and explanatory power, comprehensiveness, coherence, and simplicity for inquiries presenting a philosophical position (Sarter, 1988a, p. 189). In relation to the findings, the following questions can also be asked: Is there increased understanding of Orem's SCDNT as a result of the inquiry? Are the findings useful in terms of conceptualizing nursing and providing direction for further knowledge development?

Nature of Human Beings

Through the inquiry process the philosophical position on the nature of human beings that is foundational to Orem's SCDNT was identified. As previously stated, Orem does not clearly articulate the philosophical foundations of the SCDNT. However, she does identify views of human beings that may be useful to nurses in the conceptualization of nursing as well as in the design and production of nursing care. These specified views represent different ways of looking at or considering human beings; they are not different views regarding the nature of human beings. To promote a clearer understanding of Orem's SCDNT, it is necessary to distinguish between the philosophical position on the nature of human beings that is foundational to the SCDNT and the views of human beings that Orem claims may be taken for practical purposes.

Description of the Nature of Human Beings

A synthesis of Orem's views and positions resulted in the construction of the following description of the view on the nature of human beings foundational to the SCDNT (Banfield, 2001, p. xiii):

> Human beings are unitary beings who exist in their environments, influencing the world as well as being influenced by the world. Unitary humans are beings in process, striving to achieve their human potential and self-ideal through developmental processes. Human beings possess free will; are capable of maintaining an awareness of self and environment, attaching meaning to

what is experienced, and reflecting upon their experiences; and possess the ability to engage in deliberate action. In addition to freedom, other essential qualities of human beings include bonding together with others through human love, the unrestricted desire to know, the appreciation of beauty and goodness, the joy of creative endeavor, the love of God, and the desire for happiness.

Moderate Realism

Through the inquiry process it became evident that the philosophy of moderate realism underlies Orem's work. This philosophy is reflected in her view regarding the nature of reality and the nature of human beings. In addition, Orem's position regarding the form of nursing science is based on the moderate realist notion of practical science (1988, 2001).

Moderate realism, which is just one of a number of philosophical positions considered to be realist positions, is associated with the philosophy of St. Thomas Aquinas. According to this philosophy there is an existent world, a real world that exists independent of the thoughts of the knower. The beliefs and views of the human beings that inhabit the world do not determine the nature of reality. Realism stands in opposition to idealism, which holds that reality is mind dependent or relative to the knower. For the realist, what is real is distinguished from what is rational or logical. "The rational or logical is whatever exists in my mind in such a way that it cannot exist outside my mind. The real, on the other hand, although

in my mind when I know it, also exists outside my mind" (Wallace, 1979, p. 164).

Moderate realists believe that it is possible to gain knowledge of this existent world. Kikuchi and Simmons (1999, p. 45) state the following:

> Moderate realism takes the position that, although we view reality differently as a consequence of how we are nurtured, we can, nonetheless, attain an objective view of reality which is probably true by testing our various subjective views against reality which common sense tells us exists, and is the way it is regardless of how anyone of us views it.

Arnold (1960a) makes the point that unless we trust our senses to give us accurate information about the world, we must conclude that it is impossible to reach any kind of truth (pp. 6–7).

Nature of Reality

Although not addressed as such, a moderate realist position on the nature of reality is reflected in Orem's work. For example, Orem (2001) states that "the world of the nurse is manifested to each nurse as a system of 'qualitatively differentiable and separately locatable' persons and things" (p. 16). In relation to this statement, Orem cites the work of Harre (1970), a realist philosopher. Phrases used by Orem (2001), such as "time–place localization" (p. 17), "objectively discernible reality" (p. 27), "reality conditions in self or environment" (p. 257), and "function within a veridical (reality) frame of reference"

(p. 232), reflect a moderate realist view of reality. It is clear from these phrases that Orem sees reality as something that has an existence independent of the knower; reality is not something that is seen as relative or dependent on the knower. Orem does recognize that human beings perceive and attach meaning to the things they perceive. However, she does not support the position that reality is dependent on the perceptions and meanings held by human beings.

Four categories of postulated entities are identified as establishing the ontology of the SCDNT: (1) persons in space–time localizations, (2) attributes or properties of these persons, (3) motion or change, and (4) products brought into being (Orem, 2001, p. 141). In terms of these entities the persons in space–time localizations refer to the nurses and patients; the attributes or properties refer to the properties of self-care agency, therapeutic self-care demand, and nursing agency; motion or change pertains to the performance of self-care, the seeking of nursing assistance, the exercise of nursing agency, and the changes in properties of concern; and the products brought into being refer to the self-care and/or dependent care systems as well as the nursing systems of care provided for patients.

Unitary Beings

According to Orem (1979, 2001), human beings are unitary beings. "Men, women, and children who are patients of nurses are unitary beings with singular ways of living and singular life histories" (Orem, 2001, p. 357). The view of human beings as unitary beings is incorporated into statements pertaining to other topics. For example, in relation to deliberate action, Orem (2001) states that "persons as unitary beings act deliberately to achieve the ends or the states of affairs sought" (p. 64).

Orem's view of human beings as unitary beings reflects the moderate realist position. The phrase "rational animal" is seen in the work of those scholars associated with Aristotelian Thomism (Gannon, 1965; Wallace, 1977, 1979). Wallace (1977) states that "man, in the classical definition, is a rational animal, animal rationalis, i.e., an animal like other animals, but distinct by having the power of universal, abstract reason, and all that follows from it" (p. 80).

According to moderate realism, human beings are not made up of two things, body and soul or body and spirit. Rather, human beings are embodied beings. The human being "is a substantial unity resulting from a union between matter and spirit that is the most intimate possible" (Wallace, 1979, p. 226). "Since the body is only human through the soul, and the soul in turn determines the body, the soul-body relationship is not that of a mere juxtaposition of parts but rather the unity of substantial being" (Wallace, 1977, p. 81). Wallace (1977) makes the point that the person who is experienced in bodily presence is the same person who thinks; that person is one entity or being, not two different beings (p. 81). Macmurray (1957) also addresses this notion of unity, maintaining that the person or self who engages in action is the same self who engages in thought. Plattel (1965) claims that, due to limitations of our understanding, we often think and speak of the body and soul as two things rather than as a unity of being (p. 50). Although we may speak of body and soul as two different things, this does not make them two different things.

In relation to the notion of parts of human beings, Orem (2001) maintains that "each human being, like other living things, is a substantial or real unity whose parts are formed and attain perfection through the differentiation of the whole during processes of development" (p. 187). Acknowledging that human beings have parts or structural and functional differentiations does not negate the position that human beings are unitary beings. It is important to note that Orem does not claim that human beings are structural and functional differentiations, rather that they have these differentiations.

Human–Environmental Relationship

With regard to the relationship of human beings and their environments, Orem (1991) claims that "within the theory of self-care, person and environment are identified as a unity characterized by human-environmental interchanges and by the impact of one on the other. Person-environment constitutes a functional type of unity with a concrete existence" (p. 143). Persons exist in their environments and are never isolated from them. It is in our thinking that we often consider persons as separate from their environments.

Ongoing Developmental Process

According to Orem (1979), each human being is a dynamic unitary being in a continuing process of development (p. 122). "The existence of men, women, and children lies in their development. They are beings in process" (Orem, 2001, p. 100). Rather than being regarded as something that just happens to a person, development is viewed as an ongoing process to which the person contributes through striving to achieve his or her human potential and self-ideal. This process of development occurs throughout the lives of human beings.

Essential Humanness

In her work, Orem (1979, 2001) uses phrases such as "uniquely human qualities" and "essential humanness of individuals." She states that "a person focus will never be explicated if the uniquely human qualities of men, women, and children are ignored and not recognized as operative in nursing practice situations" (Orem, 2001, p. 28). These qualities or aspects of essential humanness, which develop as persons live, are free will, human love, desire to know, appreciation of beauty and goodness, joy of creative endeavor, love of God, and the desire for happiness. Authors whom Orem cites in relation to these human qualities include Arnold (1960a, 1960b), Fromm (1956/1989), and Rahner (McCool, 1975).

Free Will One of the essential human qualities is that of free will. In relation to free will, Orem refers to the work of Rahner, a Catholic theologian (McCool, 1975, pp. 352–353):

> If, therefore, man is personal freedom, then it follows that he is one who uses the resources of his

own innermost nature to form himself by his own free act, for by the exercise of this freedom of his he can definitively determine the shape of his life as a whole, and decide what his ultimate end is to be, the ultimate realization of his own nature, beyond all possibility of revision.

Personal freedom does not mean that a person is free to be or do anything he or she wants. Rather it means that, given the possibilities, that person is free to decide the course he or she will pursue.

The idea of self-care as deliberate action is based on the view of human beings as possessing free will. According to Macmurray (1957), the possibility of action is dependent on human beings having free will (p. 134). "Deliberate action is essentially action to achieve a foreseen result that is preceded by investigation, reflection, and judgment to appraise the situation and by a thoughtful, deliberate choice of what should be done" (Orem, 1991, p. 272). Arnold (1960b) differentiates deliberate action from instinctive and emotional action patterns and from overt reactions to feelings of pleasantness and unpleasantness (p. 193). Deliberate action involves the person making the choice to pursue a particular course of action.

In a discussion of deliberate action, Orem (2001) identifies seven assumptions about human beings. These explicit assumptions pertain to aspects of deliberate action rather than to the nature of human beings. For example, the assumption that "human beings are capable of self-determined actions, even when they feel an emotional pull in the opposite direction" (Orem, 2001, p. 65) pertains to the ability to take action. This explicit assumption rests upon the implicit assumption that human beings possess free will.

Intellectual Capabilities   Human beings are distinguished from other living things by their capacity (1) to reflect on themselves and their environment, (2) to symbolize what they experience, and (3) to use symbolic creations (ideas, words) in thinking, in communicating, and in guiding efforts to do and to make things that are beneficial for themselves or others (Orem, 2001, p. 182).

The position that these intellectual capabilities are unique to human beings, and therefore serve to differentiate humans from other living beings, reflects the philosophy of St. Thomas Aquinas. Wallace (1979) claims that "man differs from lower animals in his ability to grasp meanings or ideas or intelligible contents that become the basis for his language, literature, culture, science, and other distinctively human activities" (p. 237). He goes on to say that this capability is also associated with the will power, or free will, of humans.

According to Arnold (1960b), the desire to know exhibited by human beings is possible only in beings able to form concepts and use symbols. Lonergan (1958) identifies the desire to know as the inquiring and critical spirit of human beings (p. 348).

The position that human beings possess intellectual capabilities is foundational to the conceptualization of self-care as deliberate action as is the position that human beings have free will. The capability for deliberate action is unique to human beings (Arnold, 1960b; Macmurray, 1957; Orem, 2001). Deliberate action involves the intellectual activities of reflecting on possible courses of action, making judgments, and deciding on a course of action to be pursued. The following are two assumptions regarding human beings that Orem (2001) identifies in relation to deliberate action: (1) "human beings know and appraise objects, conditions, and situations in terms of their effects on ends being sought" and (2b) "human beings know directly by sensing, but they also reflect, reason, and understand" (p. 65). These assumptions pertain to intellectual capabilities that are regarded as uniquely human.

Human Love Another quality of essential humanness is the bonding together with others through human love. "Mature love with its element of care and concern for others develops and is expressed when individuals live in or seek communion with one another in fundamental unity as persons in community" (Orem, 2001, p. 30).

Authors whom Orem cites in relation to human love include Fromm (1956/1989) and Arnold (1960b). Fromm (1956/1989) claims that "love is not primarily a relationship to a specific person; it is an attitude, and orientation of character which determines the relatedness of a person to the world as a whole, not toward one 'object' of love" (p. 42). Arnold (1960b) maintains that human love is essential to the formation of the self-ideal and its pursuit (p. 312).

Plattel (1965) claims that human beings coexist together in the world. "It is love, the social art par excellence, which serves most

to confirm man in his value as a person" (p. 23). The quality of human love is an integral component of the nurse's ability to help others (Orem, 2001, p. 100).

Other Aspects of Essential Humanness Appreciation of beauty and goodness, joy of creative endeavor, love of God, and the desire for happiness are all regarded as aspects of essential humanness and are seen as involved in the person's ongoing development and pursuit of self-ideal. Arnold (1960b) describes the contemplation of beauty as a satisfying, perfective, and integrative human experience (p. 321). This human experience is valued not as a means to an end but as a connection to the spiritual activities of knowing and loving truth and goodness. Human beings derive satisfaction from achieving a goal. The love of God and the desire for happiness are aspects of humans' striving for their self-ideal.

The view of the nature of human beings foundational to Orem's SCDNT is that of human beings as unitary beings in the process of becoming and possessing qualities such as free will. This position regarding the nature of human beings reflects the philosophy of moderate realism. The identification of this philosophical position on the nature of human beings may not fit with the conception some people hold of Orem's SCDNT. However, unless one is carefully focusing on what Orem says, it is easy to overlook the points she makes about human beings. Because Orem does not specifically address the nature of human beings, it is possible to misinterpret the foundational view on the nature of human beings without a thorough, in-depth study of her work.

Views of Human Beings

Orem (1979, 1997, 2001) identifies five views of human beings that, when taken by nurses, serve some practical purpose: (1) person, (2) agent, (3) user of symbols, (4) organism, and (5) object subject to physical forces. These five views of human beings "are necessary for developing understanding of the conceptual constructs of self-care deficit nursing theory and for understanding the interpersonal and societal aspects of nursing systems" (Orem, 1997, p. 28).

As persons, human beings are regarded as embodied unitary beings living in coexistence with other human beings. This view reflects the philosophical position on the nature of human beings upon which the SCDNT rests. In relation to this view, Orem (1979) maintains that "the reference then is to their individuality expressed as a unity of being and becoming; of knowing, feeling, and imagining; of reflecting and judging; of valuing and willing; and to their possession of self by self" (p. 122). The view of human beings as persons is the conceptualization of human beings in the fullness of their being human. However, for practical purposes, the other views of human beings "can be taken at different times without considering all that characterizes human beings as persons" (Orem, 2001, p. 187).

The view of human beings as agent is central to understanding nursing as conceptualized within the SCDNT. From the view of agent, human beings are regarded "as persons who can bring about conditions that do not presently exist in humans or in

their environmental situations by deliberately acting using valid means or technologies to bring about foreseen and desired results" (Orem, 1997, p. 28). The person-as-agent is foundational to the SCDNT's conceptual elements of self-care, dependent care, nursing care, self-care agency, dependent care agency, and nursing agency. Self-care, dependent care, and nursing care are all conceptualized as deliberate action, action purposefully engaged in to achieve desired results. Self-care agency, dependent care agency, and nursing agency are conceptualized as powers or capabilities of persons to engage in specific types of deliberate action.

Considered from the view of user of symbols, "individual human beings are viewed as persons who use symbols to stand for things and attach meaning to them, to formulate and express ideas and to communicate ideas and information to others through language and other means of communication" (Orem, 1997, p. 29). This view of human beings is useful to nurses in understanding the interpersonal aspects of nursing situations, in understanding the communication that occurs between persons involved in nursing practice situations.

From the organism view, "individuals are viewed as unitary living beings who grow and develop exhibiting biological characteristics of Homo sapiens during known stages of the human life cycle" (Orem, 1997, p. 29). Within the view of person-as-organism, human beings are regarded as having functional and structural differentiations. Orem (2001) states that "each developmentally differentiated structure or functional system can be studied as an existent entity with its own operations, with relations to other differentiated parts and to their operations, and to the unitary functioning of individuals who coexist in a world with other human beings" (p. 187). It is important to recognize that, for Orem, health and well-being are not synonymous. Well-being refers to the person's perceived condition of existence, whereas health refers to the soundness and wholeness of human structures and functioning. The study of the functional and structural differentiations of human beings is the domain of various sciences such as human anatomy, human physiology, and psychology. Knowledge from these sciences is helpful for nurses in understanding health and well-being and is used in the design and production of nursing care.

The view of person-as-object subject to physical forces is taken in situations in which the person is unable to protect himself or herself from physical forces. For example, in a nursing practice situation in which the patient is unable to initiate and control movements, the nurse might consider the person from the object point of view in designing and providing care to protect him or her from hazards associated with the inability to move.

To summarize, Orem (1979, 1997, 2001) claims that these views may be taken by nurses for some practical purpose, be it to understand nursing as conceptualized within the SCDNT, to gain understanding of human health and well-being, and/or to design and produce nursing systems for persons in need of the human health service known as nursing. In taking the view of person as agent,

symbolizer, organism, or object subject to physical forces, the nurse considers the person from the particular view to accomplish some purpose. For example, the nurse may consider the person receiving nursing care from the perspective of organism to understand how a particular structural defect may be impacting on his or her health. Although the nurse may take a particular view to achieve some practical purpose, it is the person view that is taken by nurses in all of their interpersonal contacts with persons receiving nursing care (Orem, 1997, p. 29).

Conclusion

Because Orem does not clearly articulate the philosophical assumptions and beliefs that are foundational to the SCDNT, it is easy to misunderstand or misinterpret her position. Certainly, phrases and statements can be identified in Orem's work that do not seem to support the view regarding the nature of human beings that is presented in this chapter. However, through the philosophical inquiry process described in this chapter, Orem's assumptions and beliefs were explicated and synthesized into the presented description.

Orem's views regarding the nature of human beings and reality all reflect the philosophy of moderate realism. Human beings are unitary beings engaged in ongoing development and becoming. They possess free will as well as intellectual capabilities, which enable them to engage in deliberate action. The explication of Orem's position on the nature of human beings serves to clarify the SCDNT. Hopefully, the clarification of this view will also serve as an incentive for nurses to pursue an in-depth, comprehensive understanding of Orem's work. It is also important for nurse researchers investigating phenomena from the perspective of the SCDNT to take this foundational position on the nature of human beings into consideration when making decisions about the types of knowledge to be developed and about the appropriateness of various research approaches for the development of this knowledge.

References

Allport, G. W. (1955). *Becoming.* New Haven, CT: Yale University Press.

Arnold, M. B. (1960a). *Emotion and personality* (Vol. 1). New York: Columbia University Press.

Arnold, M. B. (1960b). *Emotion and personality* (Vol. 2). New York: Columbia University Press.

Banfield, B. E. (1997). A philosophical inquiry of Orem's self-care deficit nursing theory (Doctoral dissertation, Wayne State University, 1997). *Dissertation Abstracts International,* 58, (02), 5885B.

Banfield, B. E. (2001). Philosophic foundations of Orem's work. In D. E. Orem (Ed.), *Nursing concepts of practice* (6th ed.) (pp. xi–xvi). St. Louis, MO: Mosby.

de Montcheuil, Y. (1954). *Guide for social action.* Chicago: Fides Publishers.

Ellis, R. (1983). Philosophic inquiry. *Annual Review of Nursing Research,* 1, 211–228.

Fromm, E. (1956/1989). *The art of loving.* New York: Harper & Row.

Gannon, T. J. (1956). Emotional development and spiritual growth. In M. J. O'Brien & R. J. Steimel (Eds.), *Psychological aspects of spiritual development* (pp. 3–22). Washington, DC: Catholic University of America Press.

Gilby, T. (1970). Appendix 1 Structure of a human act. In T. Gilby (Ed. and Trans.), *St. Thomas Aquinas Summa Theologiae Vol. 17* (pp. 211–217). New York: McGraw-Hill.

Gilby, T. (1974). Introduction, Appendix 2 Prudence and casuistry, Appendix 3 Prudence and conscience, Appendix 4 Prudence and certainty. In T. Gilby (Ed. and Trans.), *St. Thomas Aquinas Summa Theologiae Vol. 36* (pp. xiv–xvii, 178–184). New York: McGraw-Hill.

Harre, R. (1970). *The principles of scientific thinking.* Chicago: University of Chicago Press.

Kikuchi, J. F. (1992). Nursing questions that science cannot answer. In J. F. Kikuchi & H. Simmons (Eds.), *Philosophic inquiry in nursing* (pp. 26–37). Newbury Park, CA: Sage.

Kikuchi, J. F., & Simmons, H. (1999). Practical nursing judgment: A moderate realist conception. *Scholarly Inquiry for Nursing Practice: An International Journal,* 13, 43–55.

Lonergan, B. J. F. (1958). *Insight a study of human understanding* (rev. ed.). New York: Philosophical Library.

Macmurray, J. (1957). *The self as agent.* New York: Harper & Brothers.

Macmurray, J. (1961). *Persons in relation.* New York: Harper & Brothers.

McCool, G. A. (Ed.). (1975). *A Rahner reader.* New York: Seabury Press.

Orem, D. E. (1971). *Nursing: Concepts of practice* (1st ed.). New York: McGraw-Hill.

Orem, D. E. (Ed.). (1979). *Concept formalization in nursing* (2nd ed.). Boston: Little, Brown, and Company.

Orem, D. E. (1980). *Nursing: Concepts of practice* (2nd ed.). New York: McGraw-Hill.

Orem, D. E. (1985). *Nursing: Concepts of practice* (3rd ed.). New York: McGraw-Hill.

Orem, D. E. (1988). The form of nursing science. *Nursing Science Quarterly, 1,* 75–79.

Orem, D. E. (1991). *Nursing: Concepts of practice* (4th ed.). St. Louis, MO: Mosby.

Orem, D. E. (1995). *Nursing: concepts of practice* (5th ed.). St. Louis, MO: Mosby.

Orem, D. E. (1997). Views of human beings specific to nursing. *Nursing Science Quarterly, 10,* 26–31.

Orem, D. E. (2001). *Nursing: concepts of practice* (6th ed.). St. Louis, MO: Mosby.

Orem, D. E., & Vardiman, E. M. (1995). Orem's nursing theory and positive mental health: Practical considerations. *Nursing Science Quarterly, 8,* 165–173.

Parse, R. R. (1987). *Nursing science major paradigms, theories, and critiques.* Philadelphia: W. B. Saunders.

Parsons, T. (1949). *The structure of social action.* Glencoe, IL: Free Press.

Parsons, T. (1951). *The social system.* New York: Free Press.

Plattel, M. G. (1965). *Social philosophy.* Pittsburgh, PA: Duquesne University Press.

Sarter, B. (1988a). Metaphysical analysis. In B. Sarter (Ed.), *Paths to knowledge: Innovative research methods for nursing* (pp. 183–191). New York: NLN.

Sarter, B. (1988b). Philosophical sources of nursing theory. *Nursing Science Quarterly, 1,* 52–59.

Sarter, B. (1988c). *The stream of becoming: A study of Martha Rogers's Theory.* New York: NLN.

Smith, M. J. (1987). A critique of Orem's theory. In R. R. Parse (Ed.), *Nursing science major paradigms, theories, and critiques* (pp. 91–105). Philadelphia: W. B. Saunders.

Soltis, J. F. (1978). *An introduction to the analysis of educational concepts.* Reading, MA: Addison-Wesley.

Uys, L. R. (1987). Foundational studies in nursing. *Journal of Advanced Nursing, 12,* 275–280.

Wallace, W. A. (1977). *The elements of philosophy.* New York: Alba House.

Wallace, W. A. (1979). *From a realist point of view.* Washington, DC: University Press of America.

CHAPTER 10

Reframing Outcomes: Enhancing Personhood

Anne Boykin, PhD

Savina Schoenhofer, PhD

The concept of "enhancing personhood" is a key aspect of the theory of nursing as caring. It is tenuously, though importantly, related to the currently popular notion of outcomes of care. While the standard connotation of outcomes as discrete economic results or end products of nursing care is incongruent with nursing as caring, the ethical professional practice of nursing requires attention to value. This article presents a theoretically congruent reconceptualization of valuing of advanced practice nursing. It offers a model for reframing the concept of outcomes within the theoretical context of enhancing personhood. *Suppose that time is not a quantity, but a quality, like the luminescence of the night above the trees just when a rising moon has touched the tree line . . . in a world where time is a quality, events are recorded by the color of the sky . . . events glide through the space of the imagination,* *materialized by a look, a desire. (Lightman, 1993, p. 123)*

Key words: *caring, education, graduate, intentionality, nursing, outcomes, personhood, values.*

A dilemma exists in advanced nursing practice today in that advanced practice nurses, having acquired an unprecedented base of knowledge on which to draw, are challenged to articulate the way in which this knowledge influences the relationship of care from a nursing perspective. The viability of advanced practice nursing is at stake as nursing professionals struggle to make a recognizably unique contribution and avoid being subsumed in the anonymity of generic primary care providers and midlevel

Source: Boykin, A., and Schoenhofer, S., Advanced Practice Nursing Quarterly, 1997, 3(1), 60–65.

practitioners. Nurse practitioners, clinical nurse specialists, and others in advanced practice nursing roles face the important challenge of advancing the discipline of nursing while simultaneously communicating with the larger world of health care. A crucial aspect of this challenge involves effective languaging of nursing outcomes of care.

While nurses claim to "know" the value added to the health care situations in which they participate, that knowing remains largely tacit. Evidence supporting this conclusion is readily apparent in nursing literature describing various classification efforts over several decades. Nursing Minimum Data Set (NMDS) (Werley & Lang, 1988), the North American Nursing Diagnosis Association (1994), Rush Medicus (Haussman & Hegyvary, 1976), and the Royal College of Nursing's dynamic standard setting system (McFarlane, 1970) are all examples of frameworks used directly or indirectly to generate statements of nursing outcomes. These and similar frameworks effectively address nursing outcomes related to medical diagnosis and treatment activities, thus serving the generic primary care provider and mid-level practitioner well. However, they fail to communicate the richness of experience gained within the context of nursing situations, falling short of specifying the "value added" of the nursing contribution to care.

Why do these existing frameworks tend to disguise rather than disclose the meaningful experiences our patients gain in their relationships with us? Two interrelated explanations are proposed: intention and language. Compliance with the health care industry standard for provider reimbursement is an underlying intention of these frameworks. Thus, the systems use language that closely mirrors outcomes of medical care. To the extent that nursing care creates a different, unique realm of experience, and thus a different and unique value, this generic approach to outcomes has impoverished our ability to advance nursing practice.

What is the nature of the unique nursing contribution to health care situations? This question may be answered from a variety of perspectives in the formal literature of nursing. For example, within the framework of Orem's (1985) self-care deficit theory, the answer is assistance with self-care. From another perspective, nursing's contribution is termed promotion of adaptation (Roy, 1984), and from yet another, it is the provision of culturally congruent care (Leininger, 1988). Although language from these and other organized views of nursing is included along with more medically oriented diagnoses and standards, statements specifying outcomes of nursing depict the contribution of our practice in rather mechanical, simplistic, and superficial language that fails to satisfy our largely unspoken understanding of the true value of nursing in the lives of those we nurse.

Assumptions underlying one's practice of nursing reflect values and beliefs. They color the lens for being in relationship and direct what one sees. Therefore, it would seem that assumptions ought to influence significantly the experience of being cared for by a nurse. If the approach to practice is grounded in the importance of normative science, with medical diagnosis as guide to prediction of successful care, the outcomes of care will likely depict cause-and-effect relationships, depersonalization, detachment, and objectification of person. Watson (1995) calls us to reflect on this perspective with the following questions, "Does modern science establish the norms and standards of reality for us? Has science determined the norms and standard of the human experience?" (p. 65). Nursing practice grounded in the importance of person-as-person, of person-as-caring, and of person-as-whole-in-the-moment would likely result in outcomes of care—or experiences of having been cared for—that are within the context of person. What is experienced as the result of care would reflect characteristics of personhood: unity—creative evolving of a unifying, consistent, whole awareness; wholeness—creative unfolding of a recognizable self; and intention—blending desire and purpose. This picture of personhood, a core value in the experience of nursing, cannot be adequately described in normative science terms such as objectivity, prediction, measurement, and control. Rather, it requires a language and structure more akin to poetry. Meaningful explication of the values that emerge within the context of a nursing situation will be more subjective than objective, descriptive than predictive, concerned more with illumination than measurement, and intention more than control.

Nursing as Caring

Nursing as caring offers a perspective in which both intention and language center around caring. While not all nurses accept Leininger's (1988) assertion that caring is the central and dominant construct of caring,

it is widely acknowledged by nurses and those we nurse that caring is an important aspect of nursing. Formal knowledge of caring as an important aspect of nursing, initiated by Leininger (1978), Watson (1985), Gaut (1983), and others, is currently incorporated into a broad range of nursing theory development (Orem, 1985; Rogers, 1986; Roy, 1988).

The theory of nursing as caring (Boykin & Schoenhofer, 1993) is grounded in several fundamental assumptions: that to be human is to be caring (Roach, 1987), that personhood is a process of living grounded in caring, and that the capacity for personhood can be nurtured in relationship with caring others. Another important underlying assumption is that persons are whole in the moment, growing from moment to moment. From this grounding, nursing as caring posits that the unique focus of nursing is nurturing persons from the understanding that they are living caring in the moment and growing in caring from moment to moment. The nurturance that is nursing involves acknowledging, affirming and celebrating persons as caring, and supporting them in their unique ways of growing in caring.

From the lens of nursing as caring, the living of values of practice and the knowing of nursing occurs within the context of the nursing situation. The nursing situation is a "hard lived experience in which the caring between the nurse and the one nursed enhances personhood" (Boykin & Schoenhofer, 1993, p. 33). The nurse and one nursed bring to this experience the fullness of their being—their wholeness. The intention of the nurse is to know and to nurture the person in his or her wholeness and to know the one nursed as a person living and caring uniquely in the moment. In the mutuality of the nursing relationship, the nurse too risks allowing self to be known as caring person.

Relationships

Relationships grounded in caring express the value of the importance of person-as-person. Imbedded in this relationship is the intention of wanting to know other, as well as a willingness to be open and receptive to other. Such relationships require the personal investment of both the nurse and the nursed. The nurse's deliberate presence creates an experience for one being cared for in which wholeness is felt. Such presence involves a way of listening and communicating through which one gives of self. It is through this connectedness, inspired by presence, that the nurse hears calls for nursing and responds with unique expressions of caring.

Reflective Practice

The knowing of person is accomplished by being open to knowing and participating in personal stories. Reflective practice (Schon, 1982) is integral to this process. As the nursing situation unfolds, the nurse, drawing on a vast and expanding knowledge base, is sensitive to gathering every cue, every sign, and every hunch, and reflects on the meaning of these in each particular situation. Upon reflection, the nurse communicates emerging understanding of the situation with the one nursed and together they engage in a dialogue to share understanding, meaning, knowing, and planning in the situation. These reflections and dialogues shape the moment and influence the nurturing response of the nurse. As Taylor (1992) states, the "shared sense of humanity helps a nurse stand back quietly, to move in to help where it is appropriate, to speak plainly and sensitively, to provide comfort at subtle levels and to be oneself in spite of professional knowledge and skills" (p. 42). Through such presence the nurse expresses humility and active patience, allowing the person the freedom to be himself or herself and to share his or her story as it is lived (Boykin & Schoenhofer, 1991).

Intention

Intention is a key aspect of nursing from the perspective of nursing as caring. Practice grounded in this perspective is not concerned with diagnosis of a problem to be addressed through nursing, but rather with participating in a mutual relationship in which the nurse seeks to know the nursed in his or her unique, unfolding expressions of caring. The nurse enters the relationship with the intention of knowing the other as caring person, creating appropriate ways of knowing and of offering nurturance that are in tune with the uniqueness of the person and the situation. The intention to know and to nurture harmoniously opens a context in which caring is allowed to surface and flourish freely and creatively.

Outcomes

The quality of the nursing relationship as described leads to possibilities that are fully nonprobabilistic and unpredictable though recognizable and patterned. The idea of outcomes of nursing care, then, must be viewed in a different way. The concept of outcomes, as it is widely employed, is static, limited to what can be "predicted" and traceable back to those predictions and the circumstances that are guided by predictions. As acknowledged earlier, this sense of outcome is workable when reflection on the nursing situation is held to a superficial understanding of the situation. However, this approach to outcome specification fails to illuminate the significance of the nursing relationship in the lives of these nursed, and thus it sells short the contribution of nursing to the larger arena of health care.

Transformation

Transformation to a richer understanding of nursing contribution requires courage—courage for nurses to reflect upon and note the meaning of their care, courage to go beyond what is currently accepted in delimiting and languaging the value experienced by persons who participate in nursing situations. Courageous discovery and explication of the full value of nursing are responsibilities of those who would wish to call their efforts advanced practice nursing. Intention, knowledge, and skill are required for the fulfillment of these responsibilities.

Knowledge

Intention is the exercise of a commitment to bring the full power of nursing to those persons seeking nursing involvement in their life situations. The basic, enduring values of nursing—respect, caring, openness, intimacy, hope—provide the content

of intention. Knowledge is in the moment, ever transforming and being transformed. It encompasses who we are, what we understand, and the challenges encountered for growth in understanding. Knowledge, or more accurately, knowing, is the convergence of many pathways—personal, empirical, ethical, aesthetic (Carper, 1978), unknowing (Munhall, 1993), and spiritual knowing. Knowing is enriched in dialogue, reflection-in-practice, and reflection on-practice, and it is characterized by humility. Skill is developed as nurses live their intention to explicate the value added through their practice knowledgeably, persistently, and in community with other nurses, those nursed, colleagues in other health care practices, and those in related economic and political arenas.

Nursing Situation

The following advanced practice nursing situation was shared by a nurse whose practice is guided by the theory of nursing as caring. It will be used to provide examples of nursing outcomes framed within that theoretical perspective.

> Nurses associated with a community health service for migrant worker families in south Florida went weekly to a nearby labor camp where health information and support were offered as an extension of the primary care services for the migrant community. On this particular night, the plan, by request, was to teach infant cardiopulmonary

resuscitation (CPR). Upon arriving at the designated place, three men were encountered who had just finished their evening meal after having spent the day in the fields. These men were among those who had left their families in Mexico, Guatemala, and Salvador in May and would not return until the coming April. It was now early February.

After some general conversation, the nurses worked one on one with the men, teaching and demonstrating the techniques of infant CPR. When it came time for the return demonstration, one man told a nurse why he was interested in learning. He had left two small children and a pregnant wife in Salvador, and his third child was born several weeks after he had left. He was eager to learn all he could that would be helpful to his family.

As he accepted the demonstrator doll, the nurse noticed that he cradled it in his arms and gazed into its upturned face. He was very careful and tender as he proceeded through the return demonstration. Relinquishing fears related to the possible language and cultural barriers, the nurse invited him to share his thoughts and feelings about his family, the child he had never seen, and the present experience of holding the doll in his arms. His eyes glistened with tears as he talked and rocked the child—for it was obvious that it was no longer a doll but his own newborn infant he was encountering for the first time. As the

sharing continued, the other men gathered around and talked of their own experience of leaving home and family, of their longing and their determined willingness to suffer separation to provide for their families.

What were the outcomes of this situation of nursing? What was the value added to human health and quality of life? The narrative of this nursing situation and the subsequent outcome statements reflect an explicit theory of nursing, nursing as caring, and provide an example of the value of this perspective in recognizing and languaging the richness of nursing. Included in the outcome statements drawn from this nursing situation are three sets of outcomes: one for the nursed, one for the nurse, and one for the health care agency. They are as follows:

1. Nursed
   - affirmation of self as loving father
   - affirmation of self as caring through unique expressions of hope and courage
   - acquisition of knowledge of a lifesaving technique that could be used as an expression of self as one competent in a specific way of caring
   - strengthening of a human bond with coworkers through personal openness
2. Experience of building a trusting relationship with health care providers
3. Nurse
   - confirmation that through intentionality, life stories unfold
   - confirmation that risk-taking on another's behalf facilitated beneficial

self-knowing and interpersonal connection
- sense of personal connectedness in a bicultural situation
4. Health care agency bond established between agency representative and potential consumers
  - demonstration of agency services as valuable and culturally competent
  - health teaching that is culturally congruent decreases the future likelihood of need for acute care services

It should be noted that these exemplar outcomes emerged through observation, reflection, and dialogue with other nurses. A research method is presently being developed in which the nurse, the nursed, and the nurse researcher engage in dialogue to uncover the meaning of the lived experience of nursing. This approach will allow direct input on the value of the nursing experience to the nursed. A similar approach is planned to obtain information about the value of nursing from the health care agency.

Knowledge and Skills

The knowledge and skills needed for advanced practice nursing are many and complex. The nurse uses multiple ways of knowing to create the artistry of nursing. The expert advanced practice nurse understands that knowledge and skills are global and that unless they are distilled in the context of a particular nursing situation they

are meaningless. For example, technological expertise has meaning for nursing only in the context of a particular nursing situation. Advanced practice nurses are uniquely positioned to articulate the reality that the essence of nursing lives in the context of an intentional, mutual, caring relationship, a relationship in which the nurse draws forth a breadth and depth of knowledge for the purpose of knowing person(s) and of nurturing them as they live caring.

The resultant value of our service to society would be made manifest not only by the nurse but also by those nursed, from whom we truly know the value of our care. Rather than being detached from meaning to those nursed, outcomes reframed in the perspective of nursing as caring focus on understanding the value of care to particular individuals, families, and groups. Rather than outcomes extracted from a reducible view of person and causal in nature, outcomes reframed focus on the value of person as whole and caring.

Of all the sample outcomes listed from this nursing situation, the typical framework would have produced only one, acquisition of competence in infant CPR. The value of this outcome is not to be diminished. However, the value accruing from the experience of this nursing situation as expressed in the outcome statements is only truly appreciated when framed within the intention and language of the nursing theoretical perspective of nursing as caring.

This exemplar expresses a new vision of the purpose and structure of nursing outcomes. In addition to the responsibility of seeking appropriate reimbursement for advanced practice nursing, a more comprehensive sense of quality and accountability should concern us. The outcome statements offered can lead the way to the required demonstration of economic value, that is, a cost-benefit accounting of care. However, without an appropriate perspective, coupled with suitable language, the frustration that nurses experience in their attempts to explicate the real value of our nursing will persist—nursing's contribution to care will continue to be depreciated. To paraphrase Lightman (1993), suppose that nursing is not a quantity but a quality, suppose that nursing events that are recorded by the color of the sky, that glide through the space of the imagination, materialized by a look or a desire, could be described in all their richness, clearly seen and understood. This exemplar opens the door to the possibility.

References

Boykin, A., & Schoenhofer, S. (1991). Story as link between nursing practice, ontology, epistemology. *Image: The Journal of Nursing Scholarship, 23*, 245–248.

Boykin, A., & Schoenhofer, S. (1993). Nursing as caring. New York: National League for Nursing.

Carper, B. (1978). Fundamental patterns of knowing in nursing. Advances in Nursing Science, 1, 13–23.

Gaut, D. (1983). Development of a theoretically adequate description of caring. Western Journal of Nursing Research, 5, 312–324.

Haussman, R., & Hegyvary, S. (1976). The relationship of nursing process and patient outcomes. Journal of Nursing Administration, 90(10), 18–21.

Leininger, M. (1978). Transcultural nursing concepts, theories and practice. New York: John Wiley & Sons.

Leininger, M. (1988). Leininger's theory of nursing: Cultural care diversity and universality. Nursing Science Quarterly, 1, 152–160.

Lightman, A. (1993). Einstein's dreams. New York: Pantheon Books.

McFarlane, J. (1970). Study of nursing care: The first two years of a research project. International Nursing Review, 117(2), 101–109.

Munhall, P. L. (1993). "Unknowing": Toward another pattern of knowing in nursing. Nursing Outlook, 41, 125–128.

North American Nursing Diagnosis Association. (1994). Nursing diagnosis: Definition and classification 1995–1996. Philadelphia: NANDA.

Orem, D. (1985). Nursing: Concepts of practice (4th ed.), New York: McGraw-Hill.

Roach, S. (1987). The human act of caring. Ottawa, Canada: Canadian Hospital Association.

Rogers, M. (1986). Science of unitary human beings. In V. Malinski (Ed.), Explorations of Martha Rogers' science of unitary human beings. Norwalk, CT: Appleton-Century-Crofts.

Roy, C. (1984). Introduction to nursing: An adaptation model. Englewood Cliffs, NJ: Prentice Hall.

Roy, C. (1988). An explication of the philosophical assumptions of the Roy adaptation model. Nursing Science Quarterly, 1, 26–34.

Schon, D. (1982). The reflective practitioner. How professionals think in action. New York: Basic Books.

Taylor, B. (1992). A comforting nurse–patient encounter. Advances in Nursing Science, 15(1), 33–43.

Watson, J. (1985). Nursing: Human science and human care. A theory of nursing. Norwalk, CT: Appleton-Century-Crofts.

Watson, J. (1995). Nursing's caring-healing paradigm as exemplar for alternative medicine? Alternative Therapies, 1(3), 64–69.

Werley, H., & Lang, N. (Eds.). (1988). Identification of the nursing minimum data set. New York: Springer.

CHAPTER 11

Expressing Health Through Lifestyle Patterns

Nola J. Pender, RN, PhD, FAAN

Few concepts have received more attention from health professionals and the public during the last decade than health. This is largely due to the emergence of disease prevention and health promotion as global priorities. Unfortunately, the nature of health as a positive life process is poorly understood. Theoretical formulations of health often lack specificity and existing measures almost without exception reflect a narrow clinical perspective of health as the absence of disease. The purpose of this chapter is to propose a system for classifying expressions of health of persons in their entirety and to suggest related indicators of high-level health.

During the last decade, nursing, as well as other health disciplines, has recognized the limitations of medical and technological approaches for improving the quality of life and health of the world's population. Major changes in social, political, and environmental conditions of living and the life ways of large segments of society are necessary, if significant improvements in health are to occur during the next century. Thus, disease prevention and health promotion have become global agendas with the potential for achieving health goals unattainable previously through curative interventions. The escalating commitment to health promotion among nations raises important questions concerning the nature of health. What is the critical essence of that which is to

Source: Pender, N. J. (1990). Expressing health through lifestyle patterns. Nursing Science Quarterly, 3(3): 115–122. Reprinted by permission of and copyright © 2002 Sage Publications, Inc.

be promoted? A review of relevant scientific literature confirms that health as a human life span process is poorly understood.

Historically, illness, not health, has been the primary concern of the health professions and mortality and morbidity the indicators of "health" used most frequently (Smith, 1981). Therefore, it is not surprising that in reviewing studies of health, Terris (1975) identified the following illness-related approaches to health assessment: measurement of impairment, assessment of physiological systems in relation to established norms, and measurement of performance in the context of potential decrements. The concept of health has not fared much better in nursing. Although health along with person, environment, and nursing constitute the commonly accepted metaparadigm of the discipline (Fawcett, 1984), the concept of health seems to elude clear theoretical descriptions and, to an even greater extent, useful empirical specifications. Reynolds (1988), in reviewing the measures of health used in reports of nursing research, found that, despite articulation of a holistic concept of health in dominant theoretical views within the discipline, nurse scientists tended to use indicators derived from a clinical model as the absence of disease.

Is health such a complex human process that it cannot be studied qualitatively or quantitatively? Is high-level health a utopian state, a mirage to be fantasized but never achieved (Dubos, 1965)? On the other hand, if health can be the object of systematic investigation, can it only be defined by negation, that is as the absence of disease? Unwilling to settle for such a narrow definition, various health disciplines have attempted to define health from fragmented perspectives placing primary emphasis on psychological, sociological, cultural, or spiritual dimensions. Some attempts have been made to synthesize these perspectives to achieve a complete view of health. Parse (1987) refers to this approach as the totality paradigm, in which persons are considered as biopsychosocial spiritual beings responding and adapting to their environment. A major question about this additive approach is whether the whole is equal to or greater than the sum of the parts.

Person and Health: New Views of Old Concepts

Within the past two decades in nursing, there has been a significant conceptual shift toward viewing persons as unified wholes possessing integrity and manifesting characteristics that are more than and different from the sum of the parts. According to Rogers (1970),

> The unity of man is a reality. Man interacts with his environment in his totality. Only as man's wholeness is perceived does the study of man begin to yield meaningful concepts and theories. Only as man's oneness is apprehended is it possible to identify man's distinctive attributes. (p. 44)

This shift in nursing toward a unitary view of human beings has resulted in increasing reliance on the tenets of human science in addition to the reductionistic paradigm of traditional science for understanding health. How do individuals experience health, and what meanings do they give these experiences that have emerged as central questions within the discipline? Tripp-Reimer (1984) suggested that within nursing health be reconceptualized to incorporate both etic and emic perspectives. In the etic perspective, objective observations without input from those observed are used to determine health. In the emic perspective, the meaning of health to individuals within their particular culture is ascertained. Concerns relevant in the latter perspective include these: How is health expressed? Is the expression of health universal or culture specific? Are expressions of health qualitatively different at various developmental phases throughout the life span?

In contrast to the totality paradigm based primarily on the etic perspective, the simultaneity paradigm (Parse, Coyne, & Smith, 1985) captures the emic perspective. Within the latter paradigm each person is viewed as a synergistic being in open, mutual, and simultaneous interchange with the environment. In this context, health is a wholistic unfolding of humans in interaction with the environment in which all the elements or dimensions of health are experienced as a unitary phenomenon. Based on Rogers's theory of unitary human beings, Newman (1979) defined health as the totality of the life process evolving toward expanded consciousness. Parse et al. (1985), also in the Rogerian tradition, described health as a "process of becoming uniquely lived by each individual . . . a nonlinear entity that cannot be qualified

by terms such as good, bad, more, or less. Unitary man's health is a synthesis of values, a way of living . . . a continuously changing process that man cocreates" (pp. 9–10). Definitions with similar themes have been offered by Pender (1982), who described health as the actualization of inherent and acquired human potential, and Watson (1988), who defined health as harmony with self and environment. A new approach for combining objective (etic) and subjective (emic) health perspectives is needed to avoid a conception of health in which observable physical and behavioral aspects are viewed as separate or in oppositional relationship to experiential aspects. It is the author's belief that both perspectives are valuable and can coexist within the discipline of nursing.

Along with acceptance of a unitary view of health, there is an increasing tendency in nursing to reject the health–illness continuum that Newman (1979) criticized on the grounds that it maintains a false dichotomy by polarizing health at one end of the continuum and illness at the other end. If nursing is to facilitate a client's movement toward health on the health–illness continuum, this must always be away from illness. An "either–or" dichotomy precludes the existence of high levels of health in the presence of a disability or chronic illness. This belief, if carried to its logical conclusion, would imply that health promotion efforts are futile for millions of Americans young and old who have a chronic disease incurable by existing medical means. Health promotion would only be considered appropriate for the favored few without any evidence of disease, thus disenfranchising the poor, the old, and the disabled of services directed toward optimizing their health. To address this dilemma, Newman (1979) suggested a synthesis of the concepts of diseases and nondisease into an integrative concept of health.

Taking another theoretical approach to the problem posed by the health–illness continuum, Pender (1987) described health as the primary life experience with illness superimposed on health. Health can exist without illness, but illness never exists without health as its context. When illness occurs, it is synthesized as part of the ongoing health experience modifying it in varying ways—changing the quality of the experience and decreasing or increasing overall feelings and perceptions of health. Unlike Parse (1981), who rejects the idea of health as existing to varying degrees, Smith (1981) views health as a comparative term. It has long been recognized that all persons free of disease are not equally healthy. It is the degree to which health is present from both objective and subjective points of view that should be mutually assessed by nurse and client. It is only on the basis of both perspectives that effective efforts can be directed toward appropriate health enhancement activities.

The dominant definition of health espoused by a society has profound political and economic implications because the dimensions of that definition and their associated measures often become major social concerns. Frequently, programs of national and international scope are established to bring about positive changes in the identified indicators of health (McDowell & Newell, 1987). Thus, the discipline of nursing faces one of its biggest challenges in decades—how to best articulate the dimensions of health of persons in their entirety and develop valid and reliable indicators of health as a unitary phenomenon. Such indicators must be articulated with a level of conceptual clarity that permits communication of this perspective to other health disciplines and the public. The clinical view of health as the absence of disease has been the dominant definition in the United States for decades. It is time for a paradigmatic shift to a unitary conception of health that will enable society to deal capably with the multiplicity of factors now known to have an impact on health status.

As nursing moves forward in developing a unitary concept of health, strongly influenced by the tenets of human science, the discipline should not lose sight of empiricism as a viable approach to health-related research. Some questions asked about health are best addressed within a traditional science paradigm. For example, health processes outside of conscious awareness may be observable using highly sophisticated methods and techniques (Norbeck, 1987). Nursing can provide leadership to the health disciplines in blending the approaches of traditional and human sciences. Differences between the two paradigms should not be interpreted as conflict but as integrative tension that promotes creativity in scientific endeavors (Kritek, 1989).

Health as Pattern

Rogers (1970) identified the energy field as the fundamental unit of the universe for the science of nursing. The human and environmental fields are coextensive and in an intimate relationship. Pattern is the distinguishing characteristic of an energy field, which becomes more complex throughout the life span. Persons shape their own health experiences to a considerable extent as they make choices from the options available to them (Parse, 1981). Innate to energy fields are generative powers that can facilitate positive patterning and repatterning, resulting in progressively healthier conditions of being, as objectively measured and subjectively reported.

There is no single, universal health pattern that all human beings share. Health when viewed as a lived experience, that is, within the emic perspective, represents many alternative realities. Only individuals can reveal the hidden meanings that they create for health. Although health has many different shades of meaning, there are recurring themes or commonalities that persons report as expressions of health when queried as to what health means to them. The critical question is this: What are the varying human patterns most indicative of health?

Dimensions of the Health Experience

In 1981, Smith proposed a model of health with four dimensions reflective of existing literature: the clinical dimension defining health as the absence of disease, the role performance dimension describing health as competent performance of socially defined roles, the adaptive dimension characterizing health as flexible adjustment to changing life situations, and the eudaimonistic dimension viewing health as exuberant well-being. Laffrey (1986) operationalized Smith's model in a scale intended to determine the extent to which individuals viewed health along each of these dimensions. In further research, Woods and colleagues (1988) supported the health conception model of Smith in a study of 528 women who were asked, "What do you mean when you say you are in good health?" Their work contributed to the further elaboration of the eudaimonistic view of health identifying nine images consistent with this dimension: actualizing self, practicing healthy life ways, positive self-concept, positive body image, social involvement, fitness, effective cognitive function, positive mood, and harmony.

Parse et al. (1985) conducted a phenomenological study of 400 men and women who were asked to write descriptions of a personal situation in which a feeling of health was experienced. Recurring themes were identified for persons of differing ages. As an example, the recurring themes for persons between 20 and 45 years of age as expressed within the theoretical framework of man–living–health were spirited intensity, fulfilling inventiveness, and symphonic integrity.

Classifying Expressions of Health

In this section, a system for classifying human expressions of health is proposed. Five dimensions of human health expression are organized further into 15 subcategories as shown in **Table 11-1**. This framework for

Table 11-1   Classification System for Expressions of Health

Affect

Serenity	Harmony	Vitality	Sensitivity
Calm	Close to God	Energetic	Aware
Relaxed	Contemplative	Vigorous	Connected
Peaceful content	At one with the universe	Zestful	Intimate
Comfortable		Alert	Loving
Glowing		Fit	
Happy		Buoyant	
Joyous		Exhilarated	
Pleasant		Powerful	
Satisfied		Courageous	

Attitudes

Optimism	Relevancy	Competency
Hopeful	Useful	Purposive
Enthusiastic	Contributing	Initiating
Open	Valued	Self-motivating
Reverent	Committed	Innovative
	Involved	Masterful
	Challenged	

Activity

Positive Life Pattern	Meaningful Work	Invigorating Pay
Eating a healthy diet	Setting realistic goals	Having meaningful hobbies
Exercising regularly	Varying activities	Engaging in satisfying leisure activities
Managing stress	Undertaking challenging tasks	Planning energizing diversions
Obtaining adequate rest	Assuming responsibility for self	
Avoiding harmful substances	Collaborating with coworkers	
Building positive relationships	Receiving intrinsic or extrinsic rewards	

Table 11-1   (Continued)

Seeking and using health information

Monitoring health

Coping constructively

Maintaining a health-strengthening environment

Aspirations

Self-Actualization	Social Contribution
Growth or emergence	Enhancement of global harmony and interdependence
Personal effectiveness	Preservation of the environment
Organismic efficiency	

Accomplishments

Enjoyment	Creativity	Transcendence
Pleasure from daily living	Maximum use of capacities	Freedom
Sense of achievement	Innovative contribution	Expansion of consciousness
		Optimized harmony between man and environment

studying health has emerged as a result of discussions with colleagues, review of the literature, and reflection on 5 years of quantitative and qualitative research conducted by a health promotion research team (S. N. Walker, K. R. Sechrist, M. F. Stromborg, & N. J. Pender) in which the health and health practices of approximately 2,000 adults were studied. The following assumptions undergird the proposed classification:

1. Integration of the views of clients as well as health professionals is essential to derive a useful definition of health.
2. Health is a manifestation of person/ environment interactional patterns that become increasingly complex throughout the life span.
3. Some human health patterns can be directly observed, others must be self-reported.

The five dimensions within the classification are expressed in common language and the alliteration, although originally unintended, may be useful. Each of the five dimensions of health expression—affect, attitudes, activity, aspirations, and accomplishments—should be assessed in terms of daily fluctuations as well as evolving patterns over time. The five dimensions are proposed as culture free, whereas some of the 15 subcategories and potential indicators may be culture specific. Tools already exist to measure some of the suggested indicators; for others, approaches to description and/or measurement remain undeveloped. Consistent with a unitary view of human beings, a comprehensive assessment tool could be constructed to assess all of the dimensions simultaneously.

Affect

Sensation and emotion are fundamental attributes of humanness that are expressions of wholeness or unity (Rogers, 1970). Affect as used here is intended to denote emotions and feelings as subjectively experienced. Affect can be assessed best through personal report, but facial expressions, body positions, or gestures, as well as an increasing array of technologic measures (biofeedback, electromagnetic resonance imaging), can provide some indication of internal emotional states. The link between emotions and illness has been suspected for centuries, but little has been known about feelings as an expression of health. Recent research in psychoneuroimmunology indicates that person/environment interactions and accompanying emotional responses may moderate immune function (Kiecolt-Glaser & Glaser, 1987). Certain emotional patterns such as serenity and harmony may enhance immune competence; their polar opposites may impair immune capabilities. There is also considerable evidence that physiological changes related to activity have an impact on emotions. For example, production of endogenous opiates or internal tranquilizers can contribute to emotional experiences of comfort and calm (Watkins & Mayer, 1982).

Feelings and emotions have a direct effect on the quality of the lived experience of health. The emotions identified in Table 11-1 are those frequently reported as expressions of high-level health. Serenity is a sense of tranquility, a peaceful inner state, amid life's ebb and flow. Harmony emanates from feelings of relatedness to God and/or the universe and is sometimes described as a feeling of being at peace with nature and fellow humans. Vitality is a sense of energy and power. Sensitivity is intense knowing of self and others. Feelings of serenity, harmony, vitality, and sensitivity at any moment reflect much more than the current life situation. Human beings have the unique ability to evoke emotions in response to remembered events from the past or anticipated events in the future. This capacity provides persons with the power to transcend current situations—to be unbound by time and space. Persons may be calm, content, or even joyous in the face of difficult situations because of their vision of a greater good to be attained in the future.

Exploration of emotions as important expressions of health presents many exciting challenges to the research community. Current research on the connections between emotions and illness need to be recast in a positive perspective. Research questions from this viewpoint might be these: What person/environment interaction patterns encourage positive emotions? Which emotional patterns or fluctuations in patterns are healthful, which are unhealthful, and are these effects general or person-specific? Are different emotional profiles expressive of health at different points in the life span? What interventions on the part of health professionals assist clients in achieving positive emotional patterns? What self-care strategies can increase the frequency of positive emotions? Do emotions perceived as negative detract from or at times promote health?

Emotions can be a positive integrative force (Rogers, 1970). It is the richness of emotional experience that is uniquely human. Research approaches must be used that capture this richness as well as rhythms and fluctuations in emotional patterns. Recent scientific breakthroughs in understanding emotions will fuel increased interest and expanded research efforts in this area in the next decades.

Attitudes

Language, thought, and the ability to form attitudes and beliefs characterize unitary human beings and result from innate capacities to abstract and image features of person/environment interaction. Humans not only think in concepts and relationships but also give meanings to such abstractions. According to Rogers (1970), persons seek to organize the world of experience and make sense of it and can do so because of the capacity for rational thought. Attitudes structure the way persons see their world and, like emotions, express persons' values and priorities.

Attitudes can be developed in relation to specific situations, events, or actions. Life in its entirety can be viewed as an event. As such, persons develop attitudes or beliefs about their own personal lived situation as well as the life process as a shared experience with others. It is these general attitudes or beliefs that are proposed to profoundly influence health.

Attitudes expressive of high-level health are presented in Table 11-1. These are recurring cognitive themes in the literature and in more than 75 in-depth interviews conducted by the author and her colleagues with persons considered to have stellar health behaviors. Three subcategories of attitudes have been proposed: optimism, relevancy, and competency.

Attitudes toward life, its value, meaning, and ultimate worth are reflected in the subcategory of optimism. Beliefs that all will end well despite life's changing circumstances and that there are possibilities for personal growth even in difficult situations is expressed through an optimistic outlook. Optimism is enhanced by reverence for life and trust in God or the orderliness of the universe. Optimism expands openness to creative possibilities in life patterns.

Relevancy is grasping one's place in the world with an appreciation for unique, personal contributions. Relevancy is expressed through self-respect and a feeling of acceptance by others as a useful and contributing member of society. Persons experiencing a sense of relevance are caring, committed, and involved in life. Relevancy also has an eternal time frame by which persons come to appreciate the importance of their personal existence within infinite time and space.

Competency is expressed in personal clarity about actual and potential capabilities and belief in the power to channel capabilities into meaningful patterns of work and play. Competent persons actively initiate challenging life situations. They are interactive rather than passive, challenged rather than threatened, and self-affirming rather than self-debasing. Perceptions of personal competency are transferred to fellow humans with resultant appreciation of their unique patterns and emergent potential.

Positive attitudes and beliefs express high-level wellness. They are an integral part of health as a lived experience.

Activity

Movement is an alternative to language for communicating thought (Engle, 1984). Activity reflects patterns of energy distribution as well as person/environment rhythmicity. Movement is a means whereby space and time become experienced reality (Newman, 1979). Movement augments awareness of human and environmental fields. According to Newman, the total pattern of movement reflects the organization or disorganization of the thought and feeling processes of the individual. Activity expressive of health facilitates the fuller emergence of personal potential. Three dimensions of activity considered expressive of health are positive life patterns, meaningful work, and invigorating play (see Table 11-1).

Positive life patterns go beyond isolated health practices to action patterns that are an integral part of life ways. Thoughtful patterning and repatterning of daily routines and rhythms through informed decision making based on an awareness of options enhance human capacity for optimal well-being. Clusters of behaviors with empirical support for their health-enhancing properties are the backbone of positive life patterns. Eating well, exercising regularly, obtaining adequate rest, and managing stress represent behavioral clusters comprising positive life patterns. Such patterns must be sustained over time to optimize health. Exercise as one behavioral cluster expressive of health is a good example of unitary characteristics. If exercise is to be maintained, it must be of appropriate rhythmicity, periodicity, complexity, and intensity for a given human field. Human and environmental fields must have compatible activity rhythms and patterns to optimize health.

Health is also expressed through meaningful work. More energy is expended on work than on any other human activity. Work that is health promoting has been characterized as challenging, varied, well directed, interpersonally satisfying, and both intrinsically and extrinsically rewarding. In recent years, attempts have been made to achieve greater harmony between human fields and work patterns. Child care, flexible time, job sharing, and the use of home as a satellite work site are only a few of the examples of greater awareness of the need for compatibility between person/environment patterning and work.

The rhythm between work and invigorating play changes throughout life. For most children, play constitutes the major activity in which they engage. In fact, meaningful work as an expression of health may not be relevant until the preschool or school years when confronted by the "tasks" of learning. The harmonious integration of work and play often becomes disrupted in young, middle aged, and older adult years. Young and middle-aged adults, in striving to be successful, to achieve adequate pay, and to contribute meaningfully to society, may neglect play. Some compensate for this imbalance by focusing on enjoyable aspects of work and reinterpreting work as play. Older adults often have considerable discretionary time for play but lament lack of resources for recreational pursuits or the absence of meaningful work. It is predicted that leisure time will expand for many persons in the United States in the future as efforts are made to maximize the employment rate in a large and diverse population (Bezold, Carlson, & Peck, 1986). For both younger adults on shortened work weeks and the aging population in part-time employment, meaningful hobbies, satisfying leisure activities, and energizing diversions will be increasingly important as expressions of personal health.

Aspirations

Human beings are inherently purposeful. Life is not a random series of events, but an organized unfolding of each individual in light of personal aspirations and choices. Persons choose the directions in which they evolve in light of the range of options within awareness. Unfortunately, for persons in disadvantaged groups such as the poor and some ethnic/racial minorities, the range of choices is often constricted, limiting options for self-realization. Unnecessary limitations on self-expression is dehumanizing as well as detrimental to the continuing viability and vitality of a society.

The capacity of human beings to bring about changes in human and environmental fields is important for achievement of aspirations and goals. By modifying the nature of person/environment interactions, individuals can maximize available choices. Although persons usually have considerable freedom of choice concerning the goals they will pursue, the goals selected must be compatible with those of society. Social and cultural values as well as the needs of significant others provide a context for setting goals. Inherent in humanness is the moral responsibility for the ethical selection of goals and the means used to accomplish them.

Aspirations within a society often reflect normative patterns—the usual rather than the unusual, the average rather than the exception. Fitting in to societal norms rather than exceeding them is often condoned and encouraged to the detriment of creative change. Individuals possess unique capabilities for self-transcendence (Sarter, 1988). It is only as society encourages people to achieve their uniqueness unconstrained by normative expectations that we will have instances of maximized human health potential for systematic study.

Self-actualization and social contribution are proposed as two subcategories of aspirations needing further clarification and study in relation to human health patterns.

Self-actualization is not a new term. Maslow (1970) popularized the concept in his writings as a high-level need for human organisms. Self-actualization is predicated on fulfilling a more basic need for self-preservation. Suggested empirical indicators for self-actualization are growth or self-emergence, personal effectiveness, and organismic efficiency. Self-actualization is an orientation toward being all one can be and fulfilling one's personal potential.

Social contribution enhances global harmony, creates health interdependence, and promotes an ecologically balanced environment for present and future generations. The community in which we live is a world community in which annihilation is an ever present threat. Social contribution as an expression of health is a sensitivity to the needs and potentials of all people, which results in responsible social actions within a particular life situation. It is through shared aspirations of aggregates that social changes supportive of health are realized.

Accomplishments

Accomplishments as expressions of health can be identified as the payoffs for a life well lived. They are unencumbered by time and space and may be viewed as daily achievements, life attainments, or states to be experienced only after death. Regardless of the time frame, persons need bench marks to measure their progress, their emergence as unique human beings. Accomplishments confirm a person's selfhood as well as his or her oneness with the evolving universe.

In modern society, accomplishments are often viewed as measures of worth rather than as expressions of health. Too frequently, being and becoming are sacrificed to doing, thus destroying the balance among affect, attitudes, activity, aspirations, and accomplishments. When kept in proper perspective, accomplishments contribute to the richness of human experience. Creative achievements of human beings throughout history have markedly enhanced the quality of life for others.

Enjoyment, creativity, and transcendence are accomplishments proposed as expressive of health (see Table 11-1). Enjoyment is a condition in which there is heightened aesthetic awareness of the multiple dimensions of human and environmental fields. Positive emotions and thoughts predominate. Daily experiences are sources of joy. Human unfolding, its challenges and exigencies as well as successive stages of development, provide continuing sources of pleasure.

The capacity for creativity is inherent in all human beings. It is expressed through envisioning new configurations within human and environmental fields and restructuring reality or abstractions consistent with these envisioned patterns. Creativity is experienced as performing at one's optimum, maximizing human capabilities, and accelerating diversity and complexity.

Transcendence is stretching beyond the realm of human experience toward new options and possibilities (Parse, 1981). It is experienced as freedom from constraint and expansion of human consciousness to encompass infinite time and space. It is the experience of optimum mutuality and harmony between person and environment.

Accomplishments are the expression of life purpose and thus the expression of health. Their pursuit directs human patterning and evolutionary emergence.

Concluding Comments

Health is a life span process, a largely subjective and private experience, only partially observable by traditional scientific methods. Although defining health only in terms of negation, that is, as the absence of disease, has been common practice for more than a century, this approach will no longer suffice in an era of increasing concern about the promotion of health and the quality of life for human populations. Health as an experience is not fragmented, it only becomes fragmented in the minds of health professionals with differing perspectives. A new view of health is needed that is positive, comprehensive, unifying, and humanistic. This article represents one attempt to move toward that goal. It is imperative that an increasing number of nurse scientists direct their efforts toward expanding our understanding of human health processes and the personal, social, political, and environmental factors affecting the health of differing populations if significant progress is to be made in optimizing health for a larger segment of the world population in the years ahead.

References

Bezold, C., Carlson, R., & Peck, J. (1986). The future of work and health. Dover, MA: Auburn House.

Dubos, R. (1965). Man adapting. New Haven, CT: Yale University Press.

Engle, V. F. (1984). Newman's conceptual framework and the measurement of older adults' health. Advances in Nursing Science, 7(1), 24–36.

Fawcett, J. (1984). Analysis and evaluation of conceptual models of nursing. Philadelphia: Davis.

Kiecolt-Glaser, J., & Glaser, R. (1987). Psychosocial moderators of immune function. Annals of Behavioral Medicine, 9, 16–20.

Kritek, P. (1989, April). Nursing research enterprise in clinical practice: An agenda for the future. Paper presented at Northern Illinois University Annual Research Conference, DeKalb, IL.

Laffrey, S. C. (1986). Development of a health conception scale. Research in Nursing and Health, 9, 107–113.

Maslow, A. H. (1970). Motivation and personality (2nd ed.). New York: Harper & Row.

McDowell, I., & Newell, C. (1987). Measuring health: A guide to rating scales and questionnaires. New York: Oxford.

Newman, M. (1979). Theory development in nursing. Philadelphia: Davis.

Norbeck, J. S. (1987). Empiricism and health promotion research. In M. E. Duffy & N. J. Pender (Eds.), Conceptual issues in health promotion: Report of proceedings of a Wingspread Conference (pp. 110–120). Indianapolis, IN: Sigma Theta Tau International.

Parse, R. R. (1981). Man-living-health: A theory of nursing. New York: Wiley.

Parse, R. R. (1987). Nursing science: Major paradigms, theories, and critiques. Philadelphia: Saunders.

Parse, R. R., Coyne, A. B., & Smith, M. J. (1985). Nursing research: Qualitative methods. Bowie, MD: Brady.

Pender, N. J. (1982). Health promotion in nursing practice. Norwalk, CT: Appleton-Century-Crofts.

Pender, N. J. (1987). Health promotion in nursing practice (2nd ed.). Norwalk, CT: Appleton & Lange.

Reynolds, C. L. (1988). The measurement of health in nursing research. Advances in Nursing Science, 10(4), 23–31.

Rogers, M. E. (1970). An introduction to the theoretical basis of nursing. Philadelphia: Davis.

Sarter, B. (1988). The stream of becoming: A study of Martha Roger's theory. New York: National League for Nursing.

Smith, J. A. (1981). The idea of health: A philosophic inquiry. Advances in Nursing Science, 3(3), 43–50.

Terris, M. (1975). Approaches to an epidemiology of health. American Journal of Public Health, 65, 1037–1045.

Tripp-Reimer, R. (1984). Reconceptualizing the construct of health: Integrating emic and etic perspectives. Research in Nursing and Health, 7, 101–109.

Watkins, L. R., & Mayer, D. J. (1982). Organization of endogenous opiate and monopiate pain control systems. Science, 216, 1185–1192.

Watson, J. (1988). Nursing, human science, and human care. New York: National League for Nursing.

Woods, N. F., Laffrey, S., Duffy, M., Lentz, N. J., Mitchell, E. S., Taylor, D., & Cowan, K. A. (1988). Being healthy: Women's images. Advances in Nursing Science, 11(1), 36–46.

CHAPTER 12

Healing as Appreciating Wholeness

W. Richard Cowling, III, RN, PhD

The "clinicalization" of human experience by the health care disciplines has been instrumental in denying important facets of human life and not fully accounting for the essence and wholeness of experience. A unitary conceptualization of healing as appreciating wholeness is proposed. Appreciating is actualized through a praxis approach used for research and practice—unitary pattern appreciation—created to bring the theoretical principles of unitary science into practical reality. It is essentially a praxis for exploration of the wholeness within human/environmental pattern. Healing is conceptualized as the realization, knowledge, and appreciation of the inherent wholeness in life that elucidates prospects of clarified understanding and opportunities for action. The essential features of the process of pattern appreciation are a synoptic stance toward pattern information, a participatory engagement with people in the exploration of wholeness, and the transformative nature of the process that illuminates the possibilities in wholeness. A case demonstrates the nature of the unitary pattern appreciation process and its healing qualities.

Key words: *healing, nursing practice, nursing science, nursing theory, Rogers' science of unitary human being, transformation, unitary theory.*

As nursing has moved to assume an expanded role in the clinical care of patients, nurses have participated in the creation of "clinicalization" of human experience that has been instrumental in denying important facets of human experience. The clinicalization

Source: Cowling, WR. Healing as Appreciating Wholeness. Advances in Nursing Science 2000;22(3):16–32.

of human experience takes the form of an overemphasis on diagnostic representations that do not fully account for the essence and wholeness of the experience. This clinicalization is expressed in empirical, conceptual, and theoretical approaches that yield partial, and sometimes erroneous, accounts that miss the essential wholeness, unity, and uniqueness of human existence, similar to the androcentric bias in science noted by feminist scholars.[1] This occurs in spite of our claimed holistic perspective that has embraced spiritual care and complementary healing modalities. Related manifestations of this phenomenon are an overemphasis on clinical specialization, client interventions shaped by economics rather than need, educating natural healing tendencies out of students, general subjugation of our spiritual consciousness to economics of health care, treatment protocols that do not consider wholeness of human existence, and overreliance on physical/material conceptions and models of human health and illness. A recent study[2] comparing alternative healers and nurses described healers as creating a sacredness and reverence around their work in contrast with the clinical structures and techniques of nursing. An alternative to the clinicalization perspective is the focus of healing with its attendant concern for wholeness.

A Differentiated Healing Conceptualization

It is acknowledged that there is a range of potential meanings given to healing that is extensive and diverse.[3] Kritek[3] points out that healing is a gerund derived from heal, which means whole. A gerund is a term originating from a verb but used as a noun. Consequently, the foundational meaning of the term is directly derived from the notion "to heal" or the activity of becoming whole. Therefore, healing is a process that becomes an object. Kritek's[3] comprehensive essay on the construct of healing and her reflections on the multiple meanings of the construct provide an opening and an invitation for articulating a unitary perspective of healing. She forcefully demonstrates the depth, richness, specificity, and focus that context brings to the meaning assigned to healing by persons and groups. She warns of "the anomalous situation where a sought-after wholeness is conceptualized and pursued in a manner that implicitly or explicitly denies or ignores dimensions of the human condition that are essential to achieving that wholeness."[3(pp. 11–12)] Furthermore, Kritek sheds light on the situation in which nurses are educated to attend to the subjective and objective meanings associated with wholeness and healing and to devise responses based on those meanings, yet "the ambitiousness of this intention is only superficially acknowledged, and the skills and the knowledge necessary to excel in such an effort are not yet delineated."[3(p. 14)] A unitary conceptualization of healing as appreciating wholeness responds to Kritek's concerns and cautions.

A unitary conceptualization of healing as appreciating wholeness differentiated from the synthesized view in the current literature provides an alternative to be considered as a framework for a healing science and practice.

The synthesized view of healing as a nursing construct is elaborated by Kritek.[3] In spite of the variety of meanings, there is an overarching idea of wholeness inherent in healing stemming from what Kritek refers to as "some admixture of complementary conceptualizations," as seeking or reaching for a desired wholeness. There is an understanding that wholeness is an ideal rather than a reality, "since no human is actually whole."[3(p. 14)] A goal or destination toward this ideal is implied. It also is understood that dissonant definitions of wholeness are differentiated, more or less, by their potential as confining and limiting in viewpoint and by the degree of complexity and robustness.

A unitary conceptualization of wholeness,[4] which is at the heart of healing, is clearly a departure from this synthesized view of healing. A unitary view posits that human beings are irreducible wholes and that the unitary nature of the environment also is irreducible. The concept of field is central to the unitary perspective and "provides a means of perceiving people and their respective environments as irreducible wholes."[4(p. 29)] Although Rogers did not explicate a conceptualization of healing, it is clear that a unitary conceptualization of healing, grounded in wholeness, would require an understanding of human being/environmental wholeness as unitary. Practice and science through a unitary lens would accept the reality of wholeness not as an ideal, but as a given. Human beings and their environments would be approached as integral fields within fields that could not be extracted into parts, or more specifically, in theoretical terms as unitary energy fields.

Newman puts it more succinctly and directly, "unbroken wholeness is what is real—not the fragments we devise with our way of describing things."[5(p. 37)]

While I have a deep respect for the theoretical language of the science of unitary human beings, I have an even greater reverence for the experiential nature of wholeness that supports this theoretical language. That is, my experience of being human engaged in practicing nursing with other human beings suggests a reality of wholeness. Newman aptly points out that we are embedded in what we want to study, and the nature of nursing requires that we engage in the experience of it to understand it fully.[5] My own view is that the nature of nursing is one of responding to the wholeness of human experience. I have used the practice and research enterprises simultaneously in an attempt to engage in nursing with a reverence for the wholeness humans bring to that engagement and to prepare myself for knowing and appreciating that wholeness. I have spent a considerable portion of my career developing this praxis that gives attention to the wholeness of humans and their environments and opens the possibilities for participatory, transformative change.[6–9] The approach has been refined to serve both the purposes of research and practice or can be used for either individually. I could not have sought this reverence for human wholeness or created an approach that attends to this wholeness without the conceptual system of unitary science. This is an example of what Wheeler and Chinn describe as praxis, "thoughtful reflection and action that occurs in synchrony."[10(p. 2)]

Thus, it is for me theory and experience that create the synchronous context for reflection and action and provide the grounds for the perspective I have adopted of healing as appreciating wholeness.

The Appreciating Context

The appreciating context is based on the common understanding of the meaning of appreciation and the unitary perspective of pattern. In the dominant view of healing there is a seeking to understand desired wholeness through attention to the parts and the interrelationship of the parts to one another. In the practice of healing the focus is "on establishing, achieving, or regaining a sense of cohesion" among the parts.[3(p. 17)] In the unitary view of healing as appreciating wholeness, the attention is on the pattern that emerges in human experiences, perceptions, and expressions occurring in unity and arising from human and environment mutual process. In the practice of healing, the focus is on appreciating the wholeness within this pattern. Pattern, in unitary terms, is the distinguishing characteristic of a field and gives identity to the field.[4] Each unitary human field pattern is considered to be unique along with its own unique environmental field pattern. In human terms, the pattern gives identity to and distinguished one person from another. It is the essence of being who you are; thus, pattern appreciation is reaching for this essence in each individual and seeing the wholeness within pattern. In summary, rather than knowing the parts to know wholeness, the unitary scientist/practitioner seeks knowing the pattern to know wholeness.

The elemental characteristics of appreciation were derived from reviewing the Oxford English Dictionary definitions of appreciation: perception of the full force; sensitive to and sensible of delicate impression and distinction; perception, recognition, and intelligent notice; expression of one's estimate; sympathetic recognition of excellence; and gratefulness, enjoyment, and understanding.[11] Appreciating means "perceiving, being aware of, sensitive to, and expressing the full force and delicate distinctions of something while sympathetically recognizing its excellence as experienced in gratefulness, enjoyment, and understanding."[7(p. 130)] The something in unitary healing science and practice terms is the wholeness inherent in field pattern as manifest in human experiences, perceptions, and expressions, or in simpler terms, the wholeness inherent in human life.

Unitary pattern appreciation reaches for the wholeness within pattern in the following six ways:[7]

1. It seeks a perception of the full force of pattern.
2. It requires sensitivity to and sensibility of the manifestations that give identity to each person's unique pattern.
3. It involves perception, recognition, and intelligent notice of human expressions that reflect pattern.

4. It takes the form of an estimate of unitary energy field pattern as a meaningful representation of the pattern called a profile (often emerges as story, metaphor, and music).
5. It implies sympathetic recognition of excellence of energy field pattern meaning that pattern is significant regardless of characteristics.
6. It is approached with gratefulness, enjoyment, and understanding that reaching for the essence of pattern has potential for a deepening understanding in service to the individual and knowledge development for practice and science, and ultimately transformation of participants.

These characteristics or features provide the context for establishing an appreciating endeavor with clients or participants

The Appreciating Process

Unitary pattern appreciation was developed for the purpose of creating a unitary art and science that would bring theoretical principles into practical reality.[6,7] It consists of a process, orientation, and approach that can be used for research, practice, or combined research and practice intentions (praxis). Through its use over the past 2.5 years with participants in a praxis enterprise, I became aware of the healing nature of appreciation turned toward wholeness. Three critical features of pattern appreciation create the

conditions for healing: synoptic, participatory, and transformative.

Synoptic

The synoptic orientation provides an alternative to the process of analysis for understanding information. Murphy[12] employed an approach to his research on transformation known as synoptic empiricism. It was used in unitary pattern appreciation. According to Broad, "Synopsis is the deliberate viewing together of aspects of human experience which for one reason or another, are generally kept apart by the plain man and even by the professional scientist or scholar. The object of synopsis is to try to find out how various aspects are interrelated."[13(p. 8)] In the practice of appreciation, there is shift away from the attention on the interrelatedness of aspects and a focus on sensing an emerging pattern that reflects the wholeness of human life. Thus, aspects of human life, namely the experiences, perceptions, and expressions associated with living, are viewed together in an inclusive way to reveal the fullest picture of the inherent wholeness.

The scientist/practitioner may look for themes and commonalities in the pattern information or may use an assortment of ways of knowing that reveal a compelling sense of wholeness amidst the variety of phenomena of life. The synoptic process requires an inclusive view of what counts as pattern information. Pattern manifestations or phenomena that are labeled by participants as physical, emotional, mental, social, and spiritual are included as pattern information.

They are understood contextually as arising from wholeness, not reflective of parts that do not exist in the unitary perspective. Observations by the scientist/practitioner of physical phenomena also are included as pattern information.

Ensemble is a useful concept to consider when thinking about the process of synopsis as a way of appreciating wholeness. Phenomena or features of human life are viewed as an ensemble that reflects pattern and wholeness. The definition of ensemble is "all the parts of anything taken together so that each part is considered only in relation to the whole."[11] In the case of unitary pattern appreciation, the term facets is substituted for parts since facet implies an aspect of something that is whole rather than something that is divisible into separate entities. The ensemble of phenomena of human life represents the facets of a pattern reflecting wholeness. As in the musical notion of ensemble, which means "the united performance of all voices or instruments in a piece of concerted music,"[11] the scientist/practitioner of pattern appreciation listens for the united concert of voices in the phenomena conveying the essence of the pattern and thus the wholeness, of human living. "The multiple, and sometimes seemingly disparate, manifestations of the field pattern form an ensemble of information that conveys a singularity of expression."[6(p. 140)] Developing one's ability to sense the pattern and wholeness is the goal of the synoptic process that supports healing.

Participatory

Appreciative inquiry and practice are fundamentally participatory inquiry and practice. People seek to participate in the research or practice based on an invitation and/or knowledge of the work of the nurse. Although my work has been primarily in the community and participants come to engage in the appreciating process from knowing about my research/practice, it is possible that clients of health care institutions might have access to this type of engagement through expert nurses who have developed the requisite knowledge and skills. Regardless of setting, it is critical that there be mutual understanding between the nurse and the participant from the beginning as to the nature of the appreciating process, the egalitarian ideal inherent in the relationship, the openness to emergent discovery in the work, the potential for negotiation, and the fact that potential outcomes are not predicted or prescribed.

The participatory orientation capitalizes on one of the major tenets of the science of unitary human beings: the capacity of humans to knowingly participate in change and in patterning.[4] It is this capacity that provides the opportunity for mutual discovery of possible avenues of action. The actions chosen emerge from the knowledge of wholeness that comes from exploration of one's pattern. The exploration and discovery mode of the process is created through a partnership. In this partnership, the nurse provides a contextual process of appreciating pattern, which is open to modification depending on the desires of the participant. The participant is viewed as an expert on his or her own life and the source of his or her own power and knowledge. Each encounter in the appreciating process is primarily in the form of a dialogue with content focused on life experiences, perceptions, and expressions. However, the use of music, imagery, or movement also might serve the dialogue and the emergence of useful pattern information to understand the person's wholeness.

The appreciative inquiry aspect has been developed over time using knowledge of participatory modes of inquiry.[14] Recently, I discovered a field of participatory inquiry in organizational life known as appreciative inquiry,[15] which has features similar to unitary pattern appreciation. In relation to the organizational context, "more than a method or technique, the appreciative mode of inquiry is a way of living with, and directly participating in, the varieties of social organization we are compelled to study."[15(p. 131)] Likewise, unitary pattern appreciation is a way of participating in the varieties of human life experiences that reflects the wholeness of human existence. It aims to use this participation as a way of bettering the lives of human beings and to grasp a deeper understanding for developing knowledge of human wholeness and healing.

The life process system practice model described by Schaef[16] has served to inform the refinement and development of aspects of the unitary pattern appreciation practice approach. This model of practice advocates for practitioner receptivity to the client's life process, embraces honoring this process, and acclaims the inherent healing capacity of the client. Likewise, in unitary pattern appreciation praxis the scientist/practitioner is receptive to the person's life experiences, perceptions, and expressions and honors the uniqueness of each individual life. The

healing capacity is acclaimed through respect for the client's ability to participate knowingly in change. In the life process system model, as in unitary pattern appreciation, "Diagnosis is not the foundation for practice; wisdom arising from participation with clients is the foundation. In its denial of the primacy of diagnosis, the model implies a rejection of a dualistic view of illness (ill and not-ill) and of judgment as a critical attribute for the potential of healing."[7(pp. 139–140)] The ideal of control is inconsistent with the notions of unitary science predicated on acausality and unpredictability. Thus participation becomes central to the appreciating process of healing.

Transformative

The transformative potential of unitary pattern appreciation is the cornerstone of healing. By giving attention to the wholeness of human existence through appreciating pattern, phenomena are seen in a new context. For example, my praxis involves helping individuals who are experiencing despair. When the experiences of despair, the perceptions of despair, and the ways in which despair are expressed in one's life are placed in the context of the wholeness of one's life there are revelations that go beyond the tendency to treat and/or understand the despair as a symptom of a disease or a single condition. Returning to the organizational brand of appreciative inquiry, there is a similar perspective that relates to healing. In organizational appreciative inquiry "serious consideration and reflection on the ultimate mystery of being engender a reverence for life that draws the researcher to inquire beyond superficial appearances to . . . the life generating essentials and potentials of social existence."[15(p. 131)] Likewise, in the case of unitary pattern appreciation, the inquirer/practitioner reaches for the essentials and potentials within the wholeness of human life, and like the organizational appreciative inquirer who is "drawn to affirm, and thereby illuminate, the factors and forces involved in organizing that serve to nourish the human spirit," the unitary nurse is drawn to affirm and illuminate the factors and forces that nourish awareness of the richness and potentialities in the wholeness of human life.[15(p. 131)] This creates a condition and context ripe with possibilities for transformation.

Unitary pattern appreciation also invites participants to consider the possibilities of seeing change within the consciousness of pandimensionality, which is a unitary view of time, space, and movement. However, this is a concept introduced in the context of the participant's life concerns and not imposed as the only way of viewing the realities of change. Thus, it is provided as one way of viewing change amidst many others. Ultimately, the participant's choice of viewing change is acknowledged and embraced as an aspect of the participatory and exploratory nature of unitary pattern appreciation. Pandimensional consciousness, a complex and abstract concept, is akin to Moss' spiritual concept of "unitive consciousness."[17] Unitive consciousness occurs when individuals become referent to infinity, meaning that they realize infinite potential and infinite time–space–movement–change. Moss[17] described unitive consciousness in ways similar to those Martha Rogers[4] used to conceptualize a pandimensional universe.

Two descriptors best convey this pandimensional or unitive consciousness where we are "in a great sea of being infinite in all directions."[17(p. 65)] The first descriptor is "where feeling, sensation, and thinking are a unified continuum that is not limited by the boundaries of the body."[17(p. 65)] The second is "every moment is a new birth and what is being born is not merely the product of the past, not merely the cause of some earlier effect, but rather part of a ceaseless cosmos of revelation."[17(p. 66)] The transformation potential of pandimensional awareness is the same as that of unitive consciousness as Moss described it—that is, "to become referent to infinity is to not have our identity located in any finite notion of ourselves. We are movement and flow. Our careers, our health, our families and possessions may temporarily represent a harbor of our sense of self, but ultimately we are always far more."[17(p. 67)]

Finally, the transformative potential for scientists/practitioners rests within the way in which they learn to use themselves as instruments for pattern appreciation. Because the quest for pattern knowledge requires attention to all realms of data, one must develop data acquisition skills that allow the data to reveal themselves. This is very similar to the quest for data acquisition and verification in religious life described by Wilber.[18] A person must be developmentally adequate to a disclosure or the data will not reveal themselves. In meditative knowing, injunctive tools of Zen are used for this disclosure. Injunctive tools also are used for the disclosure. Injunctive tools also are emerging from the quest for understanding unitary pattern. The inquiry process associated with unitary pattern appreciation calls for a willingness to use injunctive devices that will open one to the revelation of unitary pattern data. Likewise, this inquiry process calls for the scientist/practitioner to use these data in ways that are responsive to the unique pattern of the individual in designing unitary nursing practice strategies. For most nurses, this would mean at least a relative transformation toward being a more sensitive instrument of awareness.

In summary, the healing potential of appreciating wholeness rests with these three foundational features of the process that are integrated within the context of an appreciating attitude. The nurse invites people to engage in a participatory exploration of the wholeness within life using a pattern lens that avoids the fragmentation of other ways of viewing experiences. By using a synoptic framework, all phenomena are considered relevant and are embraced as an ensemble of information that helps both the nurse and the participant see the wholeness within this pattern. Spiritual phenomena are considered along with physical, emotional, mental cultural, and social phenomena in an inclusive way. In contrast to the interpretative paradigm that seeks "to understand and derive meaning from the human experience,"[19(p. 71)] unitary pattern appreciation seeks to represent the wholeness within human experience by attending to pattern. In the unitary way of thinking, healing is not seeking a desired wholeness but rather is realizing, knowing and appreciating an inherent wholeness that illuminates potentials of understanding and possibilities of action.

A Case of Healing as Appreciating Wholeness

The following is a sketch of a case from my ongoing praxis project that demonstrates healing as appreciating wholeness. Karen, an early participant in the unitary pattern appreciation project, came in response to a flyer distributed in the community. She was in her early 50s, had three grown children, had been married and divorced twice, and was working as a legal secretary. She came to see me because of "ongoing despair." She said that when she saw the flyer she identified closely with the word despair. "I just feel like I'm in a lot of despair. I probably don't look it, but I am. I am broken spiritually. . . . It's not a psychological problem, but spiritually I need healing. . . . That's why I wanted to come—to heal that."

The process of pattern appreciation with Karen involved asking questions about the nature of her experiences, the perceptions she had of these experiences, and the ways in which despair was being expressed in her life. Some of the questions were contemplated in preparation, but most often they emerged from the content of the dialogue. The dialogue focused on past, present, and future, and it covered topics related to relationships, family, work, play, beliefs, spirituality, physical sensations, health, dreams, feelings, and aspirations, in addition to whatever topics Karen raised. During the dialogue, I attempted to position myself in a stance of openness to hear the wholeness within Karen's portrayal of life. My emphasis was not only on listening to the words but also on being sensitive to and sensible of the variety of information that came forth in dialogue—the ways in which words were stated, the expressions, the movements, and the posture as well as my own reactions. I did not take notes because I wanted to be fully present to the experience of the dialogue.

I have tried to capture the unitary pattern appreciation process by describing the experiential, perceptual, and expressive aspects of Karen's life phenomena and by explaining the ways in which the synoptic, participatory, and transformative features were integrated. It is important to clarify that experience, perception, and expression are sources of pattern information and are considered facets of pattern, not parts. A person experiences, perceives, and expresses all at once or contiguously. "Experience is the raw encounter of living loaded with sensation."[7(p. 133)] Experience involves sensing and being aware as a source of knowledge.[11] "Perceiving is the apprehending of experience or the ability to reflect while experiencing."[9(p. 202)] Experiencing and perceiving cannot be disentangled from one another. Perception is conscious knowing in the midst of experience. To express is to manifest.[11] Expression is manifesting the experience and perception of living that is the unique pattern of the individual. Expressions of pattern are the avenues to knowing pattern and thus wholeness. In the dialogue and the resulting text, the facets of experience, perception, and expression

come forward in a unified way. They are disentangled here only as a simpler way of portraying the facets. There is a risk of violating the sense of wholeness involved in creating this representation of Karen's life as only excerpts can be portrayed from transcripts.

Experience

Karen recounted a childhood of instability and feelings of not being acknowledged. "I went to six schools by the time I was in the sixth grade. I mean there must have been a reason why we moved so much. I don't know what it was. It seemed like my father was under more and more stress and became more and more distant. . . . He was physically not available. His emotions weren't available. Then when my mother died, he remarried and became even more distant." After her mother died, her father never discussed the death.

Karen told of one incident in her childhood that for her symbolized the essence of being unacknowledged. She was in elementary school and was being chased and taunted by a little boy. She asked for help from the teacher, but the teacher told her not to worry. One day the little boy pushed her down on the playground, and she got a deep cut on her chin. When she went to the teacher, the teacher laughed and told her the little boy just liked her and that was his way of showing her. Karen's mother was called, and Karen was taken to the doctor. The doctor painted a big red Mercurochrome smile on her face, and her mother and the doctor laughed.

Karen married a man who was so involved with his career that he gave her very little attention. He criticized her appearance and what she chose to wear. He had to approve of her clothing purchases or he would not give her money to buy clothes. She married a second time and experienced a similar situation: "Both husbands . . . I kept hearing how much they loved me and yet it is not my definition of love or they're not available." She recounted a situation where as a young married woman she had a cat that had only one kitten. When she was away with her husband, her mother-in-law gave the kitten away without asking her even though the kitten was still nursing. When she became upset about it, her husband defended his mother. She portrayed this event as symbolic of this theme of not being acknowledged or recognized.

Karen went on to describe a recent time in her life after the end of the second marriage. She was being sexually harassed by a supervisor in a company for which she was working. This harassment went on for about 6 months. "He was married to a daughter of one of the founders, and he had a great deal of money." She finally had the courage to report him to her employers, and she was given a new assignment. Later she left the company because of the discomfort she felt.

Karen had read many self-help books and tried many alternative modes of healing, including workshops on energy, music, and color. She was making efforts at integrating exercise and diet changes in her lifestyle. She also was participating in a motherless daughter support group. None of these efforts had helped her in a deep way, but she expressed the feeling that the despair would have been worse if she had not done these things.

Perceptions

In relation to the death of her mother, Karen felt that no one ever recognized the pain she experienced. She brought this topic up in relation to parenting her own adult children. "I lost my mother when I was 19, so I'm real confused with what my role is. This has been a real issue for me. I don't know how an adult child relates to his or her parents." She went on to describe how she experienced parenting: "I do perceive them as draining the life right out of me. I even say that to them. I do feel I don't get very much back. I wish someone would take care of me." Karen recounted the physical tiredness and physical constraints of her life experience.

Karen perceived her situation as spiritual in nature. Her biggest spiritual concern for the future was one of being punished for her involvement with the man who had sexually harassed her in the workplace. "Yes, even though I know there wasn't anything I could do. I understand how it happened and I didn't have any evil with him. Still, I think I participated—being weak or doing something so despicable." Shame was a dominant theme in her life and expressed itself in her feelings about herself and in her dreams. She described herself as invisible during the sexual harassment. "I left my body. I think of the experience just like children do. I felt very much like a child. Who could I tell? Nobody would listen to me. He had all the power. I felt just like a child. The one thing was that he knew me so well. We had known each other for a year before this started. I trusted him." She added, "I think the first person I told did shame me and that was like my worse fear."

During the second session with Karen, I asked her if she could identify any ongoing trend in her life. This was an attempt to reach for the essence of her life experience. She described feeling as if she were being punished and went on to clarify what she meant. "I guess there is a theme—people who should care about me, take care of me, or help me, letting me down or abandoning me—falling short." Karen perceived her life as lonely and lacking any sense of belonging. In this regard, she depicted this as searching for a home. She demonstrated it with the example of her mother's death and her sense of not belonging in her father and stepmother's home and then getting married and hoping to find safety and security with her husbands. "I think I was looking for that place where they have to take you when you come home. Home is where they have to let you come in when you come home. I don't have that." I asked her if it was like shelter, and she said, "If I draw it it's like a cave with a fire." She described the lack of a sense of belonging as an ongoing theme in her life and gave multiple examples from relationships with family members, spouses, and friends.

Expressions

There were multiple expressions of the underlying pattern and wholeness of Karen's life. These included her choices of words and phrases. It also included the tone of her voice; her posture; her reactions and responses to questions; the way she walked; her clothing; her affect; her likes and dislikes; her favorite activities, books, and movies; her behaviors; her personal belongings; and her home and work environments. Three examples of expressions were dreams, stories describing events, and drawings depicting her experiences and perceptions. She spoke about the relevance of her dreams in understanding her situation. "I do pay a lot of attention to my dreams. It's reflected in my dreams of futility, of working for how to accomplish something." Her dreams were filled with painful images of her futile efforts to clean herself or get out of entanglements or mires while surrounded by taunting and laughing groups of people. In one dream, Karen is in a bathtub that is in a room open to viewers. She is filthy and dirty, but the more she tries to clean herself, the more muddy she becomes and the more everyone laughs at her.

In another dream she is at a dance and the room is very cold. Everyone at the dance is wearing warm clothes. She is trying to put on a sweater when somehow her dress is pulled away. In another dream sequence she attempts to make a speech. While preparing her speech, the spiral of her notebook pops open and strikes her in the face. She went in front of the audience with a red, swollen cheek. "The man came in who was going to help me and I was so relieved. I kept trying to turn it over to him, but whatever I did it just wasn't good enough, and I got really distressed about presenting myself to someone who was an expert and then not really following through—winging it. That's sort of how I'm looking at my life when I'm telling you that. I feel like I'm winging it and I should know better, but I don't. Yes, that's sort of how I feel about myself right now."

One of the stories she wrote expressed the experience and perceptions of the event in her childhood where she was harassed and pushed by the little boy. This is an excerpt:

> Well, the little girl was very confused. She felt like she was falling down a deep dark hole, watching the tall teacher, laughing at her as she disappeared. Something was terribly wrong. She was really and truly afraid! She had asked for help but no one was listening. What she thought was frightening, apparently everyone else just thought was funny—very funny. What could she do? Her friends just disappeared and the only adult only laughed. So she convinced herself that she must be mistaken and decided she would just do her best to avoid the mean little boy.
>
> The next day at recess, the little boy seemed to know the teacher wasn't going to do anything to help the little girl, and he ran up to her when she was standing near the merry-go-round and pushed her so that she fell and got a deep cut on her chin. Her worst fears had been realized. Her mother was called and came to take her to the doctor. Certainly now someone would do something about this awful situation.
>
> But instead of comforting her and making plans to punish the mean little boy, the doctor started to laugh too and painted a big red circle on the little girl's face with Mercurochrome. Her mother started to laugh too, and the little girl felt herself falling down that hole again, watching people she loved and trusted laughing at her. Everything seemed topsy turvy and very, very scary. Who could she trust? Where was she really safe? What was the matter with her that she was terrified and everyone else seemed to be enjoying a good joke? Was she so worthless that her fear was laughable? Either they were wrong or she was. And this scared her the most.

Karen had drawn pictures as a child and teenager, but her father had told her to stop because there was no future in being an artist. She used drawings to express her life and supplement a journal that she kept as part of her recovery from the abuse of the sexual harassment experience. She shared her drawings with me. She described what the drawings meant as she displayed them. One image depicted a woman with a big hole in her chest and someone standing on her shoulders. Karen described the picture. "That was me. That was how I was feeling Sunday night. I feel like there is some protection, but I feel so empty. This is my heart. There is promise of good things, but I don't have any way of getting them. I am tired." One image showed her straining to pull herself out of a crack. Another image showed a figure on a hillside with a gleaming and glittering town in the distance. Karen said that this represented her being away from happiness and wanting to reach it but not being able to go that far. Still another image was a figure crouched in a cave with a fire. Karen explained that she was trying to stay warm in her dark spot of life.

Karen also had a drawing of a figure next to a door. She explained,

> And this is pretty much despair. But then it gets better. And here I am and here I come. I'm all shaped up and I'm ready for things to get better. I'm all patched up. I'm trying to find a way out because the doorknob fell off. There is no way out. My only alternative is to bust down this door. I want to go, but it's not possible.

Karen described a series of drawings done when she was going through the problem with the sexual harassment: "[H]ere I am in the comforting arms. But then she walks away and leaves me. I will be dropped at any minute. Here I am in a hollow again. The tip of my iceberg."

In explaining the essence of the drawings, Karen made the following remarks: "Yes, I'd like to feel, what you said, I'd like to feel my life is moving. I guess I'm tired of life . . . like that first drawing was about comforting arms dropping. The universe comes and gives me a hug and then forgets me. I feel forgotten. And I think I said before that we were talking about if Jesus came back and he would say, 'Hi, Richard. How are you? Who's that? Do I know you?'"

Synopsis, Participation, and Transformation

The synopsis, which replaces data analysis in conventional research, occurred in the unitary pattern appreciation process by looking at all facets of the data as a unit. In the beginning of my project I used a form that contained columns for experience, perceptions, and expressions and began looking across these facets for themes. I soon realized that disentangling the information was not necessary and as I read the transcripts and used a synoptic perspective the wholeness and pattern became evident. Synopsis also occurred in the unfolding dialogue that explored Karen's experience along with her perceptions and the ways in which these were expressed in her life. It was very important to acknowledge and honor the spiritual aspects of Karen's life in the process. The story that was written synthesizing the information was the most distinctive source of synopsis in the process.

Participation with Karen happened through setting the stage for the process to be negotiable and responsive to her needs, desires, and concerns. I talked with Karen about creating a partnership for this exploratory journey. Although I asked questions, Karen also asked my opinion, and I often shared my own experiences. There was a higher degree of freedom to share experiences, mutuality, and negotiation than in counseling sessions I had conducted using an interpersonal framework. When I presented the story that I created as Karen's profile, I asked her to consider whether or not it was an accurate representation of her life and to reject it, accept it, or alter it on her own terms. Throughout the entire process, Karen was viewed as the person who had the final decision on our process.

The transformation was experienced during the dialogues, at points of reflection on the process and content, in the creation of the story profile, and when I presented the story to Karen. In most cases, the dialogues led to deeper understanding of the nature of her experience in its fullest sense. She used a strategy that I suggested—to rewrite the endings of dreams. She adapted this strategy to rewrite the endings of actual events that had taken place in her life. These events were ones in which her pain or distress was not acknowledged and she was not supported. She reported that this activity created a greater sense of power that was useful to her in dealing with current life situations.

Story, Metaphor, and Music

After 3 weeks of dialogue I started to create a profile of Karen's pattern. I looked at the information from the transcripts and recalled my own experiences with her during our sessions. During my review of the transcripts I discovered that the most powerful metaphor in the text was the image of being in a cave with a fire, except Karen could not build a fire and often found trouble finding any shelter at all. I thought this image symbolized her life most clearly. The image of the cave and building fires became the source of inspiration for a story that I started writing as the pattern profile that would represent the wholeness of Karen's life. It took me approximately 3 weeks to develop the story. I also decided to include music as a way of conveying the themes within the story.

The story is a dream-like account of the life of a little girl as she grows up and becomes a woman. The girl starts out with a wonderful life with loving parents.

There was once a beautiful child . . . a bright and loving child . . . born into the world and belonging to the world . . . a world of love and of light and wonder . . . of stars and moons and playfulness . . . a world of laughter and joy. The child, a girl, was sheltered and cared for by two loving and adoring parents . . . parents of the universe with wisdom and compassion and with a deep understanding of children and what they needed to grow and blossom.

As the child grew older life became colder and harsher. Her parents became more preoccupied with life and preparing for changes in each season, but her mother had begun to teach the girl to build fires to keep herself warm. One day the child came home and her mother was gone and she never knew what happened. Her father did not want to talk about anything but his work, and he never had time to help the girl cultivate the building of fires. The father saw that she was growing up and thought she should be able to build her own fires.

Her father was working on one of his projects. He was always making things . . . interesting things . . . the girl wanted to know something about this, but she also sensed she could not interfere with her father's work. It was particularly cold that day and she decided to ask her father to build a fire. "Father," she said, "I am so cold. Would you build the fire?" The look in her father's eyes was more chilling than any cold air . . . or icy temperature she had ever felt before. Her father scolded her for asking. "It is time you learned to take care of yourself. You are old enough. If one is cold one finds warmth of his or her own will and action."

Her life after that became a series of attempts to find warmth in caves, to build fires, or to find someone to help her build fires. But after many disappointments she came to realize that there would be no help.

She built her own fires and it was easier this way—even if she was alone. The woman occasionally thought of her mother building fires and she missed that. No one ever built her a fire. They promised, but it never happened. She was alone except for her children. They needed many fires built because life was very cold.

At this point in her life, the woman meets a man who promises to build her fires. He tells her about a new kind of warmth that can be generated by the two of them being together. In the end, she suffers from her trust of this man.

The man taught her that she did not need fires to keep warm . . . he could give her warmth . . . and it would be better than fires . . . and she would not have to give anything in return. The woman wanted to learn about this new warmth . . . she did . . . and she paid a heavy price for this new warmth. The man taught her how they could use each other to stay warm . . . how they could use the heat in their bodies . . . he didn't tell her the price. The price was a dear one . . . she must keep

their warmth a secret . . . and if she told anyone she would suffer. The woman would have said no when she learned the price, but she was afraid of not being warm. You see the man had also found a way to take her fires away from her . . . and when she tried to build a fire there was no warmth.

This is where a song is introduced in the story. It conveys the sense of being trapped after being involved with the sexual harassment. The song is "Paralyzed" by Rosanne Cash. It conveys a sense of hopelessness that then leads to moving beyond the event. In fact, Karen had in her real life finally faced her abuser and brought charges against him. The words convey the story of a woman who is paralyzed by a relationship. It describes her running from the bedroom with her legs paralyzed. She attempts to carve out her future acknowledging that she is both a prophet and blind. She realizes that it is nobody's business and that no one is to blame. She believes that she will meet the man sometime in the future with a new identity. She knows she has lifted the veil and walked through the flames and she will move on.[20]

In the story, after this experience, the woman learns that she has lost her power to build fires and finds herself at the mercy of her destiny. This experience is captured in a song by Nanci Griffith entitled "Southbound Train." This is the story of a woman who is riding a train headed south. She describes herself as staring at the sky and thinking about her childhood while she is holding back her tears. She says that a stranger is sleeping beside her and it feels to her as if she is his wife. It is probably her husband. She notices the towns and cities going by and thinks about them as passing like the pages in the story of her life. Most poignantly, she characterizes her heart as being on the baggage rack, very heavy, and she is yearning for someone to carry it for her. She longs to have someone pay attention to it and to handle it with care, noting that it has been damaged from being dropped and that it needs repair.[21]

As the woman pondered her situation she remembers the power she had as a child and the sense of belonging and she also becomes aware of angels. A song is introduced here, "Calling All Angels," sung by Jane Siberry. This song begins with some beautiful chanting of religious and spiritual incantations leading to the continuous chant of calling all angels. The singer describes her journey as full of tears and hurt and uncertainty. She yearns not to be left alone. She questions her life situation and why it exists. Yet at the same time, she notes the beauty of the sunset and nature, which brings love and intensity into life. The singer appears to have a revelation in understanding as she thinks about the beauty and realizes that even if she could crack the code that would explain her life, she would not give up the pain and suffering that goes with all the beauty. In other words, she knows that she needs to embrace all of life, including the harshness and the loveliness. The song ends with a chant about the features of life and the discovery of the reality of uncertainty.[22]

The last part of the story is about the girl awakening from the dream (the story) as a woman and realizing her own possibilities. This final part of the story was written to convey and portray the sense of hope and the woman's spiritual beliefs that are aspects of her life that keep her moving onward. In this sequence, she discovers a connection to a light and radiance that are sources of warmth. The light also takes the form of the presence of two beings who are guides and sources of support.

> They both spoke simultaneously and said, "Sweet, perfect one . . . you are not alone . . . you belong to the universe . . . just like the stars and the plants and all the creatures. We are here to help you on your journey . . . you can count on us. Never again will you need to search for fires in caves . . . or build fires . . . for we will help you learn to keep the fire in you alive and strong . . . and you will always find warmth in this fire." And the woman knew   she belonged . . . and she would take her own journey and write her own story.

The ending served two purposes: to suggest the possibilities inherent in realizing the wholeness of life and to acknowledge Karen's own power.

Karen was tearful after I presented the story and music. Excerpts from the transcripts that day capture her response: "Wonderful! Thank you. I loved it! The music was just great!" "I think you did a wonderful job! It's so wonderful. I hate for it to end. It's so great to be understood!" "This is such a gift." "This is so much better than being diagnosed." "I was thinking that while you were doing that. You make it so you validate my experience.

That's something I've never had. It's always been wanting to change or what I did wrong. This felt a whole lot more about what went on instead of, 'Oh, Lord. I have to change that now,' or 'If I would only. . . .'" A critical feature of the unitary pattern appreciation process, and also of healing through appreciating wholeness, is a willingness on the part of the scientist/practitioner to let go of expectation about change.

The story that was created represents a pattern profile specific to Karen. Karen was asked to review the story and determine if she thought it reflected her life experience and the underlying pattern of wholeness. One aspect of the participatory nature of pattern appreciation is to collaborate on the creation of the profile so that it represents the perspective of the participant. In some cases, an individual has created his or her own profile. In one case, it was a series of photographs with an essay about the person's philosophy. In other cases, individuals have altered aspects of the story profile to capture more accurately the wholeness of their life pattern. The profile becomes a referent point for considering one's life situation and possibilities for integration and/or change as well as a source for nursing knowledge arising from praxis.

Summary

It is difficult to convey the essence of the praxis of pattern appreciation and to portray the wholeness found in a human life pattern.

The scientist/practitioner is not meant to capture this fully—this praxis is really about seeking to represent the wholeness within pattern as a healing project knowing that, at best, this is a representation of the wholeness and not the wholeness itself. It is my experience that as I reach with another for this representation of wholeness we are led to revelations that far exceed our current clinical diagnostic representations. The process itself—the actual engagements of participatory exploration—serves revelatory awareness as well as the products of the story, the metaphor, and the music.

Healing is the realization, knowledge, and appreciation of the inherent wholeness in life that elucidates prospects of clarified understanding and opportunities for action. The unitary scientist/practitioner seeks knowing the pattern to know wholeness. The appreciation context orients the practitioner/scientist to perceiving, being aware of, and being sensitive to the unique manifestations of wholeness available in human encounters. It challenges him or her to express the full force and delicate distinctions of unitary pattern and its wholeness in representing the human experience. It requires a sympathetic recognition of the excellence of wholeness as experienced in gratefulness, enjoyment, and understanding. The essential features of the process of pattern appreciation are a synoptic stance toward pattern information, a participatory engagement with people in exploration of wholeness, and a transformative process that illuminates the possibilities in wholeness—the embodiment of healing.

References

1. Reinharz S. Feminist Methods in Social Research. New York: Oxford University Press; 1992.

2. Engebretson J. Comparison of nurses and alternative healers. Image J Nurs Schol. 1996;28(2):95–100.

3. Kritek PB. Healing: A central nursing construct—reflections on meaning. In: Kritek PB, ed. Reflections on Healing: A Central Nursing Construct. New York: National League for Nursing; 1997.

4. Rogers ME. Nursing science and the space age. Nurs Sci Q. 1992;5:27–33.

5. Newman MA. Experiencing the whole. ANS. 1997;20(1):34–39.

6. Cowling WR. Unitary case inquiry. Nurs Sci Q. 1998;11:139–141.

7. Cowling WR. Unitary pattern appreciation: The unitary science/practice of reaching for essence. In: Madrid M, ed. Patterns of Rogerian Knowing. New York: National League for Nursing; 1997.

8. Cowling WR. Unitary practice: Revisionary assumptions. In: Parker MS, ed. Nursing Theories in Practice, Vol. 2. New York: National League for Nursing; 1993.

9. Cowling WR. Unitary knowing in nursing practice. Nurs Sci Q. 1993;6:201–207.

10. Wheeler CE, Chinn PL. Peace and Power: A Handbook of Feminist Process. Buffalo, NY: Margaret-Daughters; 1984.

11. Oxford English Dictionary [CD-ROM]. New York: Oxford University Press; 1994.

12. Murphy M. The Future of the Body: Explorations into the Further Evolution of Human Consciousness. San Francisco: Tarcher Press; 1992.

13. Broad CD. Religion, Philosophy and Psychical Research. New York: Harcourt Brace & Company; 1953.

14. Reason P. Three approaches to participative inquiry. In: Denzin NK, Lincoln YS, eds. Handbook of Qualitative Research. Thousand Oaks, CA: Sage; 1994.

15. Cooperrider DL, Srivastva S. Appreciative inquiry in organizational life. Res Organ Change Dev. 1987;1:129–169.

16. Schaef AW. Beyond Therapy, Beyond Science. New York: HarperCollins; 1992.

17. Moss R. The Second Miracle: Intimacy, Spirituality, and Consciousness. Berkeley, CA: Celestial Arts Publishing; 1995.

18. Wilber K. The problem of proof. Revision J Consciousness Change. 1982;5(1):80–100.

19. Monti EJ, Tingen MS. Multiple paradigms of nursing science. ANS. 1999;21(4):64–80.

20. Cash R. Paralyzed. From Interiors [CD]. New York: Columbia Records; 1988.

21. Gold J, performed by Griffith N. Southbound train. From Flyer [CD]. New York: Elektra Entertainment; 1994.

22. Stewart JC. Calling all angels. From When I Was a Boy [CD], performed by Siberry J. Burbank, CA: Reprise Records; 1993.

CHAPTER 13

Thinking Upstream: Nurturing a Conceptual Understanding of the Societal Context of Health Behavior

Patricia G. Butterfield, RN, MS

This chapter addresses the issue of overreliance on theories that define nursing in terms of a one-to-one relationship at the expense of theoretical perspectives that emphasize the societal context of health. When individuals are perceived as the focus of nursing action, the nurse is likely to propose intervention strategies aimed at either changing the behaviors of the individual or modifying the individual's perceptions of the world. When nurses understand the social, political, economic influences that shape the health of a society, they are more likely to recognize social action as a nursing role and work on behalf of populations.

Despite acknowledgment that an understanding of population health is essential in professional nursing, descriptions of one-to-one relationships predominate in the literature read by most nurses. Such portrayals often emphasize the evolution of the relationship between nurse and client with minimal attention to forces outside the relationship that have been paramount in shaping the client's health behaviors. Yet for most people, their cultural heritage, social roles, and economic situations have a far more profound influence on health behaviors than do interactions with any health care professional. Examination of nursing problems from a "think small" perspective[1(p. 504)] fosters inadequate consideration of these social,

---

Source: Butterfield, PG. Thinking upstream: Nurturing a conceptual understanding of the societal context of health behavior. Advances in Nursing Science 1990;12(2): 1–8.

environmental, and political determinants of health. This perspective results not only in a restricted range of intervention possibilities for the nurse, but also in a distorted impression of clients' behaviors. An understanding of the complex social, political, and economic forces that shape people's lives is necessary for nurses to promote health in individuals and groups. If nurses are not given an opportunity to appreciate the gestalt of populations and societies, they will be unable to develop a basis for analyzing problems.

This chapter addresses the issue of overreliance on theories that define nursing primarily in terms of a one-to-one relationship and the inherent conflict between these theories and the goal of enabling nurses to promote health through population-based interventions.

Nursing's Role in Pushing Upstream

In his description of the frustrations of medical practice, McKinlay[2] uses the image of a swiftly flowing river to represent illness. In this analogy, physicians are so caught up in rescuing victims from the river that they have no time to look upstream to see who is pushing their patients into the perilous waters. The author uses this example to demonstrate the ultimate futility of "downstream endeavors,"[2(p. 9)] which are characterized by short-term, individual-based interventions, and he challenges health-care providers to focus more of their energies "upstream, where the real problems lie."[2(p. 9)] Upstream

endeavors focus on modifying economic, political, and environmental factors that have been shown to be the precursors of poor health throughout the world. Although the analogy cites medical practice, it also aptly describes the dilemmas of a considerable portion of nursing practice, and although nursing has a rich historical record of providing preventive and population-based care, the current American health system, which emphasizes episodic and individual-based care, has done woefully little to stem the tide of chronic illness, to which 70 percent of the American population succumbs.

What is the cost of a continued emphasis on a microscopic perspective? How does a theoretical focus on the individual preclude understanding of a larger perspective? Dreher[1] maintains that a conservative scope of practice often uses psychologic theories to explain patterns of health and health care. In this mode of practice, low compliance, broken appointments, and reluctance to participate in care are all attributed to motivation or attitude problems on the part of the client. Nurses are charged with the responsibility of altering client attitudes toward health, rather than altering the system itself, "even though such negative attitudes may well be a realistic appraisal of health care."[1(p. 505)] Greater emphasis is paid to the psychologic symptoms of poor health than to socioeconomic causes; "indeed the symptoms are being taken as its causes."[1(p. 505)] The nurse who views the world from such a perspective does not entertain the possibility of working to alter the system itself or empowering clients to do so.

Involvement in social reform is considered to be within the realm of nursing practice.[3] Dreher[1] acknowledges the historical role of public health nurses in facilitating social change and notes that social involvement and activism are expected of nurses in this area of practice. The American Nurses' Association (ANA) Social Policy Statement delineates, among other social concerns, the "provision for the public health through use of preventive and environmental measures and increased assumption of responsibility by individuals, families, and other groups"[3(p. 4)] and addresses nursing's role in response to those concerns. However, in her review of the document, White[4] notes an incongruence between nursing's social concerns, which clearly transcend individual-based practice, and the description of nursing as "a practice in which interpersonal closeness of the professional kind develops and aids the investigation and discussion of problems, as nurse and patient (or family or group) seek jointly to resolve those concerns."[3(p. 19)] White[4] also notes the document's neglect of the population focus and possibilities for modifying the environment. Clearly, nursing has yet to reconcile many of the differences between operationalization of a population-centered practice and policies that define nursing primarily in terms of individual-focused care.

Three theoretic approaches will be contrasted later here to demonstrate how they may lead the nurse to draw different conclusions not only about the reasons for client behavior, but also about the range of interventions available to the nurse.

The Downstream View: The Individual as the Locus of Change

The health belief model evolved from the premise that the world of the perceiver determines what he or she will do. The social psychologists[5,6] who outlined this model were strongly influenced by Lewin and the view that a person's daily activities are guided by processes of attraction to positive valences and avoidance of negative valences. From these inceptions evolved a model that purports to explain why people do or do not engage in a preventive health action in response to a specific disease threat. The model places the burden of action exclusively on the client; only those clients who have distorted or negative perceptions of the specified disease or recommended health action will fail to act. In practice, this model focuses the nurse's energies on interventions designed to modify the client's distorted perceptions. Although the process of promoting behavior change may be masked under the premise of mutually defined goals, passive acceptance of the nurse's advice is the desired outcome of the relationship.

Although the health belief model was not designed to specify intervention strategies, it can lead the nurse to deduce that client problems can be solved merely by altering the client's belief system. The model addresses the concept of "perceived benefits versus perceived barriers/costs associated with taking a health action."[6(p. 563)] Nurses may easily interpret this situation as a need to modify the client's perceptions of benefits and barriers. For example, clients with problems accessing adequate health care might receive counseling aimed at helping them see these barriers in a new light; the model does not include the possibility that the nurse may become involved in activities that promote equal access to all in need.

True to its historical roots, the model offers an explanation of health behaviors that, in many ways, is similar to a mechanical system. From the health belief model, one easily concludes that compliance can be induced by using model variables as catalysts to stimulate action. For example, an intervention study based on health belief model precepts sought to increase follow-up in hypertensive clients by increasing the clients' awareness of their susceptibility to hypertension and of its danger.[7] Clients received education, over the telephone or in the emergency department, that was designed to increase their perception of the benefits of follow-up. According to these authors, the interventions resulted in a dramatic increase in compliance. However, they noted several client groups that failed to respond to the intervention, most notably a small group of clients who had no available child care. Although this study demonstrates the predictive power of health belief model concepts, it also exemplifies the limitations of the model. The health belief model may be effective in promoting behavioral change through the alteration of clients' perspectives, but it does not acknowledge responsibility for the health-care professional to reduce or ameliorate client barriers.

In fact, some of the proponents of the health belief model readily acknowledge the limitations of the model and caution users against generalizing it beyond the domain of the individual psyche. In their review of 10 years of research with the model, Janz and Becker[8] remind researchers that the model can only account for the variance in health behaviors that is explained by the attitudes and beliefs of an individual. Melnyk's[9] recent review of the concept of barriers reinforces the notion that, because the health belief model is based on subjective perceptions, research that adopts this theoretic basis must take care to include the subjects', rather than the researchers', perceptions of barriers. Janz and Becker[8] address the influence of other factors such as habituation and nonhealth reasons on making positive changes in health behavior, and they acknowledge the influence of environmental and economic factors that prohibit individuals from undertaking a more healthy way of life.

The health belief model is but a prototype for the type of theoretic perspective that has dominated nursing education and thus nursing practice. The model's strength—its narrow scope—is also its limitation: One is not drawn outside it to those forces that shape the characteristics that the model describes.

The Upstream View: Society as the Locus of Change

Milio's Framework for Prevention

Milio's framework for prevention[10] provides a thought-provoking complement to the health belief model and a mechanism for directing attention upstream and examining opportunities for nursing intervention at the population level. Milio moves the focus of attention upstream by pointing out that it is the range of available health choices, rather than the choices made at any one time, that is paramount in shaping the overall health status of a society. She maintains that the range of choices widely available to individuals is shaped, to a large degree, by policy decisions in both governmental and private organizations. Rather than concentrate efforts on imparting information to change patterns of individual behavior, she advocates national-level policy making as the most effective means of favorably affecting the health of most Americans.

Milio[10] proposes that health deficits often result from an imbalance between a population's health needs and its health-sustaining resources, with affluent societies afflicted by the diseases associated with excess (obesity, alcoholism) and the poor afflicted by diseases that result from inadequate or unsafe food, shelter, and water. In this context, the poor in affluent societies may experience the least desirable combination of factors. Milio notes that although socioeconomic realities deprive many Americans of a health-sustaining environment, "cigarettes, sucrose, pollutants, and tensions are readily available to the poor."[10(p. 436)]

The range of health-promoting or health-damaging choices available to individuals is affected by their personal resources and their societal resources. Personal resources include one's awareness, knowledge, and beliefs, including those of one's family and friends, as well as money, time, and the urgency of other priorities. Societal resources are strongly influenced by community and national locale and include the availability and cost of health services, environmental protection, safe shelter, and the penalties or rewards given for failure to select the given options.

Milio notes the fallacy of the commonly held assumption in health education that knowing health-generating behaviors implies acting in accordance with that knowledge, and she cites the lifestyles of health professionals in support of her argument. She proposes that "most human beings, professional or nonprofessional, provider or consumer, make the easiest choices available to them most of the time."[10(p. 435)] Therefore, health-promoting choices must be more readily available and less costly than health-damaging options if individuals are to be healthy and a society is to improve its health status.

The opportunities for a society to make healthy choices have been a central theme throughout Milio's work. In a recent book she elaborated on this theme:

> Personal behavior patterns are not simply "free" choices about "lifestyle," isolated from their personal and economic context. Lifestyles are, rather, patterns of choices made from the alternatives that are available to people according to their socioeconomic circumstances and the ease with which they are able to choose certain ones over others.[11(p. 76)]

Milio is critical of many traditional approaches to health education that emphasize knowledge acquisition and consequently expect behavior change. In addressing the role of public health in primary care, Milio voices concern that "health damage accumulates in societies too, vitiating their vitality . . . [and charges nurses to redirect energies] so as to foster conditions that help people to retain a self-sustaining physiological and social balance."[12(pp.188,189)]

One cannot help but note the similarities between Milio's health resources and the concepts in the health belief model. The health belief model is more comprehensive than Milio's framework in examining the internal dynamics of health decision making. However, Milio offers a different set of insights into the arena of health behaviors by proposing that many low-income individuals are acting within the constraints of their limited resources. Furthermore, she goes beyond the individual focus and addresses changes in the health of populations as a result of shifts in decision making by significant numbers of people within a population.

Critical Social Theory

Just as Milio uses societal awareness as an aid to understanding health behaviors, critical social theory employs similar means to expose social inequities that prohibit people from reaching their full potential. This theoretic approach is based on the belief that life is structured by social meanings that are determined, rather one-sidedly, through social domination.[13] In contrast to the assumptions of analytic empiricism, critical theory maintains that standards of truth are socially determined and that no form of scientific inquiry is value free.[13,15] Proponents of this theoretic approach posit that social discourse that is not distorted from power imbalances will stimulate the evolution of a more rational society. The interests of truth are served only when people are able to voice their beliefs without fear of authority or retribution.[13]

Allen[14] discusses how nursing practice can be enriched by enabling clients to remove the conscious and unconscious constraints in their everyday lives. He states that women and the economically impoverished are especially vulnerable to being labeled by pseudodiseases that are rooted in social formations, such as hysteria and depression. Health care providers often frame such problems only within the context of the individual or, at best, the family. But critical social theory can enable a nurse to reframe such an interpretation to gain an understanding of the historical play of social forces that have limited the choices truly available to the involved parties. Through exploration of the societal forces, traditions, and roles that have created the meanings of health and illness, clients may be freed of the isolation and alienation that accompany individual problem ownership.

At the collective level, Waitzkin asserts that the current emphasis on lifestyle diverts attention from important sources of illness in the capitalist industrial environment; "it also puts the burden of health squarely on the individual rather than seeking collective solutions to health problems."[16(p. 664)] Salmon[17] supports this position by noting that the basic tenets of Western medicine promote the delineation of individual factors of health and illness, while obscuring the exploration of their social and economic roots. He states that critical social theory "can aid in uncovering larger dimensions impacting health that are usually unseen or misrepresented by ideological biases. Thus, the social reality of health conditions can be both understood and changed."[17(p. 75)]

Because the theory holds that each person is responsible for creating social conditions in which all members of society are able to speak freely, the nurse is challenged, as an individual and as a member of the profession, to expose power imbalances that prohibit people from achieving their full potential. Nurses versed in critical theory are equipped to see beyond the perpetuation of status quo ideas and may be able to generate unique ideas that are unencumbered by previous stereotypes.[14]

Other Examples of Upstream Thinking

Recent nursing literature provides several other examples of upstream thinking. In a thought-provoking commentary on an intervention program for middle-aged women experiencing subclinical depression, Davis[18] (cited in Gordon and Ledray) notes a lack of congruence between the study's portrayal of depression as a problem with societal roots and its instruction in coping strategies as the intervention program. While recognizing the merits of the intervention program, she comments that, "if our principal task as progressive nurses is to develop and utilize interventions that will ameliorate these social problems, then the emphasis in nursing education and practice might well be on those social actions that aim to change basic social factors such as ageism and sexism."[18(p. 277)]

Chopoorian[19] takes a different tack, emphasizing the concept of environment and suggesting that nurses develop a consciousness of the social, political, and economic aspects of environment. She maintains that a static portrayal of the environment precludes nurses from acting as advocates for people who lack adequate housing and health care and live in intolerable circumstances. She charges nurses to move beyond a psychosocial conceptualization of the environment into a sociopolitical–economic conceptualization. Through this reconceptualization, nurses will see that human responses to health and illnesses "are related to the structure of the social world, the economic and political policies that govern that structure, and the human, social relationships that are produced by the structure and the policies."[19(p. 46)]

The Need for Alternative Perspectives

The danger of the conservative perspective lies not within its content, but rather in the omission of other, larger theories that enable nurses to view situations from both a microscopic and a macroscopic perspective. In discussing the dilemmas of "studying health behavior as an individual phenomena [sic], rather than in the context of a broader social change phenomena [sic]," Cummings[20(p. 93)] reminds us that the approaches are complementary, and both are necessary to a comprehensive understanding of health promotion. The strengths and utility of each theoretic approach are most clearly revealed through an understanding of alternative approaches.

Nursing needs conceptual foundations that enable its practitioners to understand health problems manifested at community, national, and international levels as well as those at the individual and family levels. The continued bias in favor of individual-focused theories robs nurses of an understanding of the richness and complexity of forces that shape the behavior of populations. The omission of theories that relate nursing to the social context of behavior may leave nurses with a minimal understanding of their responsibilities to facilitate change at this level and without the tools to promote such change in an effective and systematic manner.

Maglacas[21] provides a global perspective on the health conditions of societies throughout the world and draws attention to the gaps in service access between the rich and the poor. She then charges nurses within each society and culture to act in response to the inequities in health within that society. If nurses are to be able to enact change at the societal level, they need to be provided with theoretic frameworks that are consistent with such ends and with theoretic perspectives in which social, economic, and political forces are given equal weight with the interpersonal aspects of nursing. Through these means, nurses gain insight into the social precursors of poor health and restricted opportunities and learn rationales for engaging in social action. By tipping the scales of nursing back toward consideration of theories that address health from a societal perspective, nurses can receive not only a richness of understanding but also the means by which to enact this kind of change.

References

1. Dreher MC. The conflict of conservatism in public health nursing education. Nurs Outlook. 1982;30:504–509.
2. McKinlay JB. A case for refocussing upstream: The political economy of illness. In: Jaco EG, ed. Patients, Physicians, and Illness, 3rd ed. New York: Free Press; 1979:9–25.
3. American Nurses' Association. Nursing: A Social Policy Statement. Kansas City: American Nurses' Association; 1980.
4. White CM. A critique of the ANA social policy statement. Nurs Outlook. 1984;32:328–331.
5. Rosenstock IM. Historical origins of the health belief model. In: Becker MH, ed. The Health Belief Model and Personal Health Behavior. Thorofare, NJ: Charles B. Slack; 1974:1–8.
6. Becker MH, Maiman LA. Models of health-related behavior. In: Mechanic D, ed. Handbook of Health, Health Care, and the Health Professions. New York: Free Press; 1983:539–568.
7. Jones PK, Jones SL, Katz J. Improving follow-up among hypertensive patients using a health belief model intervention. Arch Intern Med. 1987;147:1557–1560.
8. Janz NK, Becker MH. The health belief model: A decade later. Health Educ Q. 1984;11:1–47.

9. Melnyk KM. Barriers: A critical review of recent literature. Nurs Res. 1988;37: 196–201.

10. Milio N. A framework for prevention: Changing health-damaging to health-generating life patterns. Am J Public Health. 1976;66:435–439.

11. Milio N. Promoting Health Through Public Policy. Philadelphia: F.A. Davis; 1981.

12. Milio N. Primary Care and the Public's Health. Lexington, MA: Lexington Books; 1983.

13. Allen D, Diekelmann N, Bennet P. Three paradigms for nursing research. In: Chinn P, ed. Nursing Research Methodology: Issues & Implementation. Rockville, MD: Aspen Publishers; 1986:23–28.

14. Allen DG. Nursing research and social control: Alternate models of science that emphasize understanding and emancipation. Image: The Journal of Nursing Scholarship. 1985;17:58–64.

15. Allen DG. Critical social theory as a model for analyzing ethical issues in family and community health. Fam Commun Health. 1987;10:63–72.

16. Waitzkin H. A Marxist view of health and health care. In: Mechanic D, ed. Handbook of Health, Health Care, and the Health Professions. New York: Free Press; 1983:657–682.

17. Salmon JW. Dilemmas in studying social change versus individual change: Considerations from political economy. In: Duffy ME, Pender NJ, eds. Conceptual Issues in Health Promotion: A Report of Proceedings of a Wingspread Conference. Indianapolis, IN: Sigma Theta Tau; 1987:70–81.

18. Davis AJ. Cited by Gordon VC, Ledray LE. Growth-support intervention for the treatment of depression in women of middle years. West J Nurs Res. 1986; 8:263–283.

19. Chopoorian TJ. Reconceptualizing the environment. In: Moccia P, ed. New Approaches to Theory Development. New York: National League for Nursing; 1986:39–54. Publication 15-1992.

20. Cummings KM. Dilemmas in studying health as an individual phenomenon. In: Duffy ME, Pender NJ, eds. Conceptual Issues in Health Promotion: A Report of Proceedings of a Wingspread Conference. Indianapolis, IN: Sigma Theta Tau; 1987:91–96.

21. Maglacas AM. Health for all: Nursing's role. Nurs Outlook. 1988;36:66–71.

CHAPTER 14

Environmental Paradigms: Moving Toward an Ecocentric Perspective

Dorothy Kleffel, RN, MPH, DNSc

This article examines a taxonomy of three environmental paradigms. The egocentric paradigm is grounded in the person and is based on the assumption that what is good for the individual is good for society. The homocentric paradigm is grounded in society and reflects the utilitarian ethic of the greatest good for the greatest number of people. The ecocentric paradigm is grounded in the cosmos, and the environment is considered whole, living, and interconnected. Historically, nurses have adhered primarily to the egocentric paradigm and to a lesser extent to the homocentric paradigm. However, because the world has become a global community, contemporary nurse scholars are shifting to the ecocentric paradigm.

Key words: *ecocentric, environment, paradigm, philosophy.*

The environmental focus of nursing has traditionally been centered on clients' immediate surroundings in the hospital or other institution, home, or community. This circumscribed environmental worldview of nursing is undergoing change as nurses become aware of the adverse effects of environmental disasters and degradation on human health. Regional catastrophic environmental events like the Bhopal chemical leak, the Chernobyl nuclear disaster, and the Exxon Valdez oil spill have had immediate and lasting consequences. Global dimensions of the decline of the planet's environment include worldwide temperature rise, ozone depletion, destruction of the world's forests, human overpopulation, depleted fish

Source: Kleffel, D. Environmental paradigms: Moving toward an ecocentric perspective. Advances in Nursing Science, 1996;18(4):1–10

populations, soil erosion, worldwide hunger, homelessness, and massive species extinction.[1,2] These are not isolated environmental problems that can be addressed by individual effort; they require the coordinated effort of people across the entire planet. Nurses are beginning to understand the scope of environmental threats that threaten everything that exists, living and nonliving. Nurses' enhanced consciousness of the environment has caused the profession to question its current assumptions about the environmental domain of nursing knowledge.

Nursing scholars are becoming cognizant that the existing environmental paradigm does not provide the knowledge and theoretical base to account for environmental conditions that compromise health promotion and interfere with optimum health. Nurses in general do not understand the interrelations between social, political, and economic structures and the origins of health and illnesses.[3] Nursing theory does not adequately describe the concept of the environment. Almost all nursing research conducted in the domain of environment involves only the immediate milieu of the client, family, or nurse.[4] Nursing's care theories do not allow for nonhuman interchange of care or caring because of their anthropocentricity. Anthropocentrism results in the subjugation of nonhuman nature, which jeopardizes the quality of the physical world and causes other forms of oppression and domination.[5]

These critiques of nursing's environmental assumptions indicate that the profession is experiencing an environmental paradigm shift. A paradigm is the body of values, commitments, beliefs, and knowledge shared by members of a profession. Research guidelines, questions, and methodology emanate from the paradigm. When new knowledge is discovered that no longer fits the paradigm or when the paradigm no longer provides model problems and solutions, an anomaly exists. When anomalies become so numerous and significant that they can no longer be ignored, investigations are initiated by the profession. Theories are explored and rejected until a new paradigm emerges that leads to a new basis for practice.[6]

Contemporary nursing scholars are exploring a variety of new environmental ideas and theories as the profession changes its environmental worldview. To contribute to this dialogue, I examine a taxonomy of three environmental paradigms—egocentric, homocentric, and ecocentric—that summarize the assumptions of Western culture regarding the natural world since the 17th century.[7,8] I propose the inclusion of the ecocentric environmental perspective into a central position in nursing's body of knowledge. This mainstreaming of a global view would encourage and support nurses to act with others in averting worldwide environmental disaster.

Egocentric Approach

The egocentric approach is grounded at the personal level and assumes that what is best for the individual is best for society. It is concerned with liberty, rights, and independent action of the individual. It is the dominant Western worldview. Its philosophical foundation is individualistic and mechanistic and includes the thought of Plato, mainstream Christianity, Descartes, Hegel, George Berkeley, Hobbes, Locke, Adam Smith, Malthus, and Garrett Hardin.[8] The egocentric approach is a mechanistic paradigm and assumes that matter is composed of atomic parts, the whole is equal to the sum of the parts, causation is a matter of external action on inactive parts, quantitative change is more important than qualitative change, and there is dualistic separation of mind–body and matter–spirit.[7] In the egocentric approach, the individual is the focus of change.

Most practicing nurses adhere to the egocentric worldview. Their approach is individualistic. They regard the environment as the immediate surroundings or circumstances of the individual or as an interactional field that individuals adapt to, adjust to, or control.[5] The environment is defined in relation to the individual person rather than in terms of its own essence and intrinsic value.

Because the egocentric approach has been the dominant perspective in the Western world, many nurse theorists incorporated those ideas into their theories. An example of a nurse theorist who adhered to the egocentric paradigm was Roy.[9] She defined the environment as all internal and external conditions, circumstances, and influences surrounding and affecting the development and behavior of individuals and groups. Stimuli emanate from the environment and are categorized as focal (immediately confronting the person), contextual (all other stimuli present), and residual (beliefs and attitudes that impinge on the situation). The purpose of nursing is to enhance the adaptation of the patient to environmental stimuli. Roy[10] believed that the science of nursing focuses on human life processes as the core knowledge to be developed. Roy's theory is considered egocentric because of its emphasis on individual adaptation to the environment and on human beings to the exclusion of the rest of nature.

Egocentrism has been the guiding ethic of private entrepreneurs and corporations whose goal is maximization of profit from the development of natural resources. The egocentric approach is limited because of its assumption that the individual good is the highest good that will ultimately benefit society as a whole and that humans are fundamentally different from other creatures, which they are to dominate and control.[7]

Homocentric Approach

The homocentric approach is the utilitarian ethic and is grounded at the social level.[7,8] Social justice, rather than individual progress, is the key value. Decisions are made based on the common good, which is the greatest good for the largest number of people. Humans are considered stewards and caretakers of the natural world. The philosophical foundations of homocentrism are both materialism and positivism. Its assumptions are that humans have a cultural heritage in addition to their genetic inheritance that results in their being qualitatively different from animals, that the determinants of human affairs are social rather than individual, and that culture is a cumulative progress that can continue indefinitely. All social problems are viewed as ultimately solvable. Exponents of the homocentric approach include John S. Mill and Jeremy Bentham (utilitarian theorists), Barry Commoner (socialist ecology), Karl Marx and Mao Tse Tung (political theorists), and Jørgen Randers and Donella and Dennis Meadows (limits-to-growth theorists).

The body of knowledge derived from epidemiology serves as an information base for the practice of public health nursing. Public health nurses use epidemiology in diagnosing, planning, treating, and evaluating community health problems. The nurse who interacts with individual clients and families uses the information for assessing, planning, intervening, and evaluating at the community level.[11] Epidemiology is considered homocentric because of its emphasis on the health of populations rather than individuals.

In the homocentric view, the environment is the focus of change rather than the individual. The homocentric approach to the environment is basically anthropocentric in that humans are to manage nature for the benefit of humans. The management of nature for the intrinsic benefit of other species is not considered in this paradigm.[7]

Ecocentric Approach

The ecocentric approach is grounded in the cosmos. The whole environment, including inanimate elements such as rocks and minerals, along with animate animals and plants, is assigned intrinsic value. It is rooted in holistic rather than mechanistic metaphysics. It assumes that everything is connected to everything else, that the whole is greater than the sum of its parts, that meaning is dependent on context, that biological and social systems are open, and that humans and nonhumans are one within the same organic system. Exponents of the ecocentric approach include most traditional Eastern systems of thought, traditional Native American philosophies, Thoreau, Gary Snyder, Theodore Rozak, Aldo Leopold, Rachel Carson, Fritjof Capra, deep ecology, the holographic model, and ecofeminism.[7,8]

Within the ecocentric paradigm are four contemporary nursing theorists. Sarter[12] compared the philosophical perspectives of fellow nursing theorists Rogers, Neuman, Watson, and Parse and found common shared holistic themes of process, evolution of consciousness, self-transcendence, open systems, harmony, relativity of space and time, pattern, and holism. Process is the evolutionary change of human consciousness; self-transcendence is the method of the evolution of human consciousness through higher and higher levels toward unity with the universe. Open systems are the dynamic and continuous interactions between the person and the world and are essential for the evolution of human consciousness. Harmony is considered to exist both within the person and between the person and the environment. Space and time are considered nonlinear, relative, and fluid, with the past and future merging into the present. Pattern is information that represents the whole.

Pattern recognition is nursing action that looks for patterns representing the whole rather than parts of the whole. Sarter noted that each of these theorists has been influenced, either directly or indirectly, by Eastern philosophies. She believed that the foundation of a commonly held nursing worldview has been laid.

Watson[13] has continued to develop her ecocentric perspectives, moving toward a unitary–transformative viewpoint. This model has eliminated the subject–object and mind–body duality. It acknowledges unity and integrality between humans and the environment; thus conceptualized, human beings and their worlds are not separated.

Other modern nursing scholars also adhere to the ecocentric paradigm. Schuster[14] advocated for a conscious choice of earth dwelling through self-identification and interconnectedness with all beings, which lead one naturally to care for the world in day-to-day living. It is a way of being in the world that allows for all of creation, not just humans, to emerge.

Kleffel,[15] during a qualitative research study, identified[17] distinguished scholars whose work has addressed broad environmental dimensions related to nursing. All except two explicitly reflected the ecocentric paradigm and perceived the environment to be alive, whole, interconnected, and interacting. These scholars add strength to the idea of the united nursing worldview described by Sarter.[12]

The ecocentric approach has some philosophical difficulties. The central problem is finding a philosophically adequate justification for the intrinsic value of nonhuman nature. In mainstream Western thought, only humans have intrinsic worth, although the rest of nature has instrumental value as a resource for humans. It is not considered wrong to kill the last of a species or use the last mineral if human survival is at stake.[7]

Ecocentrism in the World's Traditions

The egocentric paradigm has been the dominant worldview of most practicing nurses working in hospitals and other health institutions and is ascribed to by the greatest number of nurses in the profession. The homocentric perspective has influenced far fewer nurses, traditionally those practicing in the field of public health nursing, although there are signs of a shifting of the profession toward the homocentric approach in the form of aggregate and population-based nursing.[16] The ecocentric view is only beginning to inform the profession and has not yet achieved significant prominence in nursing scholarship or practice.

Embracing an ecocentric viewpoint has exhilarating potential for transforming nursing scholarship and practice beyond its traditional boundaries. We are now living in a global culture that is united by economic interdependence, international air transportation, and worldwide communications networks. Contemporary environmental degradation and disasters that adversely affect humans have moved into the global arena. Actions stem from worldviews, and the worldview of nursing has been mostly egocentric. Moving to the ecocentric paradigm will encourage nurses to address worldwide environmental problems that affect the health of everything that exists.

Solving global environmental problems will entail international efforts from a variety of disciplines and from many cultures. Such an approach will entail collaborative problem solving by people with differing traditions and cultural backgrounds. To work together, a common global environmental worldview that can incorporate these diverse perspectives is needed. The ecocentric paradigm, which is compatible with elements of Native American traditional ideas, Eastern philosophies, and contemporary Western thought, holds great promise for a unified worldview to which all humans can subscribe.

Native American Tradition

There are difficulties in universalizing the Native American belief system because it comprises so many different cultures. However, some generalizations can be made.[17] The Native American attitude was to regard all entities in the environment as having consciousness, reason, and volition as intense and complete as humans. These entities included the earth itself, the sky, the winds, rocks, streams, trees, insects, birds, and animals. This pervasive spirit in everything was considered a part of the Great Spirit, which fostered the perception of humans and nature as being unified and akin. The Native American's social circle or community included all nonhuman natural entities as well as other humans.

The consequences of the Native American inspirited worldview of nature produced a harmony between them and their environment that restrained their killing of animals and gathering of plants to what was necessary for survival. Although there were occasional examples of destruction of nature during periods of enormous cultural stress, the overall and usual effort was conservation of resources. The Native American cultural traditions were not altruistic; they considered it in their own self-interest to defer to nature, which they believed would withhold its sustenance or actively retaliate if provoked.[17]

Eastern Systems of Thought

Similar themes of a unified, living, conscious, and interacting world are found in almost all Eastern systems of thought. With the exception of Islam, these systems are antihierarchal and anthropocentric. Although Islam maintains that humans are dominant over nature, a view similar to the Judeo–Christian tradition, it instructs its adherents to prevent environmental deterioration because the world is God's creation.[18] Other Eastern philosophies emphasize harmony and balance. All aspects of the environment interact, with the parts being within the whole and the whole being within the parts. Humans are a part of the whole and admonished to live in equilibrium with all other parts of the planet.[19]

Some examples of Eastern thought include the law of Karma of the Advita Vedanta, which binds humans together in continuity with the natural world.[20] The wu wei of Taoism is an awareness that allows one to maximize creative possibilities of oneself as a dimension of the environment.[21] The Chi of Chinese thought is a vital force that is the basic structure of the cosmos and exists in all things. Nature is the result of fusion and merging of vital forces to form the "great harmony."[22]

A popular image for portraying the manner in which things exist is described from the Hua-yen school of Buddhism.[23] From the great god Indra there hangs a marvelous net that stretches out infinitely in all directions. There is a jewel in each eye of the net. Because the net is infinite in dimension, the jewels are infinite in number. When one jewel is selected and carefully looked at, all of the other jewels in the net are reflected. In addition, each of the jewels reflected is also reflecting all of the other jewels, so that an infinite reflecting process occurs.

This image symbolizes the cosmos, in which there is an infinitely repeated interrelationship among all of the members of the cosmos. Thus, the part and the whole are one and the same, for what we identify as a part is merely an abstraction from a unitary whole. There is no part-and-whole duality as in Western thought. This totalistic world is a living body in which each cell derives its life from the other cells and in return gives life to the others.

Western Approaches

The ecocentric environmental themes found in Eastern and traditional Native American worldviews originated in ancient times. Several modern Western ecocentric environmental approaches reflect these ideas.

The science of ecology, along with relativity and quantum theory, is creating a postmodern scientific worldview. This emerging worldview is in congruence with the traditional and indigenous environmental paradigms of preindustrial cultures.[24] Naess criticized traditional ecology (an egocentric approach), which he dubbed "shallow ecology,"[25(p. 95)] as being concerned only with pollution control and resource conservation in the interests of people in developed countries. He argued that there are deeper concerns (hence the phrase "deep ecology," also called "radical environmentalism") that touch on the principles of diversity, complexity, autonomy, decentralization, symbiosis, egalitarianism, and classlessness. Deep ecology derives its essence from some Eastern and Native American ideas as well as from feminism, John Muir, and other naturalist literature.[26]

The modern Gaia hypothesis is reminiscent of the ancient living organic theory. This view of the environment was proposed by Lovelock,[27,28] an atmospheric chemist. Lovelock saw the evolution of the species of living organisms as being so closely coupled with the evolution of their physical and chemical environment that together they constitute a single and indivisible evolutionary process. No clear distinction is made between living and nonliving material. The planet's organisms act together as a unity to regulate the global environment by adjusting the rates at which gases are produced and removed from the atmosphere. Lovelock warned that the earth's ability to self-regulate is affected by natural or human activity, which could force the climate into a new and different stable state that would result in the elimination of all living organisms.

The idea of the planet's stable state in the modern Gaia hypothesis reflects the idea of harmony in ancient Taoist thought. In both notions, the balance of the environment of the planet must be maintained, or ecological disaster will result.

Bohm,[29] a physicist and one of the early pioneers of the holographic model, believed that the universe is organized along holographic principles. Everything in the universe is part of a continuum, a seamless extension of everything else. There are no separate parts, just as a geyser in a fountain is not separated from the water from which it flows. However, the universe is not an undifferentiated mass. Things can have their own unique qualities and still be part of an undivided whole. Similarly, consciousness is present in all matter in various degrees. The universe cannot be divided into living and nonliving things. All things are interconnected; like a hologram, every portion of the universe contains the whole.

There are similarities of imagery between the holographic model and Indra's net. The giant hologram and Indra's net symbolize the cosmos. All parts of the hologram are interconnected; each jewel in Indra's net is connected with every other jewel. The parts of the hologram and each jewel of Indra's net reflect the whole. The whole of the hologram and the whole of Indra's net reflect each part or jewel. Bohm believed that fragmentation is the cause of most present-day problems. Applied to the environment, one portion of the planet cannot be harmed without resulting damage to the entire planet.

Another modern Western ecocentric view is ecofeminism. Ecofeminism is a theory that women and the environment are interconnected as both share and have been subjected to the same patriarchal domination.[30] A failure to understand these connections will result in the continued exploitation of both women and environment at the theory, policy, and practice levels. Ecofeminists recognize the interconnectedness of women and the environment and recognize the necessity of uniting feminism and ecology. However, feminist theory is not environmentally sensitive. Deep ecology and the Gaia hypothesis share themes of unity and wholeness to which ecofeminists can subscribe; however, both are oriented toward a patriarchal culture. Ecofeminists hold the view that the connections between the twin dominations of women and nature require a feminist theory and practice informed by an ecological perspective and an environmentalism informed by a feminist perspective.[31]

Ecofeminism is against domination of all kinds, including ageism, sexism, and the exploitation of nature. It is contextual and relational and includes consideration of nonhuman relationships with each other, humans, and the community. Ecofeminism identifies human nature within the historical context. It is antireductionist and pluralistic, centralizing on diversity of humans and nonhumans, yet affirming that humans are a part of the ecological community. Ecofeminism provides a central place for values that are typically underrepresented or ignored in our society such as care, love, friendship, and appropriate trust. Ecofeminism views theory building, objectivity, and knowledge as historically and contextually situated and as changing over time.[31,32]

Implementing the Ecocentric Paradigm

Understanding that the environment is alive, whole, interconnected, and interacting and that humans are one with the environment will encourage nurses to practice in an environmentally sensitive manner in whatever setting they work. Nurses working in local settings will understand the relationships between organizational resource use and the worldwide environment. Using the adage "think globally, act locally," they will act within their sphere by doing such things as calling for institutional audits of their work environment, taking client environmental histories, counseling clients regarding the effects of ozone depletion on the incidence of skin cancers and cataracts, reducing the use of toxic materials, purchasing recycled materials and supplies, using products with environmentally friendly packaging, saving water, managing waste safely, using both sides of the paper when copying reports and forms, using reusable products, reducing the use of disposable items, buying rechargeable batteries,[33] and questioning animal experimentation.[34]

Moving to the ecocentric paradigm will mean extending the concept of the nursing client to include the planetary environment.

Some nurses will choose to work in the global environmental arena and address international environmental causes of illnesses. For instance, the alarming increase of breast cancer worldwide is an area where nurses could make a difference. In the United States, the risk of breast cancer has increased from 1 in 20 in 1960 to 1 in 8 today. Other industrial countries have similar rates. The incidence in developing countries is also rising, but at a slower rate. Risk factors and lifestyle account for only 20% to 30% of breast cancer cases. Some experts believe that pollutants and chemicals that duplicate or interfere with the effects of estrogen are a possible cause. They point to the fact that in Israel, breast cancer mortality in premenopausal women declined by 30 percent following regulations to reduce levels of DDT and carcinogenic pesticides in dietary fat.[35] Other experts believe that low-level radiation and synthetic chemicals such as chlorines are responsible for the increase in breast cancer in women.[36]

Mainstream medicine and science have ignored the possible environmental causes of breast cancer, focusing on the identification of women with risk factors, early case finding through breast self-examination, routine mammograms, and changing lifestyles (smoking cessation, exercise, and lowering dietary fat intake). In contrast, groups like the Women's Environment and Development Organization and Greenpeace are advocating for public attention to the possible links between the environment and breast cancer.[37] Nurses have followed medicine's lead by emphasizing compliance with breast self-examination, counseling women with risk factors associated with breast cancer, and providing education regarding healthy lifestyles. However, they have not directed their attention toward the relationships between breast cancer and the environment, which are being ignored by most research organizations. Using a global, multidisciplinary perspective, nurses could network with other researchers throughout the world to coordinate investigative efforts to identify environmental causes of breast cancer.

Emerging strains of recurring infectious diseases is another area where nurses could make a difference. AIDS, Lyme disease, the Hanta virus, the deadly Ebola virus, the recurrence of plague in India, and the increases in cholera, tuberculosis, and malaria worldwide are examples of conditions related to environmental alterations, climate changes, rapid international travel, and other human activity.[38] Although these diseases are causing illnesses and the deaths of millions of people, nurses generally do not regard scholarship or action in this arena as part of their domain. It is predicted that the epidemics will get worse as the displacement of wild populations and their habitats caused by development activities continue. International multidisciplinary efforts are required to keep ecosystems intact, minimize habitat alterations, require planners to prepare for unanticipated consequences of development, and establish a reliable global surveillance system. Acting internationally in concert with other nurses, other disciplines, and other organizations, nurses could, if they had a global vision, bring their unique skills and perspectives to addressing this type of global environmental phenomenon.

Moving toward an ecocentric perspective will give nurses a common worldview, already held by a great proportion of the world's peoples, of oneness with a living planet, harmony, balance, interconnectedness, and transcendence. It will empower nurses to move beyond their present domain boundaries to align their efforts with other disciplines and organizations worldwide to address the devastating environmental problems affecting the earth and threatening all of existence.

References

1. Brown LR, Flavin, French H. State of the World 1995: A Worldwatch Institute Report on Progress Toward a Sustainable Society. New York: Norton; 1995.
2. Brown LR, Nicholas L, Kane H. Vital Signs 1995: The Trends That Are Shaping Our Future. New York: Norton; 1995.
3. Chopoorian TJ. Reconceptualizing the environment. In: Moccia P, ed. New Approaches to Theory Development. New York: National League for Nursing; 1986.
4. Kleffel D. Rethinking the environment as a domain of nursing knowledge. ANS. 1991;14(1):40–51.
5. Schuster EA. Earth caring. ANS. 1990;13(1):25–30.
6. Kuhn TS. The Structure of Scientific Revolutions. Chicago: University of Chicago; 1970.
7. Merchant C. Environmental ethics and political conflict: A view from California. Environ Ethics. 1990;12(1):45–68.

8. Miller AS. Gaia Connections: An Introduction to Ecology, Ecoethics, and Economics. Savage, MD: Rowman & Littlefield; 1991.

9. Roy C. Roy's adaptation model. In: Parse R, ed. Nursing Science: Major Paradigms, Theories, and Critiques. Philadelphia: W.B. Saunders; 1987.

10. Roy C. An explication of the philosophical assumptions of the Roy Adaptation Model. Nurs Sci Q. 1988;1(1):26–34.

11. Shortridge L, Valanis B. The epidemiological model applied in community health nursing. In: Stanhope M, Lancaster J., eds. Community Health Nursing: Process and Practice for Promoting Health, 3rd ed. Chicago: Mosby/YearBook; 1992.

12. Sarter B. Philosophical sources of nursing theory. Nurs Sci Q. 1988;1(2):52–59.

13. Watson J. Nursing's caring–healing paradigm as exemplar for alternative medicine? Altern Therapies. 1995;1(3):64–69.

14. Schuster EA. Earth dwelling. Holistic Nurs Pract. 1992;6(4):1–9.

15. Kleffel D. The Environment: Alive, Whole, Interacting, and Interconnected. San Diego: University of California, San Diego; 1994. Dissertation.

16. Moccia P. A Vision for Nursing Education. New York: National League for Nursing; 1993.

17. Callicott JB. Traditional American Indian and Western European attitudes toward nature: An overview. Environ Ethics. 1982;4(4):293–318.

18. Zaidi IH. On the ethics of man's interaction with the environment: An Islamic approach. Environ Ethics. 1981;2(1):35–47.

19. Callicott JB. Toward a global environmental ethic. In: Tucker ME, Grim JA, eds. Worldviews and Ecology: Religion, Philosophy, and the Environment. Maryknoll, NY: Orbis Books; 1994.

20. Deutsch E. A metaphysical grounding for natural reverence: East-West. Environ Ethics. 1986;8(4):283–299.

21. Ames RT. Taoism and the nature of nature. Environ Ethics. 1986;8(4):317–350.

22. Wei-Ming T. The continuity of being: Chinese visions of nature. In Callicott JB, Ames RT, eds. Nature in Asian Traditions of Thought: Essays in Environmental Philosophy. New York: State University of New York Press; 1989.

23. Cook FH. The jewel net of Indra. In: Callicott JB, Ames RT, eds. Nature in Asian Traditions of Thought: Essays in Environmental Philosophy. New York: State University of New York Press; 1989.

24. Callicott JB. Earth's Insights: A Survey of Ecological Ethics from the Mediterranean Basin to the Australian Outback. Los Angeles: University of California Press; 1994.

25. Naess A. The shallow and the deep, long-range ecology movement: A summary. Inquiry. 1973;16:95–100.

26. Devall B, Sessions G. Deep Ecology. Salt Lake, UT: Perigrine Smith; 1985.

27. Lovelock J. Gaia: A New Look at Life on Earth. New York: Oxford University Press; 1979.

28. Lovelock J. The Ages of Gaia: A Biography of Our Living Earth. New York: Norton; 1988.

29. Bohm D. Wholeness and the Implicate Order. London, UK: Routledge & Kegan Paul; 1980.

30. Cheney J. Ecofeminism and deep ecology. Environ Ethics. 1987;9(2):115–144.

31. Warren KJ. Feminism and ecology: Making connections. Environ Ethics. 1987;9(1):3–20.

32. Warren KJ, Cheney J. Ecological feminism and ecosystem ecology. Hypatia. 1991;6(1):179–197.

33. Shaner H. Environmentally responsible clinical practice. In: Schuster EA, Brown CL, eds. Exploring Our Environmental Connections. New York: National League for Nursing Press; 1994.

34. Todd B. An ecofeminist look at animal research. In: Schuster EA, Brown CL, eds. Exploring Our Environmental Connections. New York: National League for Nursing Press; 1994.

35. Platt A. Breast and prostate cancer rising. In: Vital Signs 1995: The Trends That Are Shaping Our Future. New York: Norton; 1995.

36. Women's Environment and Development Organization. Does the breast cancer epidemic have environmental links? News & Views. 1992;6(1): 1,9.

37. Women's Environment and Development Organization. Women's coalitions battle breast cancer and other environmental health problems. News & Views. 1995;8(1–2):2.

38. Platt A. The resurgence of infectious diseases. World Watch: Working for a Sustainable Future. 1995;8(4):26–32.

CHAPTER 15

Nursing Science: The Transformation of Practice

Rosemarie Rizzo Parse, RN, PhD, FAAN

World-wide transformations in nursing practice are evolving as more nurses are embracing extant nursing theories and frameworks in order to fortify their unique contributions to the healthcare system. This article specifies the importance of and the ethical considerations arising when using nursing knowledge from within the school of thought of the discipline to guide practice.

The ideas set forth are in stark contrast to the general nursing process with its medical model-driven diagnostic systems now proliferating in nursing practice in the global healthcare community. Both challenges and opportunities are present in the transformation of practice to a nursing knowledge base.

Introduction

Transformations are evolutionary; they are gradual and incremental. The word transformation comes from the Latin transformation (Oxford English Dictionary, 1986), which means to change or metamorphose in the structure and form of something familiar. Form refers to the distinguishing characteristics that shape something, and structure refers to the whole configuration of relationships in a system. Nursing has begun to transform from traditional medical science-based practice, where nursing is considered an applied science, to nursing as

Source: Parse R.R. (1999). Nursing science: The transformation of practice. Journal of Advanced Nursing, 30(6), 1383–1387. Reprinted with permission of Blackwell Science Ltd.

a basic science practice. Thus, it is changing in structure and form.

The structure of nursing world-wide has been and for the most part still is connected closely to and is in fact under the purview of medicine (Parse, 1981, 1993, 1994). Although nursing is growing in stature as a unique basic-science discipline, the medical-model applied-science nursing still predominates in practice. This takes the form of a mechanistic approach to humans as biopsycho–social–spiritual beings who can be fixed through diagnostic and intervention methods that objectify the human being. The structure of this practice focuses on the nurse as an expert in guiding people on what is best for their healthcare. The form of the practice is through the general nursing process (assess, diagnose, plan, implement, and evaluate).

This diagnostic process is reductionistic; it places on human beings labels that arise from objective judgments by nurses. Health-promoting actions are often taken by nurses based on the labels rather than on individual descriptions given by the persons themselves. The configuration of relationships revolves around clearly defined tasks embedded in a view that posits nursing as an applied science, one that combines physiology, psychology, sociology, and other sciences but has no specific knowledge base of its own (Parse, 1987; Cody, 1994b). In other words, nursing knowledge is a collection of ideas from other sciences (Huch, 1988, 1995). How can this be so, when nursing knowledge is, in fact, specified in the extant theories and frameworks?

Some nurse authors (Rogers, 1970; Parse, 1981, 1998; Phillips, 1996) take issue with this traditional stance of nursing as an applied science and posit nursing as a basic science embracing a unified body of knowledge with the human–universe–health process as the phenomenon of concern to the discipline. The notion of basic-science nursing as a guide to practice is a relatively new one, and the impetus to embrace it is now unfolding in light of the global healthcare reformation (Parse, 1987, 1992; Paplau, 1987). The unsettledness in health care delivery systems provides nurses with opportunities to fortify their unique contributions to the healthcare of society by deliberately and explicitly continuing to transform nursing practice. This transformation or metamorphosis happens through the use of nursing knowledge based on a unitary perspective of the human being (Parse, 1995, 1998; Rogers, 1994).

Basic-science nursing in the simultaneity paradigm has two schools of thought: the human becoming school (Parse, 1987, 1997b, 1998) and the science of unitary human beings (Rogers, 1970). This paradigm espouses the belief that the human is unitary in mutual process with the universe and that health is a process and a set of values (Parse, 1981, 1998; Rogers, 1994). The notions of unitary, mutual process, and health as a process are unique and different from traditional applied-science nursing beliefs (Parse, 1995, 1997a). Unitary refers to the human as whole, recognized through patterns, whereas the notion of biopsycho–social– spiritual refers to an applied-science view based on a separation of the biological, psychological, sociological, and spiritual parts of the human being (Parse, 1987, 1992).

The focus of this article, the human becoming school of thought (Cody, 1994a; Parse, 1997a, 1997b, 1998) within the simultaneity paradigm, has an ontology and methodologies. The ontology contains philosophical assumptions and the principles. The principles (described in detail in Parse, 1981, 1998), often referred to as the theory (Parse, 1998, p. 34), follow:

1. Structuring meaning multidimensionally is co-creating reality through the languaging of valuing and imaging.
2. Co-creating rhythmical patterns of relating is living the paradoxical unity of revealing–concealing and enabling–limiting while connecting–separating.
3. Cotranscending with the possibles is powering unique ways of originating in the process of transforming.

The methodologies are the research and practice processes congruent with the ontology. The phenomena for research with this method are universal lived experiences of health surfacing in the human–universe process reflecting being–becoming, value priorities, and quality of life, such as joy–sorrow, grieving, persisting while wanting to change, and hope. The findings are structures of the remembered, the now-moment, and the not-yet, all-at-once. The structures are the lived experiences as described by participants, and these structures enhance understanding of human becoming (Parse, 1987, 1997a, 1999). The understandings gained from research expand the knowledge that nurses use in practice.

With the human becoming principles (Parse, 1981, 1992, 1995) as a guide to practice, nurses are with persons as they enhance their own quality of life. Nurses do not focus only on persons who are ill, as is often the case with the practice of traditional nursing (Cody, 1994b; Parse, 1997a). The structure of human becoming nursing occurs within nurse-person and nurse-group configurations. Nurse–group situations may be with families or communities (Parse, 1987, 1996). Family refers to those persons with whom one is closely connected, not just nuclear family members, as is usually the case in traditional nursing (Parse, 1981).

Community refers to the universe, the galaxy of human connectedness present through face-to-face engagement, reading of printed material, use of telecommunication networks, and through imaginings with people, ideas, objects, and situations (Parse, 1996). Again, community here is defined differently than in applied-science nursing. The nurse may participate with person, family, and community for a variety of reasons arising from the specific desires of the persons in the situation. The participation of the nurse is not guided by traditional societal norms. The setting may be a home, hospital, hospice, day care center or health center, in the context of telephone conversation or computer e-mail, and wherever else persons and nurses meet.

If documentation is required as part of the structure in the specific setting where nurses and persons meet, the reporting includes the person's descriptions of their experiences, the situations from their views, and the hopes, dreams, and intents related to what is most important to them at the moment. This type of documentation is quite different from standard assessment forms that usually focus on the illness process rather than the meaning of the situation from the person's own view. The person's meanings of situations are shown in the descriptions. For example, the person's own words are used to provide a health description. Emerging paradoxical patterns of preference in living health are apparent in the descriptions and may be documented by the person and nurse. Activities and plans may also be documented but always from the persons', families', or communities' perspectives.

The form of nursing in the transformational practice guided by the human becoming principles is true presence: a non-routinized way of being with others that honors the others' views and choices on changing health patterns and quality of life (Parse, 1995, 1996, 1997a). Honoring the person's views means abiding by their wishes and not forcing a standardized plan of care on them (Parse, 1981, 1987, 1992). True presence is lived by nurses whose beliefs are consistent with the principles of human becoming—that is, persons know the way and choose their health situation and their quality of life (Parse, 1990). True presence arises in the living of the principles as the nurse is with person, family, or community. To be in true presence, the nurse centers and prepares to attend to the other through the process of coming-to-be-present, gentling down, and lifting up to focus on others as they illuminate

meaning, synchronize rhythms, and mobilize transcendence (Parse, 1990). The nurse readies himself or herself to be available to the other without judging or intending to label the other. The nurse is available to be with the person as the person changes his or her health patterns. This is very different from the traditional practice of nursing where the nurse as an expert on health informs persons what to do to achieve certain health norms. The dimensions and processes of the practice methodology in the human becoming school of thought (Parse, 1998, pp. 69–70) are as follows:

- Illuminating meaning is explicating what was, is, and will be. Explicating is making clear what is appearing now through languaging.
- Synchronizing rhythms is dwelling with the pitch, yaw, and roll of the human–universe process. Dwelling with is immersing with the flow of connecting–separating.
- Mobilizing transcendence is moving beyond the meaning moment with what is not-yet. Moving beyond is propelling with envisioned possibles of transforming.

This means that the nurse in true presence goes along with persons as they make choices about changing health priorities (illuminating meaning, synchronizing rhythms, and mobilizing transcendence). In illuminating meaning, synchronizing rhythms and mobilizing transcendence, persons share only what they wish with the nurse, and the nurse respects what is said as the persons' structured reality. No effort is made by the nurse to tell persons what to do—but the nurse does listen carefully and answers questions and refers persons to other healthcare providers when appropriate. Health teaching is not a predetermined process where all persons receive the same information, as it often is in traditional nursing practice. Rather, the teaching arises as persons indicate readiness to learn by asking questions or indicating curiosity about something of importance to them. In human becoming practice, there are no standardized teaching plans such as those in traditional practice (for example the plans for persons with diabetes or heart disease).

Clearly, nursing practice takes on a unique identity when guided by the human becoming theory, which specifies for those within and without the discipline how nurses contribute to healthcare delivery in a way different from professionals in other disciplines (Parse, 1993). There is not effort to emulate medicine; nursing is a unique discipline when lived from a human becoming perspective. For example, the nurse does not place a diagnostic label on the person as physicians do. The uniqueness lies in what nurses know; what nurses know about human beings and health always guides what they do. The activities of nurses reflect their belief systems, and if these are in concert with human becoming theory, then nursing as a basic science and performing art is recognized, as other disciplines are, by its unique knowledge base. In this case, the unique knowledge is the belief system that encompasses views of humans as

unitary and health as a continuously changing process chosen by the person.

It is logical to conclude, then, that if unique nursing knowledge really guides research and practice, the practice modalities must flow from the ontology of the schools of thought and cannot be the general nursing diagnostic system which is commonly known as the nursing process (assessing, diagnosing, planning, implementing, and evaluating). The nursing diagnostic system was a useful way to organize practice in the 1950s and 1960s when nurses had not yet specified the knowledge base of nursing, but it is not acceptable in the 21st century to utilize an outmoded system that is based on medical rather than nursing science. There are a number of nursing diagnostic systems that are offspring of the North American Nursing Diagnostic Association system vying for attention in the global nursing community. In fact, there are not only computerized nursing diagnoses but also intervention strategies and expected outcomes now prescribed and tested that further categorize people as objects. These systems did not arise from the schools of thought within the discipline but have been modeled after medicine's diagnostic system and do not support the advancement of nursing science-based practice (Barrett, 1993; Hall, 1996; Parse, 1987). The nursing diagnostic systems tend to be reductionistic and dehumanizing (Parse, 1992, 1995; Taylor, 1988).

Yet, some nurses say they wish to be eclectic and use the diagnostic system and whatever general or nursing theory seems most appropriate for the situation. This belies the whole notion of nursing knowledge-based practice. To say that nursing frameworks or theories can be used whenever the appropriate occasion arises relegates nursing knowledge to someplace outside the nurse as person. For example, following the person's perspective only when it is convenient and making demands toward a goal emanating from the nurse on other occasions mixes paradigms and confuses the person receiving nursing care.

Nurses as unitary beings live their beliefs about the human–universe–health process, and therein lies the knowledge upon which they practice. Nursing knowledge-based practice is not something "I put on." It shows itself in "what I am" to the other. The performing art of nursing is based on its science and is the explicit and tacit articulation of beliefs about the human–universe–health process. What one believes about human beings and health permeates one's actions consistently; thus, the human becoming nurse lives a different practice from nurses who believe in other views of humans and health. Eclecticism in nursing practice is scientifically unsound, serves to foster confusion, and undermines the notion of nursing as a discipline with its own knowledge base, as well as raising some issues for ethical consideration.

Ethical Considerations

What responsibility do nurses have to practice within a school of thought of the discipline? If nursing is indeed a discipline focusing on the human–universe–health process with its own unique body of knowledge concerning health services for people, then do not nurses have an ethical responsibility to offer the services guided by that knowledge? Should not nursing practice be governed by the principles of the extant theories and frameworks in the discipline instead of by procedures or diagnoses emanating from medical science? Conversely, if nursing does not have a unique knowledge base, is it a discipline, and should doctor of philosophy degrees in nursing continue to be granted? Or should the substantive content of nursing remain primarily with medical science and nurses practice from a medical-model base as assistants to physicians?

If the body of knowledge guiding the nurse is the human becoming school of thought, then the ethical responsibility flows from the values that constitute the ethic of that belief system. These values flow from the ontology; thus, the performing art of nursing brings to life the ethic of this school of thought. For example, a fundamental belief in the human becoming theory is that humans choose health in mutual process with the universe, consistent with their own value priorities, and only they can change their patterns of health as their values change (Parse, 1990, 1997a). The inherent ethic here requires that the person's value priorities be respected. The human becoming nurse, then, would not label, diagnose, plan care for, make judgments about, or exert pressure to change a person's way of living, as is often true with other guides to nursing practice. Thus, the ethic embedded in the ontology of the human becoming school of thought is lived out in the nurse's practice. This way of nursing practice is an alternative to the traditional one.

Challenges and Opportunities

Living basic-science nursing from a human becoming perspective is a weighty challenge with opportunities. The challenge arises in two main areas: (a) the human becoming school of thought requires a shift in belief systems from traditional applied science-based nursing to basic science-based nursing and gaining this knowledge requires the nurse's desire, time, and effort; and (b) the healthcare settings are often not prepared for this unique nursing practice but continue to foster the notion of nursing as part of medical science rather than nursing as a unique discipline guided by extant nursing theories and frameworks. Nurses with the desire are willing to take the time and effort to learn a different way to enhance human quality of life, and some of these nurses have conducted research studies with the human becoming perspective as a guide to practice (Jonas, 1995; Mitchell, 1995; Santopinto & Smith, 1995). These evaluation studies have shown that human becoming is a viable mode of practice.

Nurses, persons, families, and other healthcare providers state that they are more satisfied with human becoming nursing care, and these findings are substantiated in the published works of several nurses whose practice is guided by the human becoming theory (Mitchell & Pilkington, 1990; Quiquero et al., 1991; Rasmusson et al., 1991). For example,

in the research studies on human becoming practice (Jonas, 1995; Mitchell, 1995; Santopinto & Smith, 1995) persons and their families remarked that they felt listened to and respected (which they had not felt before); human becoming nurses did not tell people what they had to do but, rather, discussed with them what their own desires and goals were regarding health. They were not labeled with diagnoses or forced to follow a preplanned regime, but rather, their own desires were honored (Quiquero et al., 1991; Rasmusson et al., 1991). The persons in the research studies recognized the differences between human becoming nursing practice and traditional practice (Jonas, 1995; Mitchell, 1995; Santopinto & Smith, 1995). Thus, evidence from research shows that the nontraditional practice of human becoming is successful. Although this is remarkable, further research must be done to illustrate more clearly the value of human becoming nursing practice.

Nurses must also assume responsibility to educate healthcare systems about the meaning of a practice based on human becoming views. The opportunities involved in guiding nursing practice from a human becoming perspective are afforded to nursing, nurses, and humankind. Through practice guided by the human becoming school of thought, nursing is enhanced and can be recognized as a discipline with a unique knowledge base. This fortifies nursing's position in university and healthcare settings. Nurses have opportunities to contribute uniquely to the health of humankind by focusing on quality of life from the person's, family's, and community's perspectives. People are afforded the opportunity to be treated with dignity by having their values respected without judgment by others.

Recommendations

The transformation of nursing requires a true metamorphosis underpinned with the commitment of nurses throughout the world to practice differently and conduct research to ensure that the practice of nursing serves people in a unique way. The possibilities are unlimited when basic-science nursing guides the practice, as the form and structure will change for the betterment of humankind. The metamorphosis of nursing resides with nurses who accept the responsibility to learn and live basic-science nursing practice so that it blossoms and grows in the 21st century and beyond.

References

Barrett, E. A. M. (1993). Nursing centers without nursing frameworks: What's wrong with this picture? Nursing Science Quarterly, 6, 115–117.

Cody, W. K. (1994a). The language of nursing science: If now when? Nursing Science Quarterly, 7, 98–100.

Cody, W. K. (1994b). Nursing theory-guided practice: What it is and what it is not. Nursing Science Quarterly, 7, 144–146.

Hall, B. A. (1996). The psychiatric model: A critical analysis of its undermining effects on nursing in chronic mental illness. Advances in Nursing Science, 8, 16–26.

Huch, M. H. (1988). Theory-based practice: Structuring nursing care. Nursing Science Quarterly, 1, 6–7.

Huch, M. H. (1995). Nursing science as a basis for advanced practice. Nursing Science Quarterly, 8, 607.

Jonas, C. M. (1995). Evaluation of the human becoming theory in family practice. In Illuminations: The Human Becoming Theory in Practice and Research (Parse, R. R., ed.). New York: National League for Nursing Press, pp. 347–366.

Mitchell, G. J. (1995). Evaluation of the human becoming theory in practice in acute care setting. In Illuminations: The Human Becoming Theory in Practice and Research (Parse, R. R., ed.). New York: National League for Nursing Press, pp. 367–399.

Mitchell, G. J., & Pilkington, B. (1990). Theoretical approaches in nursing: A comparison of Roy and Parse. Nursing Science Quarterly, 3, 81–87.

Oxford English Dictionary. (1986). Oxford: Oxford University Press.

Paplau, H. E. (1987). Nursing science: A historical perspective. In Nursing Science: Major Paradigms, Theories, and Critiques (Parse, R. R., ed.). New York: Saunders, pp. 13–29.

Parse, R. R. (1981). Man-Living Health: A Theory of Nursing. New York: Wiley.

Parse, R. R. (1987). Nursing Science: Major Paradigms, Theories and Critiques. Philadelphia: Saunders.

Parse, R. R. (1990). Health: A personal commitment. Nursing Science Quarterly, 3, 136–140.

Parse, R. R. (1992). Human becoming: Parse's theory of nursing. Nursing Science Quarterly, 5, 35–42.

Parse, R. R. (1993). Nursing and medicine: Two different disciplines. Nursing Science Quarterly, 6, 109.

Parse, R. R. (1994). Charley Potatoes or mashed potatoes? Nursing Science Quarterly, 7, 97.

Parse, R. R. (1995). Illuminations: The Human Becoming Theory in Practice and Research. New York: National League for Nursing Press.

Parse, R. R. (1996). Community: A human becoming perspective. Illuminations: The Newsletter of the International Consortium of Parse Scholars 5, 1–4.

Parse, R. R. (1997a). The human becoming theory: The was, is, and will be. Nursing Science Quarterly, 10, 32–38.

Parse, R. R. (1997b). The language of nursing knowledge: Saying what we mean. In The Language of Theory and Metatheory (Fawcett, J., & King, I. M., eds.). Indianapolis, Indiana: Sigma Theta Tau Monograph, pp. 73–77.

Parse, R. R. (1998). The Human Becoming School of Thought: A Perspective for Nurses and Other Health Professionals. Thousand Oaks, CA: Sage.

Parse, R. R. (1999). Hope: An International Human Becoming Perspective. Sudbury, MA: Jones and Bartlett.

Phillips, J. R. (1996). What constitutes nursing science? Nursing Science Quarterly, 9, 48–49.

Quiquero, A., Knights, D., & Meo, O. (1991). Theory as a guide to practice: Staff nurses choose Parse's theory. Canadian Journal of Nursing Administration, 4(1), 14–16.

Rasmusson, D., Jonas, C. M., & Mitchell, G. J. (1991). The eye of the beholder: Parse's theory with homeless individuals. Clinical Nurse Specialist, 5(3), 139–143.

Rogers, M. E. (1970). An Introduction to the Theoretical Basis of Nursing. Philadelphia: Davis.

Rogers, M. E. (1994). The science of unitary human beings: Current perspectives. Nursing Science Quarterly, 7, 33–35.

Santopinto, M. D. A., & Smith, M. C. (1995). Evaluation of the human becoming theory in practice with adults and children. In Illuminations: The Human Becoming Theory in Practice and Research (Parse, R. R., ed.). New York: National League for Nursing Press, pp. 309–346.

Taylor, S. C. (1988). Nursing theory and nursing process: Orem's theory in practice. Nursing Science Quarterly, 1, 111–119.

CHAPTER 16

A Dialectical Examination of Nursing Art

Joy L. Johnson, RN, PhD

Literature relevant to the art of nursing is immensely diverse and fragmented. This state is problematic in that progress in understanding nursing art cannot be made until the subject of nursing art is clearly delineated. In light of the need for conceptual clarity regarding nursing art, a dialectical study was undertaken to identify the distinct conceptions of nursing art that are represented in the nursing literature. The examined discourse was that contained in the works of 41 nursing scholars published between 1860 and 1992. The analysis revealed five distinct conceptualizations that can be identified as the art of (1) grasping meaning in patient encounters, (2) establishing a meaningful connection with the patient, (3) skillfully performing nursing activities, (4) rationally determining an appropriate course of nursing action, and (5) morally conducting one's nursing practice.

It is often said that nursing is an art and a science. Unfortunately, what is meant by the term nursing art is not well delineated or understood. In examining the theoretical issues nurses have concerned themselves with, it is clear that the majority of time and effort has been spent considering the nature of nursing science. Although numerous descriptions and definitions of nursing art have been suggested, little effort has been expended to analyze those definitions or to enter into a dialogue regarding the nature of nursing art.

Science alone will not solve all of the problems of nursing. Nursing is, after all, a practice discipline. Guidance regarding the use or application of scientific findings does not emanate from nursing science itself.

Source: Johnson J. L. (1994). A dialectical examination of nursing art. ANS, 17(1):1–14.

As Ellis indicated, nursing is much more than the application of scientific findings. The practitioner cannot just "select from a rack of ready-to-wear theories."[1(p. 1434)] It is therefore essential that the manner in which knowledge, judgment, and skill are used in the clinical setting be carefully considered. These phenomena fall generally under the rubric of the art of nursing. Ultimately, an understanding of nursing art will further an understanding of how excellence can best be pursued and achieved in nursing practice.

The characterization of nursing as an art is not a recent development, and the literature relevant to the art of nursing is immensely diverse. It includes works such as Nightingale's[2] Notes on Nursing and Benner's[3] From Novice to Expert. Despite the abundance of writings on the topic of the art of nursing, there have been few instances in which nursing scholars have addressed one another's positions. This failure is due in part to the fact that nursing scholars have tended to pursue their conceptions of nursing art in isolation and have not considered other conceptions. Nursing scholars have not confronted one another in light of their differences, resulting in the current situation in which a plethora of diverse views concerning the art of nursing are relatively unquestioned and unexplored.

Schlotfeldt[4] pointed out that the future of the nursing profession depends on the ability of its members to identify and resolve issues. Yet nurses will be unable to resolve issues related to the art of nursing unless the subject at issue is clearly set forth. Walker identified the need for such an analysis when she argued that the controversy regarding the art of nursing "has been difficult to resolve for the point of contention has not been clearly set forth."[5(p. 118)] The tremendous diversity of ideas regarding the art of nursing expressed in the nursing literature will remain a source of confusion unless the diversities are put in order and rendered intelligible. When differences of opinion remain implicit, or even concealed, as in the nursing discourse relevant to the art of nursing, they cannot serve as the basis for the collective effort required to further thought.

In light of the state of fragmentation that characterizes the nursing literature relevant to the subject of nursing art, a philosophic study was undertaken to discover the common ground that underlies the differences of opinion regarding the art of nursing and to transmute the current diversity into rational and intelligible controversy. This study sought to render the existing diversity more intelligible so that a rational debate of fundamental issues can proceed and a better understanding of nursing art can be attained.

Method

The approach that was taken for this study was a critical examination and systematic analysis of the nursing discourse concerning the art of nursing. The method is one developed by Adler[6] and his colleagues at the Institute for Philosophical Research in Chicago to examine the controversies that surround such philosophic ideas as freedom, love, and equality. The aim of this method, which Adler[6] referred to as a dialectical approach, is to outline and clarify the structure of a controversy, and it involves a process of constructive interpretation. The goal of this philosophic method is to explicitly formulate patterns of agreement and disagreement. The challenge of the dialectical method is to achieve a nonpartisan treatment of positions or views. The dialectical task, therefore, involves rendering an objective, impartial, and neutral report of a many-sided discussion. Using this approach, the dialectician examines and clarifies what is implicit in the discourse. By way of constructive interpretation, the researcher attempts to find similarities and dissimilarities among the various conceptions.

Although the works examined in this study are historical in the sense that they date to a specific time and place, the intent of this study was to examine the ideas contained in them apart from their historical context. The study was in no way historical in its aim or its method. Therefore, for the purpose of this study, it was assumed that the authors concerned with the art of nursing are engaged in a continuing dialogue, even though they belong to different historical periods.

The point of departure for this study was the manifold and often confusing diversity that exists on the subject of nursing art. The general subject of nursing art includes a broad field of discourse and covers a variety of themes. Rather than seeking to include the work of every nursing author who has written on the subject of nursing art, a sample of works was required that was representative of the existing diversity of views regarding the art of nursing. Literature that was broadly related to the topic of nursing art was included in the study. In total, the works of 41 authors composed the examined discourse. The findings reported here are part of a larger study[7] that examined the issues and controversies that exist regarding nursing art.

Distinct Conceptualizations of Nursing Art

Based on an examination of the nursing literature related to the art of nursing, it was concluded that there are diverse answers to the question "what is the art of nursing?" The use of the term art of nursing in no way ensures that those involved in the discourse refer to the same subject. Part of the dialectical task involved determining whether there are distinct conceptions of the subject within the examined discourse. The questions that guided this determination included "is art being used in the same sense?" and "does the discussion involve one subject or several distinct subjects?" To identify the distinct conceptualizations of nursing art, each work was carefully read, and relevant passages believed to be germane to the topic were noted. Ties of relevance that connected the various authors were sought, and points of agreement were established. These points of agreement served to delineate each distinct conceptualization.

In examining the discourse, it was found that there were five separate senses of "nursing art." They can be described as

1. The nurse's ability to grasp meaning in patient encounters
2. The nurse's ability to establish a meaningful connection with the patient
3. The nurse's ability to skillfully perform nursing activities
4. The nurse's ability to rationally determine an appropriate course of nursing action
5. The nurse's ability to morally conduct his or her nursing practice

It should be pointed out that although the authors who have written about nursing art provide evidence for the construction of these conceptions, the identification of these conceptions is not theirs per se. It should also be noted that although these subjects are mutually exclusive, most authors have conceptualized nursing art as consisting of more than one ability therefore, these authors are viewed as addressing more than one conception of nursing art. Finally, it cannot be concluded that an author's apparent silence on a particular conceptualization of nursing art indicates a denial of that conceptualization. The descriptions that follow focus primarily on the similarities of thought regarding each conception, rather than the issues, or points of disagreement, that exist regarding these conceptions.

Ability to Grasp Meaning in Patient Encounters

The situations that confront nurses are often characterized by uncertainty, ambiguity, and indeterminacy.[8] This is due in part to the fact that nursing practice situations are complex. The complexity of a patient's situation can be further compounded when patients are unable to articulate their needs, either because they are unaware of the needs or because they are incapacitated.[9] Consequently, the nurse must grasp the meaning of each particular patient situation and determine what in the situation is relevant. For select authors,[3,8–33] nursing art involves the ability to grasp meaning in patient encounters. According to these authors, the artful nurse, as compared with the nurse who lacks art, can grasp what is significant in a particular patient situation. The term grasping meaning is used here to describe the process of attaching significance to those things that can be felt, observed, heard, touched, tasted, smelled, or imagined, including emotions, objects, gestures, and sounds.

Although marked variation can be found among the descriptions of the authors who have been construed to conceptualize nursing art as the grasping of meaning, several points of agreement can be found. First, nursing art is seen as based in an immediate perceptual capacity and is not affected by the intellect. This capacity to grasp meaning is often referred to as intuition. Rather than being based in reflection, or reasoning, the art of nursing according to this view is based in an immediate perceptual capacity that is more integrated than simple sensation and more concrete than intellection it is based in a capacity that involves the external senses as well as the imagination.

Using this capacity, the artful nurse attributes meaning to things that are felt, observed, or imagined. It is the artful nurse who can sense the meaning or significance of a situation, such as when a patient is distraught, perceive patterns, such as the set of signs and symptoms that indicate when a patient is going into cardiogenic shock, have a feel for what he or she is doing or sense what should be done, such as knowing when to use humor to help relieve the tension of a situation. Thus, Chinn and Kramer stated, "Esthetic knowing is what makes possible knowing what to do with the moment, instantly, without conscious deliberation."[14(p. 10)] Nursing art is thought to involve the direct apprehension of what is to be done, or what is the case, and is unmediated by concepts. The immediacy of the art of grasping meaning was emphasized by Benner and Wrubel, who argued that "the person does not assign meanings to the situation once it is apprehended because the very act of apprehension is based on taken-for-granted meanings embedded in skills, practices, and language."[9(p. 42)]

A second point of agreement is that the art of grasping meaning results in a form of understanding that defies accurate or complete description. The insights gained by this perceptual ability are thought to be tacit, nonpropositional, personal, and as such incommunicable. Carper, for example, argued that esthetic knowing is gained by "subjective acquaintance, the direct feeling of an experience"[13(p. 149)] and that this knowing defies discursive formulation. The meanings that the artful nurse grasps are concrete and individual, pertaining to a particular patient situation (e.g., this particular patient that I am nursing and can observe in front of me who happens to have had an appendectomy),

rather than abstract, pertaining to patients in general (e.g., appendectomy patients). Orlando emphasized this distinction when she stated that the nurse must distinguish between general principles and "the meanings which she must discover in the immediate nursing situation in order to help the patient."[25(p. 1)]

A third point of agreement to be found is that the art of grasping meaning is a perceptual ability that can be honed and developed over time. Rew,[31] for example, argued that the nurse can learn to become sensitive to the signals and feelings that he or she experiences and, over time, can learn to understand their significance. Similarly, Newman[21] argued that nurses can learn to attend to and trust their inner experiences. Benner[3] contended that perceptual abilities are formed by previous experiences and by immersion in the present perceptual environment. Consequently, the information taken in by the senses is endowed with meaning. According to Benner,[3] it is through experience that the nurse learns to immediately focus on what is relevant in a patient situation and to grasp its meaning. Using past experiences, or foreknowledge, the artful nurse has the ability to recognize patterns and can therefore make sense of ambiguous, unstructured situations. According to Benner, "Past concrete experience . . . guides the expert's perceptions and actions and allows for a rapid perceptual grasp of the situation."[3(pp. 8–9)]

Finally, according to those who affirm this first conception of nursing art, the art of nursing is a holistic capacity. The nurse's perceptual ability allows him or her to immediately grasp the meaning of a situation, instead of piecing together an understanding of what is happening. In contrast, the nurse who is not artful must assess every minute detail, breaking down a situation into its component parts to discover what is of significance. Benner and Wrubel described the artful capacity as "a perceptual awareness that singles out relevant information from irrelevant, grasps a situation as a whole rather than as a series of tasks, and accomplishes this rapidly and without incremental deliberative analysis of isolated facts or bits of information."[10(p. 13)]

Ability to Establish a Meaningful Connection with the Patient

The connection between the nurse and the patient is considered by many authors[13–18, 21–24,26–30,34–43] to be of particular importance, particularly in the current era of increasing technology. Many emphasize that it is the artful nurse's interactions that can bridge the gap introduced by technology and that such interactions can promote "wholeness and integrity in the personal encounter, the achievement of engagement rather than detachment, and . . . [denial of] the manipulative impersonal orientation."[13(p. 156)] Connection, as it is used here, refers to an attachment, or union, that occurs between patients and their nurses. The term connection is used because, unlike the term relationship, it encompasses short-term or fleeting encounters as well as long-term associations. According to these authors, a meaningful connection between the nurse and the patient is central to the provision of nursing care, as it is through this connection that services such as physical and emotional support

are offered and accepted. Kim,[39] for example, pointed out that the core of nursing resides in human-to-human actions. Similarly, Gadow suggested that the central question in nursing is not "how can we help them [patients] to recover?" but, instead, "how can we recover them [and] overcome the distance between us?"[16(p. 12)]

The second conception of nursing art is distinguished by four major points. First, it is contended that nursing art is nondiscursive; that is, it is expressed in the nurse's actions or behaviors. According to those who hold this second conception of nursing art, the art of nursing is "unmediated by conceptual categories."[13(p. 154)] It cannot be expressed through words; instead, it is expressed in the concrete actions and gestures of the artful nurse in response to a particular patient. Paterson and Zderad argued that "nursing is an experience lived between human beings"[28(p. 3)] and that nursing art is evident in the synchronicity between the nurse and the patient.

Second, it is contended that its expressive nature constitutes an essential characteristic of nursing art. Chinn and Kramer maintained that this expression takes the form of "human actions—words, behaviors, and other symbols—that give communicable form to what we know."[14(p. 6)] Although it is agreed that nursing art is expressive, there is little agreement regarding what exactly is expressed in nursing art. For some authors, emotions play an important role in the origin of art. For example, Watson[41] argued that through their art, nurses express emotions or feelings. The work of Peplau[29] suggested that the expression of nursing art is appropriately limited to the expression of sentiments such as concern, compassion, and caring. Paterson and Zderad,[28] on the other hand, suggested that nursing art involves the expression of the nurse's state of being.

Third, it is argued that the art of nursing occurs in relation to another human being. The ideas of philosopher Martin Buber[44] are echoed frequently in the works of authors who have conceptualized nursing art as the ability to establish a meaningful connection. Buber[44] posited that relationships are of two kinds. The first is a subject-to-subject, or "I–Thou," relationship, which is a relationship of connectedness and affirmation of another person's being. The second type of relationship is subject to object, or "I–It," which arises out of a stance of separation and detachment, in which the individual is differentiated over and against a world of objects. Authors who hold that nursing art is establishing a meaningful connection with the patient contend that nursing art can only occur when the nurse stands in a subject-to-subject relationship with the patient. For example, Paterson and Zderad stated, "If she enters into genuine relation with the patient (I–Thou) her effective power (caring, nursing skills, hope) brings forth form (well-being, more-being, comfort, growth)."[28(p. 92)]

Finally, the authors who support the view that nursing art is the ability to establish a meaningful connection are in agreement regarding the necessity of authenticity on the part of the nurse. Bishop and Scudder argued that "the inauthentic nurse merely plays the role of nurse rather than really being a nurse."[34(p. 102)] It is held that the artful nurse must be genuine, any attempt to mask or hide feelings will serve only to distance the nurse from the patient, thereby threatening the relationship between the nurse and the patient. Parse[26] referred to this authenticity as genuine or true presence. Similarly, Watson asserted that "the degree of transpersonal caring (in this sense of unity of feeling) is increased by the degree of genuineness and sincerity of the nurse."[41(p. 69)]

Ability to Skillfully Perform Nursing Activities

The conceptualization of nursing art as the skillful performance of nursing activities is one of the earliest conceptions of nursing art found in the nursing discourse.[2,3,5,9–12,45–59] It is from this view that we see in early nursing curricula the attainment of nursing skills being referred to generally as the "nursing arts." Price contended that nursing art involves the ability to "recognize the nursing needs of the patient and to develop skill, through practice, in various procedures designed to answer those needs."[54(p. 19)] According to the authors who hold the view that nursing art is the ability to skillfully perform nursing activities, the artful nurse is one who has a demonstrable capacity to effectively carry out nursing procedures and techniques. Skill, as it is used here, refers to a developed proficiency or dexterity. Nursing activities are all those tasks, procedures, and techniques that a nurse carries out in his or her practice.

The focus of these authors' conceptualizations of nursing art is an array of activities both manual and verbal in nature. For example, we see in the work of Nightingale[50] a list of behaviors that the good nurse must demonstrate. These behaviors include such things as moving silently through the sickroom, keeping constant watch over the sick, and airing out the sickroom on a regular basis. Nightingale[50] expected the artful nurse to do more than understand these edicts. She expected these behaviors to be instantiated in the nurse's practice. The artful nurse knows more than what is to be done, she knows "how to do it."[50(p. 1)] Wiedenbach[58] numbered among the skills the nurse must possess the ability to perform back rubs, to take a pulse, and to help a patient walk as well as the ability to handle necessary equipment, such as a cardiac pacemaker and the circular–electric bed: "These skills involve manipulations and techniques—executed with finesse to achieve desired results."[58(p. 28)]

Those who hold this third conception of nursing art were found to be in agreement regarding three central points. First, according to the authors, the art of nursing is primarily a behavioral ability that is, it involves observable actions and focuses on the process of doing, rather than the process of knowing. As such, it is concerned with the nurse's demonstrable ability, not his or her knowledge per se. Heidgerken made this distinction clear when she stated, "The principles, procedures, and technics, or science, of nursing are learned in the classroom. The art, or skill, of nursing is learned on the ward."[48(p. 9)] Although there is agreement among the authors who hold this third conception that nursing art is ultimately a behavioral ability, there is no consensus regarding the role that one's intellectual capacity plays in the art of nursing. Some theorists argue that the activities must be intelligently performed. Montag,[49] for example, contended that skill without understanding is mere imitation. Similarly, Heidgerken[48] contended that the memorization and demonstration of step-by-step procedures will not produce an artful nurse. Tracy, on the other hand, contended that "the nurse should have so mastered her procedures that the minimum of thought is needed for their use."[57(p. 29)] Similarly, Benner and Wrubel[9] argued that nurse's everyday actions are effective not because they think about them, or base them on theory, but because they have a sophisticated repertoire of reactions.

Second, those who conceptualize nursing art as skillful performance of nursing activities are in agreement about the claim that nursing art can be learned. Key to learning the art of nursing are persistent practice and repetition. Goodrich maintained that practical experience for student nurses should be "sufficiently long to allow of a constant repetition of procedures."[47(p. 42)] Heidgerken, however, warned that practice alone is not enough and that "the attitude of the learner, the will to improve, and eradication of mistakes are all equally as important as practice."[48(p. 54)]

Finally, there is also evidence of agreement regarding the fact that certain criteria can be used to judge the art of nursing. When discussing the art of nursing, these theorists inevitably use descriptors such as fluidity of movement, adroitness, coordination, and efficiency. Stewart indicated that nursing art involves "manual dexterity, lightness, steadiness, quickness of movement, strength, endurance, and that complete coordination of head and muscle which cannot be acquired except by long, directed training."[55(pp. 324–325)] Similarly, Heidgerken[48] argued that the artful nurse's activities must have the appropriate form, elimination of excess movements, appropriate timing, force, and coordination are among the qualities that characterize the activities of the artful nurse.

Ability to Determine Rationally an Appropriate Course of Nursing Action

For those[2,4,5,25,39,40,45,46,48–53,55,56,58–78] who support the fourth conception of nursing art, intellectual activity is essential to the performance of nursing care. According to this fourth conception, nursing art refers to the nurse's ability to rationally determine an appropriate course of nursing action. The term rational ability, as it is used here, refers to the intellectual ability to effectively draw valid conclusions from existing knowledge.

This fourth conception of nursing art is characterized by five points of agreement. First, it is argued that nursing art is practical in nature. According to these authors, the aim of this ability is the determination of an appropriate course of action. Nursing art, it is argued, is action oriented and not simply aimed at understanding. Beckstrand,[60] for example, contended that the aim of nursing art is the control of practice. Dickoff and James[62] concluded that nursing art is concerned ultimately with producing nursing

situations. Similarly, Orlando contended that nursing art is a rational capacity that is aimed at "helping the patient."[25(p. 70)]

Second, it is contended that there is an underlying discipline on which nursing art rests. All of the authors who contend that nursing art is a rational ability emphasize the importance of knowledge, specifically scientific knowledge, to nursing art. Orem stated, "The art of nursing is the nurse's quality or habit of reasoning and judging correctly about the design and production of the kind and amount of nursing needed according to the principles or laws of nursing itself. Science and technique are 'the first necessary conditions for honest art.' The point of view of nursing as art therefore encompasses the point of view of nursing as knowledge."[52(p. 24)]

Arguments about the importance of knowledge for nursing art are often tied to the claim that nursing is a profession. Abdellah and colleagues, for example, argued, "Professionalization of nursing requires that nurses identify those nursing problems that depend for their solution upon the nurse's use of her capacities to conceptualize events and make judgments about them. Nurses need to become skilled in recognizing both overt and covert nursing problems, in analyzing them in terms of relevant principles and in working out courses of action by applying nursing principles."[45(p. 11)] It was assumed by Abdellah et al.,[45] as it was by all of the authors who support this fourth conceptualization of nursing art, that the nursing profession possesses a distinct body of knowledge and that this body of knowledge provides the foundation for nursing practice.

Leininger[73] also contended that nursing art is based on scientific knowledge. She believed that nurses must, if they are to be effective, "scientifically care" for their patients. Scientific caring, according to Leininger, "refers to those judgments and acts of helping others based upon tested or verified knowledge."[73(p. 46)] The importance of knowledge to artful practice is echoed by all of the authors. Kim stated, "Knowledge is antecedent to action."[39(p. 146)] Diers contended that "nursing practice is done consciously, if not always with a formal plan, that it is not done mindlessly."[65(p. 31)] Finally, Rogers claimed that "the art of nursing develops only as it incorporates more and more of science unto itself. The nature of its art lies in the core of scientific knowledge it embodies."[75(p. 32)]

The third point of agreement regarding the art of rationally determining an appropriate course of nursing action is that it presupposes that nurses possess a thorough understanding of what is before them and the actions they should take. According to this perspective, the artful nurse solves problems by selecting the intervention that is best suited to the intended end. This process of instrumental problem solving involves a thorough consideration of the facts of a situation and is made rigorous by the application of scientific theory. For example, Johnson[70] argued that an artful nurse thinks "logically, soundly, and searchingly" about the causes and effects in a given nursing situation. The key point is that the artful nurse's actions are not "automatic" or "blind" but instead are grounded in an intellectual activity, in which knowledge or information of certain kinds is considered to determine which actions will result in the best possible patient outcome.

Fourth, it is contended that the art of rationally determining an appropriate course of nursing action involves a process of logical reasoning in which scientific principles and theories are applied to problems identified in practice. According to this view, the artful nurse uses evidence to reason through the best course of action to be followed. Beckstrand described this process in the following manner:

> Once the conditions requiring changes in the client's situation are determined, a practitioner examines the situation to identify the possibility of making the changes desired. First, a practitioner uses scientific knowledge of necessary and sufficient conditions to determine if desired changes are realizable. Next, a practitioner examines the situation to determine whether conditions for achieving the desired changes exist. . . . As a result, the set of realizable outcomes in practice is determined by what is scientifically possible within the exigencies of the practice situation.[61(p. 177)]

The steps of the nursing process (assessment, planning, implementation, and evaluation) are seen as the steps that an artful nurse takes to ensure quality patient care. The emphasis of this approach is on deliberate, systematic, and scientifically based care.

Finally, it is contended by those who hold the fourth conception of nursing art that the art of nursing can be judged according to certain standards. They agree that the appropriateness of a nursing action can be judged on the basis of whether the identified course of action enabled the practitioner to attain his or her identified goals or standards. For example, Henderson[37] contended that a nurse's art can be evaluated according to the degree to which the patient has reestablished independence. Some authors have suggested additional criteria for evaluation. Dickoff, James, and Wiedenbach,[63] for example, suggested that nursing art can be evaluated using the criteria of coherency, palatability, and feasibility.

Ability to Conduct One's Nursing Practice Morally

For a final group of authors,[2,3,9,11,15–18, 34,38,47,50–53,60,61,67,68,79–81] nursing art involves the ability of the nurse to practice morally: The nurse is obligated to practice in such a way that seeks to avoid harm and to benefit the patient. The term moral, as it is used here, refers to that which is good, or desirable, for human beings. These authors are in agreement regarding four central points. First, it is held that good or excellent nursing practice is, by necessity, moral in that it is directed toward the good of the patient. As Goodrich stated, "So much is nursing of the essence of ethics that it is consistent to assert that the terms good and ethical as applied to nursing practice are synonymous."[47(p. 5)] Conversely, the view that nursing art can under any circumstances be amoral or immoral is antithetical to this position. Indeed, for these authors, the moral aspect of nursing cannot be separated from the notion of excellence in nursing, either existentially or analytically. This is the case, it is argued, because unlike the fine arts, nursing is an art that deals directly with human beings. Artful nursing, Curtin[79] asserted, is inextricably entwined with human life and the achievement of particular human ends.

According to those who hold that nursing is a moral art, a nurse may be technically competent and knowledgeable, yet if he or she does not make moral choices in the performance of patient care, he or she is not artful. Lanara[81] argued that values and ideals must guide the nurse's care. In a similar fashion, Gadow[17] posited that good nursing is more than a cluster of techniques in that it involves a commitment to a moral end and is directed and judged by that end. This position is also supported by Bishop and Scudder, who argued that the artful nurse's ability consists in more than the ability to efficiently complete tasks: "[The] technician uses techniques which are evaluated by efficiency whereas, the professional makes decisions which are evaluated by the good."[34(p. 69)]

Second, it is held that the possession of skill and knowledge are necessary, but not sufficient, conditions for the moral conduct of nursing practice. Indeed, it is presupposed by many of these authors that the artful nurse must be competent in his or her practice. As Curtin[80] pointed out, the license to practice nursing does not include permission to practice poorly. In stating that one is a professional, one is claiming a certain level of competence.

Third, it is argued by those who hold that nursing art is the ability to morally conduct one's practice that nursing art involves a commitment to care competently for patients. Curtin stated that "although knowledge and skill are integral to the practice of a profession, the foundation consists of the performative declarations professed by its practitioners and the fidelity of the practitioner to these promises."[80(pp. 101–102)] The moral responsibility to nurse well involves a commitment not only to nurse a patient competently, but to "sustain excellent practice in the face of unreasonable demands and lack of appreciation on the part of patients."[35(p. 37)] The artful nurse not only must be competent, but must also consistently demonstrate competence in his or her practice, no matter how arduous the circumstances.

Finally, the notion that the artful nurse must possess moral virtues is reiterated in various forms by all of the authors who ascribe to the notion that the art of nursing is of a moral nature. Expressed in all of their works is the belief that the artful nurse must be properly motivated in his or her action. Rather than being motivated by self-aggrandizement or expediency, the artful nurse is motivated by care and concern for others. Benner and Wrubel suggested that the same act done in a caring and uncaring way may have different effects and that only a nurse who cares about his or her patients will notice small differences in their behaviors and create unique solutions to patient problems: "Caring makes the nurse notice which interventions help, and this concern guides subsequent caregiving. Caring causes

the nurse to notice subtle signs of improvement or deterioration in the patient. In fact, caring . . . is required for expert human practice."[9(p. 4)]

Accordingly, the nurse who does not care about his or her patient cannot nurse well. Lanara[81] argued that the ability to care about patients rests on the nurse's capacity to love others and that nurses, inspired by the ideal of love, will care not only for, but about, their patients. It is love, according to Lanara,[81] that allows the nurse to transcend obstacles and become heroic in his or her nursing practice.

Conclusion

Through the identification of these five conceptions of nursing art, nurses can begin to understand the structure of the discourse regarding nursing art. After one goes beyond the description of the five conceptions identified, differences of opinion can be found among the authors who affirm a particular conception of nursing art. Indeed, each of the five conceptions is a subject of controversy in that each comprises numerous conceptual, existential, and normative issues.

It is evident that although nursing scholars have written about the subject of nursing art, few have acknowledged one another's conceptions. Indeed, to date, there has been little recognition that different conceptions of nursing art exist. When one examines the discourse regarding the art of nursing, it is clear that not all of the authors agree about the nature of nursing art. This state of affairs is consistent with the state of the nursing discourse in general. Kikuchi and Simmons accurately characterized this state of affairs when they stated

> Although nursing scholars are prone to speak or write on the same topic, use the same words, or express a common interest in knowledge development, there is very little in their productions to indicate that they share to any great degree a common understanding, a coming-to-terms, that would allow for the minimal topical agreement required before questions can be commonly interpreted, controversies identified, issues debated, and answers commonly agreed upon.[82(p. 3)]

It is hoped that the identification of distinct conceptions of nursing art will facilitate productive debate and analysis among nursing's scholars.

The method employed in this research is limited in that it does not answer the question "what is nursing art?" The next step must be taken: to examine each of these conceptualizations in detail to determine which conceptualization or group of conceptualizations is sound. The findings of this study provide the groundwork for future philosophic analyses, thereby bringing nursing one step closer toward a sound conception of nursing art. It is only when a sound conception of nursing art is developed that nursing will be able to answer questions regarding how nursing art should be pursued and developed. It is hoped that nursing scholars in the future will dispute the nature of nursing art more explicitly and extensively.

References

1. Ellis R. The practitioner as theorist. Am J Nurs. 1969;69:1434–1438.
2. Nightingale F. Notes on Nursing: What It Is, and What It Is Not. New York: Dover; 1969.
3. Benner P. From Novice to Expert: Excellence and Power in Clinical Nursing Practice. Menlo Park, CA: Addison-Wesley; 1984.
4. Schlotfeldt RM. Resolution of issues: An imperative for creating nursing's future. J Prof Nurs. 1987;3:136–142.
5. Walker LO. Nursing as a Discipline. Bloomington, IN: Indiana University; 1971. Dissertation.
6. Adler MJ. The Idea of Freedom, I: A Dialectical Examination of the Conceptions of Freedom. Garden City, NY: Doubleday; 1958.
7. Johnson JL. Toward a Clearer Understanding of the Art of Nursing. Edmonton, Alberta, Canada: University of Alberta; 1993. Dissertation.
8. Tanner C. Curriculum revolution: The practice mandate. In: Curriculum Revolution: Mandate for Change. New York: National League for Nursing; 1988:201–216.
9. Benner P, Wrubel J. The Primacy of Caring: Stress and Coping in Health and Illness. Menlo Park, CA: Addison-Wesley; 1989.

10. _____. Skilled clinical knowledge: The value of perceptual awareness. Nurs Educ. 1982;7(3):11–17.

11. Benner P. The role of experience, narrative, and community in skilled ethical comportment. ANS. 1991;14(2):1–21.

12. Benner P, Tanner C, Chesla C. From beginner to expert: Gaining a differentiated clinical world in critical care nursing. ANS. 1992;14(3):13–28.

13. Carper BA. Fundamental Patterns of Knowing in Nursing. New York: Teachers College, Columbia University; 1975.

14. Chinn PL, Kramer MK. Theory and Nursing: A Systematic Approach, 3rd ed. St. Louis: Mosby–Yearbook; 1991.

15. Gadow S. Clinical subjectivity: Advocacy with silent patients. Nurs Clin North Am. 1989;24:535–541.

16. _____. Beyond Dualism: The Dialectic of Caring and Knowing. Presented at the conference "The Care-Justice Puzzle: Education for Ethical Nursing Practice" at the University of Minnesota; October 13, 1990; Minneapolis, MN.

17. _____. Nurse and patient: The caring relationship. In: Bishop AH, Scudder JR, eds. Caring, Curing, Coping: Nurse, Physician, Patient Relationships. Tuscaloosa, AL: University of Alabama Press; 1985:31–43.

18. _____. Body and self: A dialectic. J Med Philos. 1980;5:172–185.

19. Moccia PA. A critique of compromise: Beyond the methods debate. ANS. 1988;10(4):1–9.

20. _____. A Study of the Theory-Practice Dialectic: Towards a Critique of the Science of Man. New York: New York University; 1980. Dissertation.

21. Newman MA. The spirit of nursing. Holistic Nurs Pract. 1989;3(3):1–6.

22. _____. Health as Expanding Consciousness. St. Louis: Mosby; 1986.

23. _____. Newman's theory of health as praxis. Nurs Sci Q. 1990;3:37–41.

24. _____, Sime AM, Corcoran-Perry SA. The focus of the discipline of nursing. ANS. 1991;14(1):1–6.

25. Orlando IJ. The Dynamic Nurse-Patient Relationship: Function, Process and Principles. New York: G.P. Putnam's Sons; 1961.

26. Parse RR. Human becoming: Parse's theory of nursing. Nurs Sci Q. 1992;5:35–42.

27. _____. Man-Living-Health: A Theory of Nursing. New York: Wiley; 1981.

28. Paterson JG, Zderad LT. Humanistic Nursing. New York: National League for Nursing; 1988.

29. Peplau HE. The art and science of nursing: Similarities, differences, and relations. Nurs Sci Q. 1988;1:8–15.

30. _____. Interpersonal Relations in Nursing: A Conceptual Frame of Reference for Psychodynamic Nursing. New York: G.P. Putnam's Sons; 1952.

31. Rew L. Nurses' intuition. Appl Nurs Res. 1988;1:27–31.

32. _____. Intuition in decision-making. Image J Nurs Schol. 1988;20:150–153.

33. Tanner CA. The nursing care plan as an instructional method: Ritual or reason? Nurs Educ. 1968;11(4): 8–10.

34. Bishop AH, Scudder JR. The Practical, Moral, and Personal Sense of Nursing:

A Phenomenological Philosophy of Practice. Albany, NY: State University of New York Press; 1990.

35. _____. Nursing ethics in an age of controversy. ANS. 1987;9(3):34–43.

36. _____. Nursing: The Practice of Caring. New York: National League for Nursing Press; 1991.

37. Henderson V. The nature of nursing. Am J Nurs. 1964;64(8):62–28.

38. _____. Excellence in nursing. Am J Nurs. 1969;69:2133–2137.

39. Kim HS. The Nature of Theoretical Thinking in Nursing. Norwalk, CN: Appleton-Century-Crofts; 1983.

40. _____. Structuring the nursing knowledge system: A typology of four domains. Schol Inq Nurs Pract. 1987;1:99–114.

41. Watson J. Nursing: Human Science and Human Care: A Theory of Nursing. New York: National League for Nursing; 1988.

42. _____. The lost art of nursing. Nurs Forum. 1981;20:244–249.

43. _____. Caring knowledge and informed moral passion. ANS. 1990;13(1):15–24.

44. Buber M; Smith RG, trans. I and Thou, 2nd ed. New York: Charles Scribner's Sons; 1958.

45. Abdellah FG, Martin A, Beland IL, Matheney RV. Patient-Centered Approaches to Nursing. New York: Macmillan, 1960.

46. Abdellah FG, Levine E. Better Patient Care Through Nursing Research. New York: Macmillan; 1965.

47. Goodrich AW. The Social and Ethical Significance of Nursing: A Series of Addresses. New York: Macmillan; 1932.

48. Heidgerken LE. Teaching in Schools of Nursing: Principles and Methods. Philadelphia: Lippincott; 1946.

49. Montag MI. The Education of Nursing Technicians. New York: G.P. Putnam's Sons; 1951.

50. Nightingale F. Training of Nurses and Nursing the Sick [Microfiche, Adelaide Nutting Historical Nursing Collection]. London, UK: Spottiswoode; 1899.

51. _____. Suggestions for Thought to the Searchers After Truth Among the Artizans of England [Microfiche, Adelaide Nutting Historical Nursing Collection]. London, UK: George E. Eyre & William Spottiswoode; 1860.

52. Orem DE. Nursing: Concepts of Practice, 4th ed. St. Louis: Mosby-Yearbook; 1991.

53. _____. The form of nursing science. Nurs Sci Q. 1988;1:75–79.

54. Price AL. The Art, Science and Spirit of Nursing, 2nd ed. Philadelphia: W.B. Saunders; 1960.

55. Stewart IM. The aims of the training school for nurses. Am J Nurs. 1916;16:319-327.

56. _____. Practical objectives in nursing education. Am J Nurs. 1924;24:557–564.

57. Tracy MA. Nursing: An Art and a Science. St. Louis: Mosby; 1938.

58. Wiedenbach E. Clinical Nursing: A Helping Art. New York: Springer; 1964.

59. _____. The helping art of nursing. Am J Nurs. 1963;63:54–57.

60. Beckstrand J. The notion of a practice theory and the relationship of scientific and ethical knowledge to practice. Res Nurs Health. 1978;1:131–136.

61. _____. The need for a practice theory as indicated by the knowledge used in the conduct of practice. Res Nurs Health. 1978;1:175–179.

62. Dickoff J, James P. A theory of theories: A position paper. Nurs Res. 1968;17:197–203.

63. Dickoff J, James P, Wiedenbach E. Theory in a practice discipline: Part II. Practice oriented research. Nurs Res. 1968;17:545–554.

64. Dickoff J, James P. Taking concepts as guides to action: Exploring kinds of know-how. In: Nicoll LH, ed. Perspectives on Nursing Theory, 2nd ed. Philadelphia: Lippincott; 1992:576–580.

65. Diers D. Research in Nursing Practice. Philadelphia: Lippincott; 1979.

66. _____. Learning the art and craft of nursing. Am J Nurs. 1990;90:65–66.

67. Dock LL. Short Papers on Nursing Subjects. New York: M. Louise Longeway; 1900.

68. Dock LL, Steward IM. A Short History of Nursing: From the Earliest Times to the Present Day, 3rd ed., rev. New York: G.P. Putnam's Sons; 1937.

69. Donaldson SK, Crowley DM. The discipline of nursing. Nurs Outlook. 1978;26:113–120.

70. Johnson DE. A philosophy of nursing. Nurs Outlook. 1959;7:198–200.

71. _____. The nature of a science of nursing. Nurs Outlook. 1959;7:291–294.

72. _____. Theory in nursing: Borrowed and unique. Nurs Res. 1968;17:206–209.

73. Leininger M. Caring: A central focus of nursing and health care services. In: Leininger MM, ed. Care: The Essence of Nursing and Health. Thorofare, NJ: Slack; 1984:45–59.

74. _____. Care, Discovery and Uses in Clinical and Community Nursing. Detroit, MI: Wayne State University Press; 1988.

75. Rogers ME. Reveille in Nursing. Philadelphia: F.A. Davis; 1964.

76. _____. An Introduction to the Theoretical Basis of Nursing. Philadelphia: F.A. Davis; 1970.

77. _____. Nursing science and art: A prospective. Nurs Sci Q. 1988;1:99–102.

78. Schlotfeldt RM. Structuring nursing knowledge: A priority for creating nursing's future. Nurs Sci Q. 1988;1:35–38.

79. Curtin LL. The nurse as advocate: A philosophical foundation for nursing. ANS. 1979;1(3):1–10.

80. Curtin L. The commitment of nursing. In: Curtin LL, Flaherty MJ, eds. Nursing Ethics: Theories and Pragmatics. Bowie, MD: Robert J. Brady; 1982:97–102.

81. Lanara VA. Heroism as a Nursing Value: A Philosophical Perspective. Athens, Greece: Sisterhood Evniki; 1981.

82. Kikuchi JF, Simmons H. Prologue: An invitation to philosophize. In: Kikuchi JF, Simmons H, eds. Philosophic Inquiry in Nursing. Newbury Park, CA: Sage; 1992:1–4.

CHAPTER 17

A Conceptual Framework for Person-Centered Practice with Older People

Brendan McCormack, DPhil(Oxon), BScNsg(Hons), PGCEA, RGN, RMN

This paper presents a conceptual framework for person centered practice with older people. The research from which the framework was developed was guided by hermeneutic philosophy and integrated processes of conversation analysis and reflective conversation in data collection and analysis. The research findings suggested that nurses need to be able to particularize the person that the patient is, the relationship that exists between them and the patient, and the understandings and expectations implicit in the relationship. From these findings, a conceptual framework for person-centered practice was developed. In the framework, person centeredness is premised on the concept of authentic consciousness and is operationalized through five imperfect duties. The factors that enable person centeredness to operate in practice are identified as the patient's values, the nurse's values, and the context of the care environment. Considerations for implementing the model in practice are highlighted.

Key words: *caring, nurse–patient relationship, older people, person-centered, values.*

Introduction

This paper explores the issue of person-centered practice with older people. The paper presents a conceptual framework for person-centered practice that has been developed from a larger research study exploring

---

the meaning of autonomy for older people in hospital settings. The framework emphasizes partnership, which works between nurses and older people based on a "negotiated relationship." The paper presents an overview of the research from which the conceptual framework has been derived, a description of the components of the framework, and an example of the model in use. The conceptual framework presented in this paper makes a significant contribution to the growing body of knowledge that challenges the dominant emphasis on dependency in gerontology.[1–4]

Person Centeredness

In the United Kingdom, the idea of person-centered practice is now embedded in the language of multidisciplinary practice with older people (see, for example, The National Service Framework for Older People[5]). Respect for persons is central to the notion of person-centeredness and is rooted in a Kantian ideal of mutual respect and sympathetic benevolence.[6] Therefore, the rights of individuals as persons is the driving force behind person-centered health care.[4,7] It represents an attitude of respect for ordinary individuals to make rational decisions and determine their own ends. The idea of respecting the patient's right to self-determination has resulted in a shift in thinking about the role of the patient in health care decision making. Hope and Fulford suggest that this philosophical shift requires health professionals to think beyond concepts of cure based on scientific facts and technical

competence, to the adoption of a more holistic approach that also incorporates values.[8] Being person centered requires the formation of a therapeutic narrative between professional and patient that is built on mutual trust, understanding, and a sharing of collective knowledge.

Autonomy and Person-Centeredness: A Hermeneutic Study

The original research, from which this paper is derived, explored the meaning of autonomy for older people in hospital settings.[9] The overall research approach was guided by the hermeneutic philosophy of Gadamer.[10] Hermeneutic research does not attempt to interpret the data from an objective position, but instead creates a dialogue where the researcher and research participants' perceptions interact. The hermeneutic process is a dialogical process between the interpreter's understanding and the object being studied. Research participants' active involvement in this interpretative process is important so that a "meeting of understanding" can be achieved between perspectives of the research participants and the interpreter in order to create new understandings.

A convenience sample of four hospital nurses recorded discussions and conversations between themselves and patients, and with doctors and other members of the health care team, for at least three shifts per week over a 1-year period. In addition, interactions between a recognized expert gerontologic nurse (identified by using criteria derived from the work of Benner,[11] Jasper,[12] and Greenwood and King[13]) and patients in a community hospital setting were also recorded as a means of "testing out" initial themes generated from the data collected by the hospital nurses. Fourteen case studies of nurse–patient interactions were achieved. The local research ethics committee (LREC), in the health district where the research was being conducted, approved the research protocol and management plans. Patients with dementia or confusion (scoring 5 or less on a Mini-Mental Health Assessment[14]) were excluded from the study at the request of the LREC.

The data were transcribed, coded, and described using techniques of conversational analysis.[15] Conversation analysis was used as a structured approach to describing the data and deriving interpretive themes, that is, as a tool for the selection and description of the data sets. By using an established framework derived from conversation analysis, decisions about data choices for analysis would in the first instance be informed through the structure of the framework, rather than the researcher's own subjective choices as a "data interpreter." Conversation analysis identifies a limited set of conversational rules within which discourse is constructed and within which participants perform particular acts within the constraints of this rule system. Discourse is action in its own right and not a route to understanding action. Ordinary conversation is viewed as the predominant medium of action in the social world. Follow-up "reflective conversations"[16] with the nurses clarified and developed the researcher's initial descriptions of the data. Rigor in data analysis was maintained through an iterative process between researcher and research participants. Initial themes from the descriptions were developed through focus group discussions with a group of expert nurses and a group of patients. Nurses and patients identified themes from the descriptions prior to further thematic analysis by the researcher. Finally, participating nurses, the group of expert nurses and the patient group agreed on the final themes that were developed.

The research findings, which have been reported in detail elsewhere,[17] included the key issues of the effects of institutional discourse, the dynamics of power and control, patients' access to knowledge, the impact of professional authority, the constraining nature of institutions and the effect of family and careers on decision making. All of these factors were seen to act as constraints on the ability of older people to exercise autonomy. Through the interpretive process with participants, 23 "principles for action" to address these constraints were identified (Appendix 1) and further analysis of these resulted in the development of the conceptual framework for person-centered practice.

Person-Centeredness as Authentic Consciousness

The research findings suggest that nurses need to be able to particularize the person that the patient is, the relationship that exists between them and the patient, and the understandings and expectations implicit in the relationship. It is proposed that this can be achieved through an understanding of the person's authentic values.

Authenticity refers to a way of reaching decisions which are truly one's own: decisions that express all that one believes important about oneself and the world, the entire complexity of one's values.[18]

Authentic consciousness is a consideration of the person's life as a whole in order to help sustain meaning in life. Authentic consciousness is not a hierarchical ordering of possible desires, but a clarification of values to maximize potential for growth and development. Existing evidence highlights the dominance of routine and ritualized practices with older people that do not take account of individual beliefs and values.[17,19–21] When working with beliefs and values, the role of the nurse is to maximize opportunities for growth through authentic decision making, that is, decisions that are true to the person's life as a whole. It is not enough to just take note of another's beliefs, values, views and experiences. They must be integrated into the biography of that individual.

Being conscious of another's beliefs and values does not tell the nurse what to do; rather, it orientates the nurse to a particular way of being. As Gadow argues, the recognition of beliefs and values allows the patient and the nurse to have the kind of caring relationship that they want to have, appropriate to the context of care.[18] This

helps the nurse place actions in context, or as MacIntyre suggests, "The act of utterance becomes intelligible by finding its place in a narrative."[22] In the context of this research, what this means is that desires, wishes, and needs of an older person can best be understood by having a picture of the person's life as a whole. Therefore, being person-centered relies on getting closer to the older person and goes beyond traditional notions of respecting individuality and individualized care, such as choices about food and drink, hygiene, waking, and sleeping. In this framework, getting closer to the patient is achieved through consideration of the patient's authenticity, the adoption of "imperfect duties" and the consideration of contextual factors (**Figure 17-1**).

Imperfect Duties

The term imperfect duties is derived from Kant, who made a distinction between perfect and imperfect duties.[23] Perfect duties are strict and enforceable. In contrast, imperfect duties are "wide, broad and limited"—"they leave us a play-room for free choice in following the law,"[23] as there is no means of offering an exhaustive and a priori account of how the duties are to be fulfilled. Such duties as compassion, concern, benevolence, respect, and care would all be imperfect duties as, for example, one cannot force someone to be caring. Kant views such duties as imperfect because, in ethical decision making, one might have to decide between competing

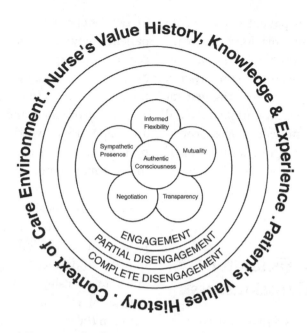

Figure 17-1 Conceptual Framework of Person-Centeredness as Authentic Consciousness

duties and account must be taken of the context in which decisions are made. This approach acknowledges the need for guiding principles that are interpreted in the context of the particular relationship. It highlights the important place of emotions in decision making by highlighting the importance of emotional factors being made explicit and acknowledged as influences on the process and outcome of decision making. Issues such as how much the nurse "likes" the patient, the individual nurse's personal experiences, and the behavior of the patient are seen as significant.

Returning to the study previously described[9] from the data analysis, five imperfect duties are considered to be important

to the operationalization of autonomy as authentic consciousness:

1. Informed flexibility: the facilitation of decision making through information sharing and the integration of new information into established perspectives and care practices.
2. Mutuality: the recognition of the others' values as being of equal importance in decision making.
3. Transparency: making explicit the intentions and motivations for action and the boundaries within which care decisions are set.
4. Negotiation: patient participation through a culture of care that values

the views of the patient as a legitimate basis for decision making while recognizing that being the final arbiter of decisions is of secondary importance.

5. Sympathetic presence: an engagement that recognizes the uniqueness and value of the individual by appropriately responding to cues that maximize coping resources through the recognition of important agendas in daily life.

The Nurse as a Facilitator of Authentic Consciousness

The imperfect duties act as guiding universal principles that are interpreted in the context of the particular care situation. Adopting a person-centered approach to practice requires nurses to recognize freedom of self-determination for patients as a fundamental and valuable human right, based on an interdependent and interconnected relationship with each other.[18] Person-centered practice holds central the knowledge and experience that each person brings to the care situation and which is necessary for decisions that will best serve the patient's well-being. Examples of this in the United Kingdom include developments in the assessment of care needs of older people,[5] models for involving older people with dementia in decision making,[4] and person-centered practices in acute care nursing.[19] At the heart of this style of nursing is the therapeutic nurse–patient relationship that requires continuity of care and the acceptance of responsibility for the outcomes

of care. Acknowledging and valuing each patient's biography and their individual perception and experience of their health care experience is fundamental to this way of nursing. Its aim is to transform the patient's experience of illness and is considered to be a therapy in its own right.[8] The role of the person-centered nurse is to be there, offering personal support and practical expertise, while enabling the patient to follow the path of their own choosing and in their own way.

However, total connectedness with a patient can lead to "ethical blindness,"[24] and in order to balance the intensity of an individual relationship with a reflective approach to decision making, the nurse needs to move between three "stances" when working with patients.[25] These stances represent different levels of engagement (connectedness) between the nurse and patient.

When engagement is present, the patient and nurse are connected in the relationship. The nurse and patient are extensions of each other and a care partnership exists. Boykin and Schoenhofer describe this as "the dance of caring persons."[26] Caring exists because the nurse and patient hold a deep respect for each other. However, a dilemma could arise in the care relationship that affects the way the nurse and patient are able to work together, such as a difficult decision and ethical dilemma or a disagreement. As a result, partial disengagement occurs while the nurse and patient take stock of the situation and formulate the problem. Such disengagement then requires a period of contemplation, and for a period of time, complete disengagement occurs. In this stance, the nurse and patient contemplate the available options from their individual perspectives. They reassess the values that underpin the relationship and decision making. Mechanisms such as supported reflective practice,[27,28] clinical supervision,[29] and case reviews[30] all help to achieve this goal. Although the nurse continues to work with the patient in seeking the most satisfactory resolution, the connectedness in the relationship is broken until such time as a resolution can be found. A skilled nurse can adopt these different stances at different times with the patient. Indeed, they were evident in the practice of the expert nurse and the clinical nurse specialist in the research underpinning this framework.[9] In contemplating options and choices, there are three important factors for the creation of an environment that facilitates person centeredness. These are the patient's values, the nurse's values and expertise, and the context of care.

The Patient's Values

Respect for values is central to person-centered practice.[4,7,9] It is important to develop a clear picture of what patients value about their life and how they make sense of what is happening. This provides a standard against which the nurse can compare current decisions and behaviors of the patient with those values and preferences made in life in general. Approaches to patient assessment that include a biographical account, using narrative and story, are one method of establishing a baseline value history. Assisting the individual to find meaning in care might help them to tolerate the incongruity of their illness and plan for a future.[31]

The complexity of many health care decisions coupled with the stresses and fears of illness, with its related anxiety, dependence and regressive tendencies, means that a patient's ordinary decision making abilities are often significantly diminished. Buchanan and Brock argue that if patients hold the ultimate responsibility for their health care decision, then their treatment choices might fail to serve their well-being, as conceived by them.[32] Thus, they argue that the same value of patient well-being that requires patients' participation in their own health care decisions might sometimes also require persons to be protected from the harmful consequences to them of their own choices.

When considered in practice, the risk to autonomous decision making by patients from paternalistic health care workers is significant. Agich asserts that the means of preventing such action is by having a clear picture of what the patient, and others important to them, really value about their life and how they make sense of the things happening to them.[33] In the exercise of their decision-making capacity, patients bring an individual approach to their concept of their own well-being. Health means different things to different people[34] and is accorded various degrees of importance by individuals. Therefore, there is no one single intervention that is best for everyone. While certain procedures might be more appropriate than others in particular cases, it is the individuality of the particular case that determines the most appropriate approach. For this reason, health care decision making ought to adopt a negotiated approach between practitioner and patient.[9]

The Nurse's Values and Expertise

Although the language of partnership is commonplace and nurses are encouraged to soften their professional presentation to the patient, it remains unusual for nurses to present their own views as a component of the array of information that patients are given to assist their decisions. Although the patient's values should be predominant,[18] the nurse's values also contribute to the process. However, these are seldom open and transparent. Indeed, it could be argued that if a mutual relationship exists between the nurse and patient, then it is especially important that the nurse's values are expressed, particularly when they conflict with the patient's values. If the nurse is truly working in partnership with the patient then there is no reason why the expression of such values should be coercive. Instead, the disclosure of the nurse's values might help the patient to understand particular negotiation positions taken by the nurse and it might offer the patient an alternative view when considering their options. However, it has been argued that despite an intention to consider patient and nursing values, the context of the care environment has a significant impact on the operationalization of person-centered practices.[35,36]

The Context of Care

The context in which care is provided has the greatest potential to enhance or limit the facilitation of person-centered practice. When facilitating person-centeredness, nurses find they not only balance competing care values but often find it necessary to consider organizational values too. Nurses are not free to fulfill a moral obligation to the patient without considering organizational and professional implications,[37] and indeed, they might find themselves having to accept a forced choice on occasion.[38] In contemporary health care, the fundamental moral predicament of nurses is that while they are expected to engage in autonomous decision making, they are often deprived of the freedom to exercise moral authority.[39] While the freedom of the nurse is a significant issue in the facilitation of person-centeredness, other characteristics of context have been found to be of equal significance,[1] such as systems of decision making, staff relationships, organizational systems, power differentials, and the potential of organization to tolerate innovate practices and risk taking. These findings have been supported in a recent analysis of the concept of context.[35]

A Composite Example

In order to illustrate the framework in use, the following example is offered. The example is derived from data extracts from the research underpinning this conceptual framework.[9] These extracts have been taken from the data of one nurse who participated in the study (Pam) and her work with one patient (Ray).

Pam is a lead nurse in a local community hospital that specializes in the rehabilitation of older people following acute illness. The unit utilizes the Burford Nursing Development Unit (BNDU) model of nursing.[40] Ray, a patient transferred from the regional general hospital, was admitted for rehabilitation following a fractured shaft of his left femur. Ray is a gypsy and values his freedom and independence. Staff in the regional hospital reported that he was "difficult," "uncooperative," and "refused to do what he was told!" When admitted, Pam used the key questions from the BNDU model: "who is this person?" and "what information do I need to know to be able to nurse him effectively?" to focus the construction of his biography, assess his care needs, and agree on a care plan. By using these questions, Ray shared his core values of personal freedom, intolerance of authority, and everyone being equal, while Pam shared her core nursing values of self-determination, honesty, and negotiation. Together, they agreed on a plan of care that encompassed these values. Pam and Ray drew up a contract of how they would work together and this was written into the care plan. The contract included the importance of them being honest with each other, that all decisions would be negotiated between them, that all prescribed interventions would be fully explained and that his lifestyle would be respected. His care plan included details of when and how he would have physiotherapy, psychosocial activities to assist his transition back to the community, and a program of self-administration of medicines. Although disagreements and challenges arose between Ray and Pam, renegotiations of his care plan occurred on a regular basis and resolutions were found. In addition, Ray attended regular case reviews with the multidisciplinary team and thus felt fully involved in treatment decisions.

This example demonstrates the centrality of values to the relationship between the nurse and patient. Ray felt part of decisions and Pam ensured that she respected his values in the way she worked with him. Pam worked with him using skills of negotiation, openness, honesty, and consultation to ensure that their agreed contract was fulfilled. The imperfect duties of informed flexibility, mutuality, transparency, negotiation and sympathetic presence are evident. The community hospital in which this case example was situated has invested much time in creating a context to support person centeredness.

Conclusions

This paper presents a framework for person-centered practice that holds as central the concept of autonomy as authentic consciousness. By viewing person centeredness in this way, an understanding of caring relationships is achieved that is not based on one person being the final arbiter of decisions but that is, instead, set within a framework of negotiation based on an individual's values base. The nurse as a facilitator of an individual's authentic consciousness engages in a process of dynamic caring that maintains autonomy at a time when for many older people, their sense of independence is under greatest threat.

References

1. Phillipson C, Biggs S. Modernity and identity. Theories and perspectives in the study of older adults. *Journal of Aging and Identity* 1998;3:11–23.
2. Kitwood T. Dementia Reconsidered: The Person Comes First. Milton Keynes: Open University Press, 1997.
3. Nolan M, Davies S, Grant G. Working with Older People and their Families: Key Issues in Policy and Practice. Buckingham: Open University Press, 2001.
4. Dewing J. From ritual to relationship: A person-centered approach to consent in qualitative research with older people who have a dementia. Dementia 2002;1:157–171.
5. Department of Health. The National Services Framework for Older People. London: HMSO, 2001.
6. Richards DAJ. Rights and Autonomy. Ethics 1981;92:3–20.
7. Williams B, Grant G. Defining "people-centeredness": Making the implicit explicit. Health Social Care in the Community 1998;6:84–94.
8. Hope T, Fulford KW. The Oxford Practice Skills Project: Teaching ethics, law and communication skills to clinical medical students. Journal of Medical Ethics 1994;20:229–234.
9. McCormack B. Negotiating Partnerships with Older People: A Person-Centered Approach. Aldershot: Ashgate Press, 2001.
10. Gadamer HG. Truth and Method. London: Sheed & Ward, 1993.
11. Benner P. From Novice to Expert: Excellence and Power in Clinical Nursing Practice. CA: Addison-Wesley, 1984.
12. Jasper MA. Expert: A discussion of the implications of the concept as used in nursing. Journal of Advanced Nursing 1994;20:769–776.
13. Greenwood J, King M. Some surprising similarities in the clinical reasoning of "expert" and "novice" orthopaedic nurses: report of a study using verbal protocols and protocol analyses. Journal of Advanced Nursing 1995;22:907–913.
14. Dick JPR, Guiloff RJ, Stewart A, Blackstock J. Mini-mental state examination in neurological patients. Journal of Neurology, Neurosurgery and Psychiatry 1984;47:496–498.
15. Drew P, Heritage J. Talk at Work: Interaction in Institutional Settings. Cambridge: Cambridge University Press, 1992.
16. Bergum V. Being a phenomenological researcher. In: Morse J (ed.). Qualitative Nursing Research: A Contemporary

Dialogue. London: Sage Publications, 1991; 55–71.

17. McCormack B. Autonomy and the relationship between nurses and older people. Aging Society 2001; 21.

18. Gadow S. Existential advocacy. Philosophical foundations of nursing. In: Spicker SF, Gadow S (eds.). Nursing: Images and ideals—Opening Dialogue with the Humanities. New York: Springer, 1980; 85.

19. Department of Health. Caring for Older People: A Nursing Priority. Report of the Standing Nursing and Midwifery Advisory Committee. London: Department of Health, 2001. No. 23668.

20. Davies S, Laker S, Ellis L. Promoting autonomy and independence for older people within nursing practice: a literature review. Journal of Advanced Nursing 1997;26:408–417.

21. Davies S, Nolan M, Brown J, Wilson F. Dignity on the Ward: Promoting Excellence in Care. London: Help the Aged, 1999.

22. MacIntyre A. After Virtue: a Study in Moral Theory. London: Duckworth, 1992.

23. Sullivan RJ. Immanuel Kant's Moral Theory. Cambridge: Cambridge University Press, 1990.

24. Benner P, Wrubel J. The Primacy of Caring: Stress and Coping in Health and Illness. Wokingham, UK: Addison-Wesley, 1989.

25. Heidegger M. Being and Time. Oxford: Basil Blackwell, 1990.

26. Boykin A, Schoenhofer S. Nursing as Caring: A Model for Transforming Practice. New York: National League for Nursing Press, 1993.

27. Johns CC. Becoming an Effective Practitioner through Guided Reflection. Unpublished PhD Thesis. Open University, Milton Keynes, 1997.

28. Johns C. Caring through a reflective lens: giving meaning to being a reflective practitioner. Nursing Inquiry 1998;5: 18–24.

29. Bishop V. Clinical Supervision in Practice: Some Questions, Answers and Guidelines. Basingstoke: Macmillan, 1998.

30. Robbins DA. Ethical and Legal Issues in Home Health and Long Term Care: Challenges and Solutions. MD: Aspen Publishers, 1996.

31. Meyers DT. Self, Society and Personal Choice. New York: Columbia University Press, 1989.

32. Buchanan AE, Brock DW. Deciding for Others: the Ethics of Surrogate Decision Making. Cambridge: Cambridge University Press, 1989.

33. Agich GJ. Autonomy and Long-Term Care. Oxford: Oxford University Press, 1993.

34. Seedhouse D. Health: The Foundations of Achievement. Chichester: John Wiley & Sons, 1986.

35. McCormack B, Kitson A, Harvey G, et al. Getting evidence into practice: the meaning of 'context'. Journal of Advanced Nursing 2002;38:94–104.

36. Rycroft-Malone J, Harvey G, Kitson A, et al. Getting evidence into practice: Ingredients for change. Nursing Standard 2002;29:38–43.

37. Johns C. Unraveling the dilemmas within everyday nursing practice. Nursing Ethics: An International Journal for Health Care Professionals 1999;6: 287–298.

38. Yarling RR, McEelmurry BJ. The moral foundation of nursing. In: Pence T, Cantrell J (eds.). Ethics in Nursing: an Anthology. New York: National League for Nursing, 1990; 335–342.

39. Holm S. Problems in Clinical Practice: The Ethical Reasoning of Health Care Professionals. Manchester: Manchester University Press, 1997.

40. Johns CC. The Burford NDU Model: Caring in Practice. Oxford: Blackwell Science, 1994.

Appendix 1

Principles for Action

1. Make explicit the care agenda.
2. Recognize that the questioning style adopted affects the ability of the older patient to contribute to the setting of the care agenda and their contribution to a conversation.
3. Be aware that actions to achieve one outcome might have an effect on a previously unrecognized need.
4. Have a repertoire of interactional approaches that will enable patient decision making and participation in the planning of care plans.
5. Pose specific and clearly formulated questions that have a clear aim.
6. Respect individuals' important routines in daily life and negotiate new components of the care agenda each day.
7. Be aware that older patients depend on professionals to minimize or prevent constraints on their autonomy.
8. Listen to patients and allow them to tell their story as a legitimate part of assessment processes.
9. Wherever possible, encourage patients to identify solutions for existing problems and care needs, set within negotiated parameters of risk taking.
10. Get to know patients and establish a negotiated level of engagement before decisions about degrees of risk taking are made.
11. For informed decision making to be facilitated in a patient-centered way, refrain from imbuing decision-making processes with one's own values.
12. Suspend the use of prior knowledge about a patient and their social context until they have been enabled to tell their story.
13. Recognize that the uniqueness of patients' experiences versus nurses' familiarity with organizational routines limits a patient-centered approach to decision making.
14. Accord the patient's perceptions of their care situation equal status as those of health care professionals.
15. Patients' subjective views of their lives should be respected in decision making.
16. To facilitate patient participation, understand and be confident with the boundaries of one's decision-making potential.
17. Adopt a patient-centered approach to risk assessment and risk taking.

18. Be explicit about the intent and motivation for action and the parameters within which decisions are set.
19. Maximize patients' independence through the balancing of patient narrative with established care policies and procedures.
20. Make decision within a framework of negotiation with clearly established care goals that are regularly reinforced and reviewed.
21. Make time to help patients to integrate new care decisions and options into their already established care program.
22. Acknowledge and facilitate patients' emotional responses as an important part of facilitating patient participation.
23. Create opportunities for reciprocity in relationships with patients.

24. Do not allow age-related perceptions of an individual's ability to limit patient participation.
25. Help patients to see beyond their own limited expectations of their involvement in care and their deference to others.
26. Continuously reinforce the value of patients' decisions.
27. Facilitate patients' emotional coping ability in order to enhance their independence.
28. Recognize that while patients want to be consulted about care decisions they do not always want to be the final arbiter of decisions.
29. Recognize that older people should have their beliefs and values considered in the making of decisions but patients being the final arbiter of decisions is not of prime importance.

CHAPTER 18

Relational Practice and Nursing Obligations

Gweneth H. Doane, RN, PhD
Colleen Varcoe, RN, PhD

Nursing relationships and the enactment of nursing values and goals in contemporary healthcare contexts are becoming increasingly challenging. Using a relational inquiry lens we examine the interface of relationships, ethics, and effective nursing practice and the way in which personal and contextual elements continuously influence and shape nursing relationships in many ways. The nursing obligations underpinning relational practice are examined, and the way in which relational inquiry can enhance nurses' ability to navigate through the highly complex, multifaceted, and contextually dependent moments of contemporary nursing practice is illustrated.

Key words: *context, difficulty, ethics, intentionality, nurse–patient relationships, reflexivity, relational inquiry, relational obligation.*

By the close of the 20th century the image of the "lady with the lamp" administering tender loving care to a wounded soul had faded. More contemporary images depict nurses rushing between too many patients, grappling with technology, paperwork, and limited resources. These changing images reflect not only a shift in the nature of nursing practice but the changing contexts of health care. Moreover, they highlight the need for broader understandings of contemporary nursing relationships, including the integral connection between "therapeutic" relationships and "ethical" relationships.

Relationships in nursing typically have been understood in congruence with liberal individualism and its companion paternalism; that is, the relationship between the

Source: Doane, G., Varcoe, C. Relational practice and nursing obligations. Advances in Nursing Science. 30 (3): 192-205. Reprinted by permission of and copyright © 2007 Lippincott Williams & Wilkins, Inc.

individual nurse and individual patient is seen as the relationship of importance. The nurse is considered as an autonomous agent with free will who is able to make choices. There is an assumption of therapeutic intent on the part of the nurse, and responsibility for achieving health outcomes through "good" relationships is vested in the nurse. As Browne[1] argues, such ideologies underpin much of the nursing theory.

Understanding relationships in this way ascribes responsibility to the nurse to foster therapeutic relationships and thus to provide better care and achieve better outcomes. Supporting this understanding is a wealth of literature focused on concepts and behaviors that have the potential to enhance relational engagement. For example, concepts such as respect, presencing, trust, mutuality, and so forth are frequent topics in the relationship literature in nursing. Less common in this literature are discussions of the multitude of factors that shape and, at times, determine the connection between any individual patient and nurse. Yet, these other personal and contextual factors frequently make trusting, respectful, and therapeutic relationships challenging. For example, work load, patient acuity, staffing ratios, and supportive (or unsupportive) collegial relationships can shape whether a nurse even views "presencing" with a particular patient as an option. Furthermore, a nurse's personal identity and social location shape his or her interpretations, willingness, and capacity to be in relation with particular patients in particular situations.

In this chapter we argue that although nurses are handed the responsibility and obligation for therapeutic nurse–patient relationships and given descriptive indicators of "good" relationship behaviors, often missing is an examination of how nurses might meet this nursing obligation within highly complex, multifaceted, and contextually dependent moments. Specifically, we wish to consider nurse–patient relationships using a relational lens that takes multiple contexts and relationships into account. Moreover, we highlight the way in which familiar relationship concepts such as trust, empathy, and respect work in concert with ethical concepts such as obligation, responsibility, and "good" action. We critically examine the concept of obligation and, using a relational understanding, suggest three obligations underlying nursing relationships. It is our contention that responsive, compassionate, therapeutic relationships and ethical and competent nursing practice are integrally connected and that relational inquiry can support the enactment of both. Our intent is to examine the way in which a relational lens of inquiry can enhance nurses' capacity and ability to navigate through the challenges and competing obligations of contemporary relationships in health care.

Connecting Relationships, Ethics, and Nursing Effectiveness

Gastmans[2] contends that relationship is "a foundational condition of nursing practice."[(p. 495)] Tschudin[3] describes relationships as "salutogenic"[(p. 35)] in the sense that they contribute to health more essentially than we often are aware. Similarly, Tarlier[4] contends that responsive relationships are one way in which nurses "make a difference" and influence clinical outcomes.

Tarlier[4] outlines that within the nursing literature, "good" relationships are conceptualized as being founded on three essential elements: respect, trust, and mutuality. Respect includes five characteristics (1) treating others as inherently worthy and equal, (2) acceptance of others, (3) willingness to listen to others, (4) genuine attempts to understand other's situation, and (5) sincerity.[5] Trust is developed through the processes inherent in respect. At the same time, trust rests on the patient's belief that the nurse will assist him or her in achieving a good outcome.[4] Baier[6] defines *trust* as "reliance on others' competence and willingness to look after, rather than harm things one cares about which are entrusted to their care." [(p. 25)] Baier[6] describes trust as involving a "reliance on another's good will not just dependable habits."[(p. 234)] Mutuality refers to a relationship as a negotiated, collaborative process where both people participate, choose, and act.

Armstrong[7] describes that nurse–patient relationships typically have been viewed in terms of human interactions, communication skills, and collaborative action. However, describing the significance of relationships to ethical nursing practice, Bergum[8] purports that in essence, relationships are a moral space where one enacts not only responsiveness but also responsibility. Similarly, Nortvedt[9] argues that nurse–patient relationships are

the site where moral responsibilities and professional duties are generated. As Gilligan[10] described, "the most basic questions about human living—how to live and what to do—are fundamentally questions about human relations, because people's lives are deeply connected psychologically, economically, and politically."[(p. 14)] Everyday interactions between patients and nurses, between nurses and other healthcare practitioners, and between nurses and their practice contexts involve complicated networks of mutual dependencies. Bergum[8] contends that "with relational space as the location of enacting morality, we need to consider ethics in every situation, every encounter, and with every patient."[(p. 487)]

A review of the literature reveals that overall being in a "good" relationship not only is considered more responsive to others in the sense of being more respectful and trustworthy but also results in more ethical and effective care. It is this integral connection of relationships, ethics, and effective nursing practice that we wish to highlight and explore further. Within both the relationship literature and the ethics literature, it is argued that nursing practice requires a deep sensitivity to what is significant to patients in particular situations. Unfortunately, there has been little integration of these different bodies of literature. Subsequently, there has been very little discussion about what is required to develop and enact that sensitivity and/or the knowledge, capacities, and skills required for ethical and responsive nursing relationships within the complexities of current healthcare milieus. For example, as social inequities deepen and neoliberal ideologies hold individuals responsible for their own health and well-being regardless of how poverty, disability, remote geographical locations, or other inequities determine health, notions of obligation, responsibility, accountability, and efficiency are as vital to nursing relationships as are notions of compassion, responsiveness, trust, and respect. Thus, nurses require a broader understanding of relationships and their significance to ethical nursing practice.

An Example: Interaction in the Emergency Department

During a long wait in the emergency waiting room to have a laceration sutured, I watched an elderly woman and her mature adult daughter get increasingly impatient "to be seen" and have the mother's injured leg attended to. At one point the daughter went to the reception window to declare in an exasperated voice that they had been waiting for close to 3 hours, she was not sure how much longer her mother could tolerate sitting in the chair, and that if they were not seen soon they would just leave. The nurse behind the window replied in an assertive voice that the emergency policy was to see patients in order of medical priority not waiting time and they would be seen as soon as it was possible. Shortly afterward I was called into the stretcher area. A few minutes later as I lay on the stretcher after having my laceration sutured, another nurse popped her head into my cubicle to say she would be with me in a minute to apply a dressing but she was first going to assist a patient onto a stretcher.

From behind the curtain I could hear the other patient was the elderly woman. As the nurse assisted her onto the stretcher the nurse exclaimed, "That's quite a gash on your leg." In response, the elderly woman began to tell the story of falling at home. The nurse quickly interjected, cutting the story off by stating, "Well at least it isn't too serious and we will be able to suture that up fine." In response, the woman ignored the nurse's words and once again began to tell the story of her fall. Once again the nurse interjected to keep the focus of the discussion on the leg wound. At this point the daughter spoke up, saying "she fell 2 days ago and just called me this afternoon—imagine she was home by herself with this and she didn't even call me."

As I lay in the next cubicle I could "hear" the nurse in that moment making an important relational decision. There were a few seconds of silence (where I believe she was weighing her promise to return to me with the more compelling obligation to listen and respond to the elderly woman and her daughter) and then she replied, "You live alone do you?" Through these few words the nurse entered into a relationship in a meaningful way, simultaneously letting the woman know she was "seen" and acknowledging the significance of her injury within the larger contextual–personal underpinnings of her life. Although the "easily fixed wound" was the physical evidence of her trauma, there were much more meaningful elements that needed attention relationally for healing to occur. As the elderly woman accepted the nurse's invitation and began to reveal the "whole" of her experience through her story, she communicated her shock in falling, her fear and vulnerability as an elderly woman living on her own, and the fierce independence, strength, and capacity she had. By creating the relational space for the woman to tell her story, the nurse provided an opportunity for the elderly woman to weave the various elements of her experience together and narrate herself and her situation into a manageable form. By the end of the story (which took a matter of approximately 2–3 minutes), the woman concluded much as the nurse had initially concluded—that the wound was easily fixed and she would be fine to return home on her own.

This story exemplifies the significance of a nurse–patient relationship and the profound difference it can make in promoting health and healing. At the same time, the story highlights the competing and, at times, conflicting obligations through which nurses find themselves navigating. Although the elderly woman had come to the emergency department to have her leg sutured, what was most meaningful and what she needed to sort through was what the fall and injury meant within the context of her life. That is, as an elderly woman living alone, the fall underscored her vulnerability and called her independence into question. Thus, for the relationship to be therapeutic and nursing practice to be effective in addressing the woman's health and healing needs, the relational space for this contextual understanding needed to be created. However, the story also highlights how personal and contextual elements (e.g.,

a nurse's sense of responsibility, feeling obligated to another waiting patient, the normative values of healthcare culture) shape what happens in any nursing moment and how the pressures of competing demands and values can lead to certain things being privileged over others (e.g., privileging treatment and procedures over the promotion of health and healing). The story also draws attention to the competing obligations that nurses may face as they try to "do good" within the competing values, demands, and expectations. The nurse in the story was obligated to both patients— yet attending to one meant not immediately fulfilling her promise to the other. At the same time, emergency department norms pressurized her to function in certain ways.

As nurses, we are obligated to ensure that our nursing actions promote health and healing and are ethical and safe. However, determining what actually constitutes "ethical," "safe," and "health/healing promoting" practices, in particular situations, can be challenging because the specific behaviors and responses are arrived at in the particularities of the relational moment—as we engage with, and respond to, specific patients in particular situations. For example, promoting the health and healing of the elderly woman in the above story required the nurse to create the relational space for the woman to reach the "outcome" that she was able to continue to function independently in her life. In contrast, as a patient in the next cubicle, the nurse's pleasant demeanor and dressing application were sufficient to address my health and healing needs.

Relationships, Ethics, and Nursing Obligations

Nursing obligations are the site where the integral connection between responsive relationships and ethical practice comes to the foreground. Peter and Liaschenko[11] highlight that proximity to others is one way nurses understand what their obligations are. "Proximity beckons moral agents to act, and therefore has an impact on moral responsiveness."[11(p. 219)]

Armstrong[7] describes that the concept of obligation "runs deep in contemporary western society"[(p. 115)] and has dominated much of existing ethical theory and practice. Subsequently, obligation-based ethics (e.g., principle approaching grounded in consequentialism and/or deontology) have been popular within nursing and remain so.[7] Within the philosophical and ethical literature, obligations have been conceptualized as external to the person[7] and most often are articulated in the form of codes or principles such as the obligations of beneficence, autonomy, and justice. As externally derived and sanctioned entities, obligations in the form of codes are expected to reinforce professional and societal values and to give coherence to professional behavior by disclosing the profession's values and duties.[12] The norms included in codes are determined by the nursing philosophy of a particular country and at the same time are influenced by the moral problems nurses face in their everyday work.[13]

One of the main criticisms of existing conceptualizations of obligation-based ethics and the principles/codes that arise from them is that they usually present overly simplistic understandings of ethical practice. For example, obligation-based ethics focus on right and wrong action[7] and theoretically assume a definitive "right" response to a situation.[12] At the same time, implying that a right answer and/or response can be determined, most existing codes that express nursing obligations do not discuss how nurses might actually enact their ethical obligations in their everyday practice.[7,12,14,15]

Codes are usually confined to idealistic prescriptions that neither explain how the concepts relate to actual practice nor provide guidance for particular nurses in particular relational moments.[12] Furthermore, within extant liberal orientations, codes of ethics tend to promote the values of individualism. In the U.S. and Canadian contexts, respectively, Bekemeier and Butterfield[16] and Kirkham and Browne[17] argue that codes of ethics encourage us to presume that Western societies are essentially egalitarian, and although we are directed to be aware of broader social issues, we are not committed by our professional values to action.

Obligations as External Entities

At the same time that existing conceptualizations of nursing obligations have been criticized for not offering practical direction, the conceptualization of obligation as an external and universal entity has been criticized for failing to address important features that shape ethical practice, including context, historical changes, culture, character, and relationship.[12] In not addressing these features, obligation-based ethics cover certain types of questions that are integral to everyday nursing practice and may also disguise the lack of agreement about values that dominate nursing situations.[12] For example, Provis and Stack[18] describe how caring work is ripe with conflicting obligations and how the interface of personal and organizational obligations can cause uncertainty about what is the "right thing to do" when these obligations run counter to each other. [(p. 6)] They offer the example of a caregiver who, interpreting her use of bath towels through the values and norms of the organization, worried that she was being "extravagant": "You're always told how much it costs for linen and that sort of thing . . . I like to put an extra towel over their shoulders to keep them warm while I dry them with the other towel, so that may not be cost conscious." Even in the smallest moments, various obligations pull us in different directions. Yet obligation-based ethics do not address what happens when nurses are obligated in conflicting ways, when, for example, their obligations to different patients are in tension and/or when their obligation to their organization is at odds with the obligations they feel to patients.

Interestingly, Pattison[14] highlights that although obligation-based ethics and, in particular, ethical codes rest on the assumption of the "thoughtful, autonomous 'ethical' practitioner who possesses independent critical judgment, practical wisdom, and the capacity to act responsibly and with regard to the hinterland of wider human values and principles,"[(p. 7)] codes of obligation may actually militate against the emergence and survival of such practitioners. For example, following a review of "the inherent ethical defects of a number of codes," Pattison[14] concluded that codes may "do little to develop or support the active independent critical judgement and discernment . . . (and) may, in fact, be in danger of engendering confusion, passivity, apathy and even immorality."[(p. 8)] Indeed, in our teaching of ethics, despite our attempts to support enactment of all values simultaneously, nursing students (both new to nursing and experienced nurses) using codes often revert to a "pick one value" mentality, wherein they use one value (e.g., such as one related to autonomy) to override other values and support their chosen direction rather than guide their choices.

Similarly, research has highlighted how viewing ethics and obligation as something that is rationally determined outside of one's own practice can lead to confusion and inaction.[19,20] Nurses have not been alone in articulating the limitations of existing conceptualizations of obligation. Within the broader field of philosophy, writers offer criticisms and alternative conceptualizations. In particular, Caputo[21,22] addresses the need for an understanding of obligation that raises questions rather than prescribes answers, opens space for the complexity and difficulty of ethical decision-making, and offers direction for how ethics and "good" relationships might be lived within the challenges of everyday life. Caputo's reframing of obligation has informed our view of obligations and relationships in nursing.

Reframing Obligation

Bauman[23] describes that within philosophy, ethics has been dominated by a modernist approach to the search for truth that has focused on looking for absolutes and universals of morality. According to Bauman,[23] modern thinkers believed that rather than being a natural trait of human life, morality was something that needed to be created and injected into human conduct. Obligation, conceptualized through this universal perspective, resulted in a decontextual, depersonalized understanding of obligation. It also resulted in ethical challenges being responded to through normative regulation.[23] In contrast, Caputo's[21] discussion locates obligation and ethics in the relational moment, for example, in the moment when a nurse finds him- or herself in the midst of people, contexts, and multiple, competing demands. Drawing on deconstructive hermeneutics, Caputo calls for a way of understanding and responding to obligations that entails both interpretation and deconstruction.

In contrast to the understanding of obligations as something external to the person, Caputo contends that obligations are local events—they are matters of flesh and blood. According to Caputo, obligation is the feeling that comes over us in very binding ways when others need our help or support and we feel bound to respond. "When I feel obliged something demands my response. It is not a matter of working through a set of principles to conclude whether one is obliged."[21(p. 22)] Caputo asks, "Does one really 'conclude' that one is obliged, or does one not just find oneself obliged, without so much as having been consulted or asked for one's consent?" Caputo's description echoes the experience of the nurse of the emergency department in the above story. Although the nurse initially attempted to extricate herself from the situation, she ultimately felt bound to listen to and create the relational space for the elderly woman to "do her healing."

Although one may find one's self obliged, one's personal values and contextual constraints may mute the sensing of those obligations. For example, initially the emergency department nurse in the above example seemed more "bound" by her obligation to the organizational norms. Similarly, how the nurse values elderly persons will shape her sense of her obligations in this case. What if the elderly woman had been, for example, intoxicated? Would the nurse's sense of obligation and her actions change? Should they change? This example highlights how determining our obligation to particular patients in particular moments of relationship involves looking carefully at our own responses, "thinking hard"[7(p. 115)] about the nursing values and obligations to which we are committed, and inquiring into the particularities of the moment and the various elements that are shaping that moment to ensure that our relational goals and behaviors are aligned with the nursing values and obligations we espouse. "Thinking hard" includes thinking about our own biases and to whom we are obligated. It is our contention that nurses are obligated to all persons, most immediately on an individual basis to all those within their care but also collectively to those who require their care. Thus, a relational conception of obligation applied to nursing relationships suggests that new conceptualizations of nursing obligations and relationships are required.

Bringing a Relational Inquiry Lens to Relationships

Although existing conceptualizations of relationships that emphasize concepts such as respect, trust, and mutuality offer a good starting point for therapeutic relationships, a relational inquiry lens expands the understanding and thereby the potential of relationships. This inquiry lens highlights that enhancing nurse–patient relationships requires more than individual nurses taking up caring attitudes or presencing behaviors. In contrast to a decontextual view of relationships that considers the nurse to be an autonomous agent who exercises free and intentional choice, relational inquiry foregrounds the way in which personal and contextual forces shape both nurses' and patients' capacities for relational connection and thereby health and healing. Relational inquiry involves a reflexive process where one is always assuming and looking for the ways in which people, situations, contexts, environments, and processes are integrally connecting and shaping each other. This inquiry process rests on the assumption that people are contextual beings who exist in relation with others and with social, cultural, political, and historical processes. Within this contextual existence, each person has a unique personal, sociohistorical location that affects and shapes that person's identity, experience, interpretations, and way of being in the world. It is assumed that the values, knowledge, attitudes, practices, and structures that dominate the sociocultural world within each person's life are passed on through relational interactions. Subsequently, people's experiences, interpretations, and actions are products of a multitude of relational interactions and processes. In this way people are both shaped by and shape other people's responses, situations, experiences, and contexts. Not only nurses but patients, their families, other healthcare providers, and actors beyond the immediate healthcare context such as policymakers and the media continuously negotiate and shape one another. Nursing practice as a process of inquiry focuses on the question "How might I most responsively and effectively be in relation to promote health and healing?"[24]

Using this inquiry lens, relationships among people are viewed as sites, opportunities, and/or vehicles for meaningful experience and response. It is possible to be in a relationship with another person without practicing responsively in the sense we are discussing. For example, one can enter into a relationship in ways that distance or objectify people ("the GI bleeding in room 8" or "at-risk youth"), as is the case in many healthcare relationships. Thus, there is an important distinction between relationships that are determined and regulated primarily by the adoption of dominant social customs and practices and relationships that are purposefully shaped through a relational inquiry where one consciously chooses within the apparent possibilities for action, or even works to create new possibilities. Overall, a relational inquiry directs a more in-depth look at the values, experiences, goals, and concerns shaping action within particular moments of practice and a conscious consideration of possibilities and intentional, responsive action.

Significance of Context

Relational inquiry requires that we move beyond the surface(s) of people, situations, and relationships—beyond the "iceberg" pattern of interaction where a substantial portion of the elements shaping the interaction is unseen and/or ignored. For example, the iceberg pattern of relationship may include a nurse engaging with a smiling, friendly demeanor while going about the tasks of morning care yet never really connecting with the patient in a meaningful way to inquire into what the patient is experiencing. Although a friendly, cheerful demeanor can certainly be responsive, it may also serve as a veneer that at best covers over and at worst does not allow space for people to be themselves, express their experience, and/or reveal what is particularly salient. A cheerful smile and a friendly demeanor can be used to effectively dismiss a patient's request for care that a nurse does not believe he or she has time to provide.

Particular contexts contribute to this iceberg pattern of relationship because the normative patterning within those contexts cues certain behaviors and responses. For example, healthcare contexts contain strong messages about what is and is not of importance. The business-driven, economic, cost-efficient values combined with the devaluing of nurses for being "too emotional" or "too involved" offer strong pressure to pattern one's actions in ways that enable the organization to work.[7] Similarly, the intricate combination of conflicting values, goals, and desires that the particular nurse brings to the relationship can serve to contribute to the iceberg pattern of interaction. For example, if a patient is in pain, the situation is ambiguous, and/or there is no clear-cut best way to respond, nurses may pull back as a result of their own vulnerability and uncertainty.[25] If they are unable to "make it better" or "stop the tears," nurses might focus their attention on other more controllable and concrete tasks. Or, as a result of the combination of practicing within a service model, "fix-it" culture, and their own compassionate desire to alleviate suffering, nurses may take up the treatment–cure values and goals and shape their relationships with patients accordingly. A nurse may focus on a laceration rather than the lacerated person. Feeling a sense of responsibility and a desire to "help," they may attempt to use relationships as a means to an end: to do, to treat and fix the patient, or to meet the needs of the organization.[2,8]

Within these dynamics, nurses may be inclined to distance themselves from situations they see as "unfixable"—such as people who under liberal ideology are seen as creating their own suffering, people with addictions, people in poverty, women in abusive relationships, and so on. Relational inquiry requires us to look beyond the tip of the iceberg when engaging with patients because, whether nurses are aware of the influence of contextual and personal elements or not and whether nurses attend to them or not, those elements shape the health and healing experience.[24,26]

Relational Inquiry and Nursing Obligations

Such an inquiry process is underpinned by three nursing obligations, all of which are predicated on the overarching obligation to all persons, regardless of their circumstances or characteristics: the obligation (1) to be reflexive and intentional, (2) to open the relational space for difficulty, and (3) to act at all levels to effect the potential for health and healing. Although for the purpose of discussion we separate these three obligations, it is important to emphasize that not only do these obligations overlap and complement each other, but they form a synergistic whole. For example, being reflexive and intentional provides the access to and a way of being in difficulty. Similarly, acting at all levels affects the contextual and personal factors that impede reflexive and intentional practice and so forth.

Obligation to be Reflexive and Intentional

Nortvedt[9] contends that "*relationship itself is a source of special responsibilities and professional qualities.*"[(p. 116)] Through relationships, nurses see patients' needs and interests

as particular reasons to act.[9] However, seeing patients' needs and interests as particular reasons to act requires conscious and intentional participation and, as we have argued, involves looking beyond the surface of people and situations. For example, in the story above the nurse did not initially respond to the elderly lady's need to tell the story of her fall. Furthermore, looking beyond the surface requires looking critically through the veil created by biases (such as ageism), structures (such as how health care is organized), and ideologies (such as individual responsibility).

Similar to Walker's[27] description of moral oblivion where there is a lack of awareness of the moral demands that are being made, when nurses are oblivious to the relational elements (e.g., the personal and contextual elements) shaping their decisions and actions, they are more likely to be at the mercy of those influences and thereby less likely to exercise their clinical judgment effectively. That is, they are more likely to be practicing *in relational oblivion*. Practicing without such awareness impacts nursing care in a very practical way and ultimately makes meeting nursing obligations all but impossible.

As Provis and Stack[18] report, sensitivity and compassion are often at odds with organizational directives. Nurses increasingly find themselves rationing their care in ways that marginalize meaningful relational engagement.[9,28] Nortvedt[9] contends that what is often central to nursing practice is not how to give the best care for one's patients but how to minimize harm to patients created by sociocontextual circumstances. For the emergency department nurse, apparently it was her believed sense of obligation that overrode the competing demands of a patient in the next cubicle and the organizational press to treat the physical injuries of patients quickly and efficiently. And, this obligation sparked the nurse to reflexively consider her options and intentionally decide to create the relational space for the woman to tell her story. As Bauman described, "when competing moral demands arise in the moment, it is the moral self which feels, moves and acts within the context of that ambiguity."[23](p. 34)

In essence, Caputo's[21] deconstructive hermeneutic approach to obligation requires nurses to be humanly involved and interpreting yet simultaneously critically analyzing and at times deconstructing the values, structures, and processes that constrain ethical nursing responsiveness. This reflexive process requires acknowledgment of the ambiguity of relationships, ethics, and nursing care. Moving beyond both prescriptive regulation and personal interpretation, it involves the nurse "activating herself as a knowledgeable practitioner"[29](p. 255) to critically examine the values, goals, and intents shaping the nursing moment and ultimately relationships. It involves using not only knowledge and information but also practical judgment, and approximates what Aristotle termed *phronesis*.[22,30]

Simply put, reflexivity enlists the moral self and simultaneously enlists nursing knowledge, experience, and judgment. In so doing, reflexive inquiry moves nurses to look at both what they are doing and how they are doing it. It creates the space for a self-conscious consideration of the relational means and ends and consideration of how nurses

are conserving, renewing, inventing, and/or changing these means and ends. For example, a nurse might more consciously weigh conserving towels in relation to conserving warmth and comfort of her patients and in relation to the consequences of providing (or not) such comfort. As such, relationships are enhanced through a reflexive process of intention, attention, interpretation, critical scrutiny, and reconstruction. That is, relational practice involves a conscious intent to act toward the espoused values and goals of nursing, attention to the particularities of people and situations, a critical consideration of one's own and others' interpretations, and very often a reconstruction of decisions, actions, and norms that may be at odds with the values and goals of nursing.

Obligation to Open Relational Space for Difficulty

As nurses respond to their obligation to be reflexive and intentional, they simultaneously find themselves obligated to "be in difficulty." As they look beyond the surface of relational encounters and begin to see people and situations through a relational lens, they find themselves in close proximity to and/or experiencing the inherent difficulties of health and healing situations. For example, they may come into closer proximity with suffering, uncertainty, and/or conflict. Similarly, they may find themselves experiencing intense emotional responses—both their own and of others. Caputo[21] describes the challenge of being in the abyss of difficulty and the suffering that is part of that experience. He describes this difficulty and suffering as something that "humbles us, brings us up short, stops us in our tracks . . . something which both strikes us down and draws us near."[21(p. 275)] At the same time, Caputo contends that within the abyss of difficulty[22(p. 29)]

> There is suffering and there is suffering. Short-term suffering may easily belong to long-term flourishing, to a larger economy of pain and suffering which is understood by anyone who understands the economy of life itself. To spare others pain, and hard work and suffering may easily mean to spare them everything that gives their life worth and a greater long-term felicity.

It is for this reason that Caputo[21] argues for the importance of being in difficulty as it presents itself and of entering the abyss of difficulty and suffering not to succumb or surrender but to be "instructed by the abyss, to let the abyss be, to let it play itself out."[(p. 278)] It is only by opening the relational space to be in the difficulty that one is able to move beyond breaking down or detaching.[31]

Along a similar vein, Mitchell and Bunkers[32] argue that the danger to nurses is not in witnessing difficulty and suffering but rather in turning away when suffering appears. In contrast to others who have argued that experiencing suffering and difficulty over time may lead to what is discussed in nursing literature variously as "burn out," "care giver fatigue,"[33–35] or, in the case of violence, vicarious trauma,[36–38] these authors

support Caputo's contention that if one enters into nursing situations without the need to fix or make the difficulty/suffering better but rather to open, be in, witness, and be instructed by it, the difficulty/suffering can be a pathway toward meeting the relational obligations to both our patients and ourselves.

Nursing has long focused on suffering, at both individual and social levels. Yet within the neoliberal dominance of Western thinking, where individualism is central and biomedicine powerful, suffering that arises from physical pathology has received greater attention. Our obligation to be in the difficulty also extends to examining and acting on suffering as it arises through relational dynamics. To return again to the situation of the elderly woman with the laceration, the example illustrates how understanding the way institutional power operates to limit the nurse's time to attend to the woman's needs allows the nurse to work against these dynamics to alleviate rather than be complicit with or further suffering. Furthermore, the nurse can inquire as to how other social forces, such as ageism or poverty or gender, might be operating in this woman's life to foster suffering and might be operating to shape the nurse's own sense of her obligations and her actions.

Difficulty and/or our experience of suffering is not separate from who we are—from our own interpretive frames and the interpretive frames that dominate the larger social world in which we live and practice.[31] How we understand any situation and how we define it and attend to it are subject to our individual and collective understandings and interpretations and the systems that shape these understandings/interpretations. There is a tendency to think of difficulty and suffering as something negative and as something to be avoided. However, difficulty is at the heart of ethically responsive nursing care. Framing difficulty as an inherent feature of nursing relationships paves the way, not only for more ethical but also for more effective and efficient nursing relationships. For example, the emergency department nurse in the story above reflexively and intentionally created the relational space for the difficulty within the situation to "play itself out" (e.g., she opened the space for the woman's fear, vulnerability, and the nurse's own competing obligations to come into relation), and in a matter of 2 to 3 minutes she not only supported the woman's health and healing but also responded to her own feelings and needs by making a nursing decision to provide the care she believed was required. Thus, she was able to conclude the encounter with her identity as an ethical "good" nurse intact.[8]

Understanding "difficulty and suffering" as windows into meaningful relationships and as the base for ethical decision-making and responsive nursing care creates the relational space for nurses to better understand multiple and competing obligations, goals, and perspectives, to raise questions and inquire into the particularities of each situation, and to ultimately develop the clarity and courage to act in health-promoting ways.

Obligation to Act at All Levels to Effect Health and Healing

Bergum[8] contends that attention to relationship as an ethical endeavor has a way of dismantling the distinctions of different levels of care: "What happens at the bedside is not cut off from the broader levels, but is part and parcel of the same system."[(p. 487)] Because each nursing moment is shaped by our own actions, by the actions and responses of others, and by the contexts within which we work, relational practice involves the nursing obligation to act at all levels, including the intrapersonal, interpersonal, and contextual levels. Developing relational nursing practice requires that we continually think through not only what it is we are doing, but also what it is that is shaping and influencing what we are doing. At the same time, it requires that we closely examine how we are responding in particular situations and intentionally act toward nursing values, goals, and obligations.

The emergency department story highlights how relational action is required at all levels. Although the nurse was able to act both intrapersonally (reflexively questioned herself and her options) and interpersonally (responded to the woman's need to tell her story) to affect the situation and possibly prevent similar situations in the future, action at the organizational level is required. For example, the policy that people are seen according to medical priority may not adequately address the needs of elderly patients. To assume that it is equitable to treat a 20-year-old in good health and an

80-year-old in frail health the same in terms of waiting time is not health promoting.

The nursing obligation to act at all levels requires accepting that we cannot control all conditions of practice and at the same time not abandoning the attempt to exert influence. Walker[27] argues that "our thinking about responsibility must encompass the reality that our impact on the world and each other *characteristically* exceeds our control and foresight."[(p. 15)] As Walker notes, our "potent but blinkered agency" requires considerable efforts and skill to achieve the understanding required to fulfill our obligations adequately. Neither fatalistic acceptance of the wider conditions of practice nor naive under-appreciation of the power of those conditions will be an adequate basis for meaningful action.

Overall, the nursing obligation to act at all levels rests on the understanding that relational concepts such as respect, trust, mutuality, and presencing require and in many ways can be enacted only through action at all levels. For example, to enact trust—to be trustworthy—requires action at all levels. Potter[39] describes a trustworthy person as someone who can be counted on to take care of those things that others entrust to that person. Selman[40] makes an interesting distinction when examining the concept of trust between trusting nurses as individual people and trusting them as representatives of nursing and of an institution. From a relational practice perspective, this distinction is an important one.

Provis and Stack[18] point out that given the nature of healthcare situations, patients,

in their vulnerability and need, are left with little choice when it comes to putting their trust in nurses. For example, when they present at an emergency department with a deep laceration that needs suturing, patients have no choice but to stay and wait to get stitched up and to put their trust in the nurses. Yet, as the emergency department story depicts, in many cases there may be a conflict between what a patient ultimately needs and what the institutional policies direct. It is at this disjuncture between individual and institutional levels of action where "the difficulty" of enacting trust and of being trustworthy also arises for nurses and where it becomes evident that the enactment of trust necessitates action at all levels. For example, if the way in which patient care is organized does not allow for nursing practice that is adequate to address the healthcare needs of patients, as was the case for the elderly woman with the laceration, how do nurses meet the nursing obligation to be trustworthy without addressing the organizational constraints? If healthcare institutions are truly about promoting health and healing, nurses' obligations/trustworthiness as individuals and as representatives of nursing and a particular institution need to be aligned. Thus, the nursing obligations to be trustworthy and "take care" of those things with which patients are entrusting nurses ultimately means that nurses are obliged to attend to issues of work load, acuity, organizational policy, availability of resources, and so on.

As Walker[27] describes, at the larger contextual level it is imperative to create active, accessible moral-reflective spaces so that ongoing inquiry and deliberation takes place. Close "relational" inspection of the contexts of practice may reveal how "good practice" is constrained. In a study we conducted with nurses in different practice settings, the fact that unmanageable workloads and high patient acuity made good practice very difficult took most of the nurses' attention and overshadowed ideas about possible actions the nurses might take. In one setting the nurses initially focused almost exclusively on how their manager made "good practice" more difficult; for example, making decisions without consulting the nursing staff led to less effective care. Changing a certain kind of intravenous tubing, a seemingly small decision, led to lengthy delays for patients and increased the nurses' workload unnecessarily. The level of frustration and anger with the manager initially overshadowed examination of other influences on practice, for example, how relationships among the nurses themselves might have contributed to an unsupportive work environment and ironically to confrontational relationships within which the manager was increasingly reluctant to consult with staff. Thus, looking critically at the context of practice *involves looking at not only wider influences, but also how we ourselves practice in relation to those influences.*

Encounters with vulnerability, pain, and suffering compel a response. "To encounter a patient's pain or the worries of a relative is to be addressed morally." [9(p. 117)] Although the close proximity of nurse–patient relationships may serve to "address us morally" and heighten the feeling of obligation, Bauman[23] argues that proximity to others can also lead to a mixture of ambiguous responses. On one hand, proximity is what calls us to action, what compels us to help. At the same time, such proximity can overwhelm and spark the flight response.

Nursing relationships and the enactment of nursing values and goals in contemporary healthcare contexts are incredibly challenging. Thus, an understanding of relationships that turns attention to the connection between attitudes, intentions, judgment, and action—one that connects responsibilities, roles, and identities to relationships—is required.[41] Such an understanding highlights not only our obligations but the ways we might better meet these obligations. By looking beyond the surface of one-to-one encounters, by considering what shapes those encounters—nurses and patients, colleagues and contexts—we can act more intentionally and direct our actions in ways that foster trust, respect, compassion, and mutuality in contexts as well as in ourselves and with others.

Conclusion

Nortvedt[9] describes that several philosophers have elucidated how relational proximity and the face-to-face encounter generate particular kinds of moral responsibilities.

References

1. Browne AJ. The influence of liberal political ideology on nursing practice. *Nurs Inq.* 2001;8(2):118–129.

2. Gastmans C. A fundamental ethical approach to nursing: some proposals for ethics education. *Nurs Ethics.* 2002;9(5):494–507.

3. Tschudin V. *Nurses Matter.* London: Macmillan; 1999.

4. Tarlier D. Beyond caring: the moral and ethical bases of responsive nurse-patient relationships. *Nurs Philos.* 2004; 5:230–241.

5. Browne A. The meaning of respect: a First Nation's perspective. *Can J Nurs Res.* 1995;27:95–109.

6. Baier A. Trust and antitrust. *Ethics.* 1986;96:231–260.

7. Armstrong AE. Towards a strong virtue ethics for nursing practice. *Nurs Philos.* 2006;7:110–124.

8. Bergum V. Relational ethics and nursing. In: Storch J, Rodney P, Starzomski R, eds. *Toward a Moral Horizon: Nursing Ethics for Leadership and Practice.* Toronto, Ontario, Canada: Pearson Education; 2004:485–503.

9. Nortvedt P. Needs, closeness and responsibilities. An inquiry into some rival moral considerations in nursing care. *Nurs Philos.* 2001;2:112–121.

10. Gilligan C. In a Different Voice: Psychological Theory and Women's Development. Cambridge, MA: Harvard University Press; 1982.

11. Peter E, Liaschenko J. Perils of proximity: a spatiotemporal analysis of moral distress and moral ambiguity. *Nurs Inq.* 2004;11(4):218–225.

12. Thompson F. Moving from codes of ethics to ethical relationships for midwifery practice. *Nurs Ethics.* 2002;9(5):522–536.

13. Dobrowolska B, Wronska I, Fidecki W, Wysijubski M. Moral obligations of nurses based on the ICN, UK, Irish and Polish codes of ethics for nurses. *Nurs Ethics.* 2007;14(2):171–180.

14. Pattison S. Are nursing codes of practice ethical? *Nurs Ethics.* 2001;8(1):5–18.

15. MacDonald H. Relational ethics and advocacy in nursing: literature review. *J Adv Nurs.* 2007;57(2):119–126.

16. Bekemeier B, Butterfield P. Unreconciled inconsistencies: a critical review of the concept of social justice in 3 national nursing documents. *Adv Nurs Sci.* 2005;28(2):152–162.

17. Kirkham SR, Browne AJ. Toward a critical theoretical interpretation of social justice discourses in nursing. *Adv Nurs Sci.* 2006;29(4):324–339.

18. Provis C, Stack S. Caring work, personal obligation and collective responsibility. *Nurs Ethics.* 2004;11(1):5–14.

19. Varcoe C, Doane G, Pauly B, et al. Ethical practice in nursing: working the in-betweens. *J Adv Nurs.* 2004;45(3):316–325.

20. Doane G. Being an ethical practitioner: the embodiment of mind, emotion and action. In: Storch J, Rodney P, Starzomski R, eds. *Toward a Moral Horizon: Nursing Ethics for Leadership and Practice.* Toronto, Ontario, Canada: Pearson-Prentice Hall; 2004:433–446.

21. Caputo J. Radical Hermeneutics: Repetition, Deconstruction and the Hermeneutic Project. Bloomington, IN: Indiana University Press; 1987.

22. Caputo J. Against Ethics: Contributions to a Poetics of Obligation With Constant Reference to Deconstruction. Bloomington, IN: Indiana University Press; 1993.

23. Bauman Z. *Postmodern Ethics*. Oxford, UK: Blackwell; 1993.

24. Hartrick Doane G, Varcoe C. *Family Nursing as Relational Inquiry: Developing Health Promoting Practice*. Philadelphia: Lippincott Williams & Wilkins; 2005.

25. Soderberg A, Gilje F, Norberg A. Transforming desolation into consolation: the meaning of being in situations of ethical difficulty in intensive care. *Nurs Ethics*. 1999;6(5):357–373.

26. Hartrick GA. Beyond interpersonal communication: the significance of relationship in health promoting practice. In: Young L, Hayes V, eds. *Transforming Health Promotion Practice. Concepts, Issues and Applications*. Philadelphia: FA Davis; 2002:49–58.

27. Walker MU. *Moral Contexts*. Lanham, MD: Rowman & Littlefield; 2003.

28. Varcoe C, Rodney P. Constrained agency: the social structure of nurses work. In: Bolaria BS, Dickinson HD, eds. *Health, Illness and Health Care in Canada*. 3rd ed. Toronto, Ontario, Canada: Nelson; 2002:102–128.

29. Purkis ME, Björnsdóttir K. Intelligent nursing: accounting for knowledge as action in practice. *Nurs Philos*. 2006;7: 247–256.

30. Flaming D. Using phronesis instead of "research-based practice" as the guiding light for nursing practice. *Nurs Philos*. 2006;2:251–258.

31. Doane G. Reflexivity as presence: a journey of self-inquiry. In: Finlay L, Gough B, eds. *Reflexivity. A Practical Guide for Researchers in Health and Social Sciences*. Oxford, UK: Blackwell; 2003:93–102.

32. Mitchell GJ, Bunkers SS. Engaging the abyss: A mistake of opportunity. *Nurs Sci Q*. 2003;16(2):121–125.

33. Taylor B, Barling J. Identifying sources and effects of career fatigue and burnout for mental health nurses: a qualitative approach. *Int J Mental Health Nurs*. 2004;13(2):117–125.

34. Bakker AB, Killmer CH, Siegrist J, Schaufeli WB. Effort-reward imbalance and burnout among nurses. *J Adv Nurs*. 2000;31(4):884–891.

35. Demerouti E, Bakker AB, Nachreiner F, Schaufeli WB. A model of burnout and life satisfaction amongst nurses. *J Adv Nurs*. 2000;32(2):454–464.

36. Rosenberg HJ, Rosenberg SD, Wolford GL, Manganiello PD, Brunette MF, Boynton RA. The relationship between trauma, PTSD, and medical utilization in three high risk medical populations. *Int J Psychiatry Med*. 2000;30(3):247–259.

37. Collins S, Long A. Working with the psychological effects of trauma: consequences for mental healthcare

workers—a literature review. *J Psychiatr Mental Health Nurs*. 2003;10(4):417–424.

38. Crothers D. Vicarious traumatization in the work with survivors of childhood trauma. *J Psychosoc Nurs Mental Health Serv*. 1995;33(4):9–13, 44–45.

39. Potter NN. *How Can I Be Trusted? A Virtue Theory of Trustworthiness*. Lanham, MD: Rowan & Littlefield; 2002.

40. Sellman D. The importance of being trustworthy. *Nurs Ethics*. 2006;13(2):105–115.

41. Bjorklund P. Taking responsibility: toward an understanding of morality in practice. A critical review of the empirical and selected philosophical literature on the social organization of responsibility. *Adv Nurs Sci*. 2006;29(2):E56–E73.

Contemporary Perspectives on Nursing

In Chapter 19, Mitchell and Cody attempt to specify the meaning of the claim that nursing is and must be a "human science." A human science, after Dilthey, they say, is one that is concerned with humanly lived experiences, meanings, patterns, beliefs, values, representations, and intentions. Its methods are qualitative, and its goal is understanding what it means to be human. Mitchell and Cody examine a range of contemporary nursing frameworks, which are described in some detail, for their adherence to basic assumptions and values of human science. A value for nursing as a human science will shape the practice of the nurse who holds this value.

In Chapter 20, Wuest provides a historical and feminist perspective on the notion of professionalism in nursing. In lieu of the received view of professionalism, which is the more familiar view, Wuest argues for value-laden feminist epistemologies and methodologies that generate and apply knowledge in a manner that values people and freedom.

In Chapter 21, Locsin and Purnell examine the consequence of increased dependence on technology, and the ways in which technological advancements affect both human life and the field of nursing. In Chapter 22, Mitchell discusses nursing's military origins and the way metaphor not only defines nursing practice, but fosters change. In Chapter 23, Ketefian and Redman offer an international perspective of nursing science and the dominance of Western (North American) perspectives therein. This chapter suggests that a value for people and their quality of life mandates a focus within the discipline that is different from that which currently obtains.

In Chapter 24, Arnold and Bruce discuss aboriginal ways of organizing and implementing health care. Beliefs and cultural differences are explored, and methods of bridging those differences are presented with the goal of providing more inclusive care.

Collectively, these six chapters' contemporary perspectives offer readers a chance to reflect on the nature of nursing itself, what constitutes nursing, and what constitutes health. All six chapters are oriented toward praxis in some way. It is incumbent on the advanced practice nurse, holding a graduate degree in nursing, to explicate the nature of the discipline and its practice and to discuss with considerable depth the nature of health, generally construed as nursing's goal. The diversity of the chapters illustrates that there is no one correct, monolithic perspective. Many views coexist and interact continually to make up the discourse of the discipline that the practitioner must master.

References

Fawcett, J. (1984). The metaparadigm of nursing: Present status and future refinements. *Image, 16*(3), 84–87.

Parse, R. R. (1998). *The human becoming school of thought: A perspective for nurses and other health professionals*. Thousand Oaks, CA: Sage.

CHAPTER 19

Nursing Knowledge and Human Science: Ontological and Epistemological Considerations

Gail J. Mitchell, RN, PhD

William K. Cody, PhD, RN, FAAN

Increasingly, nursing is being referred to as a human science (Connors, 1988; Gortner & Schultz, 1988; Melcis, 1990; Munhall, 1989; Parse, 1981, 1987; Watson, 1985). The meaning of this term as it is used in the literature, however, is not clear. Munhall (1989), Parse (1981), and Watson (1985) refer to human science as distinct from natural science and as bearing specific views, concepts, and methods. In contrast to this position, Connors (1988) and Gortner and Schultz (1988) refer to human science as the fields of biology, psychology, anthropology,

and sociology. Is human science inclusive of any inquiry about human beings, or is it a distinctive philosophical foundation for science? Is nursing currently a human science or is this an ideal to be esteemed and aspired to? The purpose of this chapter is to examine the meaning of human science as originated by Dilthey (1961, 1976, 1977a, 1977b, 1988) and explicated by Giorgi (1970, 1971, 1985) and to compare selected works from nursing's extant theoretical base with the explicit attributes that constitute "human" science.

Source: Mitchell, G. J., & Cody, W. K. (1992). Nursing knowledge and human science: Ontological and epistemological considerations. Nursing Science Quarterly, 5(2): 54–61. Reprinted by permission of and copyright © 1992 Sage Publications, Inc.

Defining Human Science

The origins of the term human science can be traced to the philosopher Wilhelm Dilthey (1833–1911). The German term for human science, Geisteswissenschaften, has also been translated as "human studies." Translators frequently note the linguistic challenge involved in capturing the meaning of freshly coined and esoteric German expressions in English. Also noted in Dilthey's works is his tendency to refer to "psychic" life in a nineteenth-century fashion while writing of the coherent whole of lived experience. Dilthey did, however, describe life as a unity, a living nexus, and he consistently referred to individuals as wholes and to human life as interconnected with others and history. The intent of the authors here is to offer an admittedly hermeneutical interpretation of Dilthey's view, in what is believed to be the unitary perspective of human beings that he intended.

Dilthey in the late 1800s was very concerned about what he called a "crisis in science," a crisis of modern consciousness, thought, and values (Ermath, 1978). The industrial society had already concretized the successes of the natural sciences, and the developing science of Anthropologie, with no other model, was rapidly abandoning any interest in human consciousness in favor of a crude "mindless" naturalism (Ermath, 1978). Dilthey (1977a) described what he saw as a sterile empiricism that disconnected life from knowledge. His fears were stoked by the growing trend to regard human behavior and culture as susceptible

to the methods of natural science, which, he thought, stripped life of human meaning and purpose (Dilthey, 1977a). He proposed that "the deepest problem of modern thought and culture is to understand life as it is lived by man" (Ermath, 1978, p. 17).

Dilthey (1977a, 1977b, 1988) believed that the development of a human science held the only hope for understanding life as it is humanly lived. He proposed that the human sciences required concepts, methods, and theories that were fundamentally different from those of the natural sciences (Dilthey, 1977a, 1988). Dilthey viewed human beings as the preeminent source of knowledge. His philosophy took as its basis the whole of lived experience, the coherent nexus of life as it is humanly lived (Dilthey, 1977a). He wrote about "living" knowledge and "reflective" life. History and culture were, for Dilthey, manifestations of patterns of human life, pervaded with meaning. The natural sciences, concerned with the elaboration of physical laws from observation and experimentation, were, for Dilthey, very different from the concerns a true human science would focus on meaning, values, and relationships within the coherent texture of humanly lived experience. The subject matter of the human sciences is "the interrelation of life, expression, and understanding" (Dilthey, 1976, p. 175).

Dilthey proposed that the lived experience should be "the basic empirical datum of the human sciences" (Ermath, 1978, p. 97). Further, the researcher, a living being too, is inexorably and unequivocally "in" and "of" what is investigated. There could be no meaningful objective/subjective dichotomy and no analytic reduction beyond experience as humanly lived. Human experience is a coherent whole to which subjectivity is fundamental; objectivity is a human creation. Dilthey maintained that life is a process, a continuous becoming that manifests itself in the dynamic unity of experience (Dilthey, 1976). Human beings were described as individual wholes with intrinsic value (Dilthey, 1977b). Dilthey (1977b) referred to the self as a "life–unity" that is free yet also determined by history. The concept of free will is a fundamental assumption of human science. On free will, Dilthey (1988) wrote, "This is an immediately given actuality. It cannot be denied. . . . [O]ne cannot explain the fact of free will, for it is precisely its hallmark that we cannot break it down in a conceptual system" (p. 270).

More recently, the psychologist Giorgi (1970, 1971, 1985) has reasserted the need for an approach to the human sciences fundamentally different from conventional empirical methods. He proposed to study human beings as persons, as experiencing participants. He challenged the prevailing positivistic methods of psychology, contending that human experience must be understood in the way that it reveals itself, and he maintained that the study of lived experience could be done scientifically (Giorgi, 1985).

According to Giorgi, understanding life experiences requires a focus on meaning within the context of the person's experience of the phenomenon. Human beings cannot be known as objects, nor as separate from their lives. Echoing Dilthey, Giorgi maintained that a person is not "a passive receiver of physical energies, but rather his or her behavior reflects intentionality" (Giorgi, 1971, p. 23). Giorgi also addressed the influence of the researcher in conceptualizing research and the impact of the researcher on study findings. For Giorgi, the most important variable in the human sciences is the meaning of the lived experience for the subject. An exposition of the major thinkers and scholars, such as Gadamer (1976), Geertz (1973), Heidegger (1962), Ricoeur (1974), Schutz (1967), and Winch (1958), who have built on the tradition of which Dilthey is the foremost progenitor, is beyond the scope of this article.

The domination of twentieth-century social science by positivistic approaches in stark contrast to human science philosophy has been well documented (Polkinghorne, 1983) and contributes to the contextual situation in which this article emerges. The philosophical stance of human science outlined here has underpinned or strongly influenced the works of the six seminal scholars mentioned above and many others in the tradition of human science. These scholars have recognized the manifest necessity for the human sciences to explore and understand lived experience, the full complexity of human meanings and values, with no more fundamental reference than the human lives which are the phenomena of concern; indeed, this formidable undertaking is the very mission of human science.

Based on the above explications of human science by Dilthey and Giorgi, specific ontological and epistemological attributes emerge as crucial to this approach for nursing science. Human science, in view of its origins and its philosophical foundations, cannot be viewed as a generic term for any and all disciplines studying human beings. It is proposed here that for a scientific discipline to be considered a "human science" logically it must incorporate the ontology and epistemology of its philosophical underpinnings, as described in **Table 19-1.**

A distinction must be made between a "humanistic" philosophy of science and "human science." According to Webster (1985), "humanism" entails a rejection of supernaturalism and asserts "the essential dignity and worth of man [sic] and his capacity to achieve self-realization through the use of reason and scientific method." Humanism thus is seen to acknowledge human values and potentialities without requiring a critique of "scientific method." Human science, in contrast, unequivocally rejects the methods of natural science (Dilthey, 1976, 1977a, 1988; Giorgi, 1985) and asserts from the outset that lived experience, the world as experienced, meaning, and understanding are all aspects of a unitary process of human life and cannot be adequately described, explained, or analyzed through objectification, measurement, or reduction.

Table 19-1   Ontology and Epistemology of the Human Science Paradigm

Ontology	Epistemology
Human beings are unitary wholes in continuous interrelationship with their dynamic, temporal, historical, cultural worlds.	Research and practice focus on the coherent experience of the person's meanings, relations, values, patterns, and themes.
Human experience is preeminent and fundamental and reality is the whole complex of—what is experienced and elaborated in thinking, feeling, and willing.	Lived experience is the basic empirical datum, as gleaned from the participant's description free of comparison to objective realities or predefined norms.
Human beings are intentional, free-willed beings who actively participate in life continuously.	The person's coparticipation in generating knowledge of lived experience is respected, and no more fundamental reference than what is disclosed by the person is sought.
The researcher is inextricably involved with any phenomenon investigated.	The researcher seeks knowledge and understanding of lived experience and is cognizant of the other's lived reality as a unitary whole.

Source: Synthesized and condensed from Dilthey (1961, 1976, 1977a, 1977b, 1988) and Giorgi (1970, 1971, 1985).

Significance of Human Science for Nursing

If nurses embrace the human science paradigm, activities in theory development, research, and practice will change to reflect the new philosophical perspective. An examination of nursing's philosophical and theoretical body of literature reveals that, in the past decade, such a change has already begun. In order to explore to what extent nurses are incorporating beliefs of the human science paradigm in theory, research, and practice, four nursing frameworks were selected for analysis. These frameworks are Paterson and Zderad's (1988) humanistic nursing, Newman's (1986a, 1990) model of health as expanding consciousness, Watson's (1985) human science and human care, and Parse's (1981, 1987, 1990a) theory of human becoming (formerly man–living–health, 1981). These frameworks were selected because all their authors claim a unitary conceptualization of human beings, thereby evincing some degree of interfacing with the human science perspective. Further, these authors have publicly renounced the natural science approach and have called for new and different methods more congruent with nursing's philosophical foundations.

Critical to the development of nursing theories underpinned by the human sciences would be the acknowledgment of human beings as individual wholes who are situated in the world and who are respected as intentional, free-willed persons. Any theoretical principles and concepts used to structure a theory would need to incorporate these

beliefs. Also essential would be approaches which view the individual's lived experience as the focus in both practice and research and which honor the person's lived experience as reality. Researchers and practitioners would be regarded as coparticipants with persons in inquiry and practice in a human science paradigm.

Analysis of the Nursing Frameworks

Inquiry into the four frameworks above revealed a definite commitment to the human science paradigm. Parse's theory of human becoming was found not only to be consistent with the human science beliefs but to clarify, expand, and develop this approach. Consequently, an in-depth analysis of Parse's theory will be offered at a later point. Analysis of the works of Newman, Paterson and Zderad, and Watson illuminated consistencies and inconsistencies in relation to the beliefs of human science. Consistencies and commonalities included affirmation, to varying degrees, of the wholeness of the human being, the significance of subjective experience, and mutual participation in the creation of reality.

The inconsistencies took two main forms. In some instances, the author(s) acknowledged an inability to reconcile traditional objectivist beliefs with beliefs congruent with human science, and consequently they incorporated conflicting beliefs in theoretical conceptualizations. Alternately, the author(s) extended and elaborated on beliefs essential to the human science tradition, leading to significant dissidence with the core philosophy. These two inconsistencies are discussed with specific examples to illustrate logical incongruencies with the human science tradition. The intent here is not to rebuke the nursing theorists for their philosophical obscurities, for obscurity engenders clarification. Rather, the intent is to illuminate the inconsistencies in order to foster clarity and further the development of nursing science.

Incorporating Diverging Beliefs

As previously noted, the nursing frameworks revealed both consistencies and inconsistencies with the foundational beliefs of the human science paradigm. Perhaps reflecting the evolutionary nature of knowledge and theory development, several of the authors incorporated diverging beliefs in their work, leaving the reader unclear as to their philosophical underpinnings. The inconsistencies arise in three main areas: the human being's wholeness, the intentionality and free will of the person, and the nature of reality. Each of these will be explored in relation to the works of Paterson and Zderad (1988), Newman (1986a, 1990), and Watson (1985).

Wholeness of Human Beings

Paterson and Zderad (1988) in their humanistic nursing practice propose that "the nurse sees the patient as a whole, a gestalt" (p. 25). Human beings are described

as "in-the-world" and nurses are guided to recognize the complexity and uniqueness of each person's relating and experiencing. Paterson and Zderad note, however, that this view of the person as a whole conflicts with the evaluative stance of the conventional nursing process. They address this conflict by positing that "both subject–subject and subject–object relationships are essential for clinical nursing" (Paterson & Zderad, 1988, p. 27) in which focusing on discrete parts rather than the whole person is sometimes necessary. This attempt to incorporate human science beliefs with biomedical traditions leads to conceptual inconsistencies. It is suggested here that nurses cannot switch their very beliefs according to the nature of the practice situation. What seems to be overlooked by Paterson and Zderad is that nurses can live according to human science beliefs and still perform tasks related to the execution of medical orders. There need not be the subject–subject, subject–object dilemma as espoused by these authors. Although Paterson and Zderad reflect on the inadequacy of the labeling process for capturing lived experiences, they accept the linear, causal nursing process and the diagnosing of human responses as necessary evils, required for economic reasons. Paterson and Zderad maintain that the natural science tradition is inappropriate for nursing, yet they do not reconcile the inconsistencies between reductionistic and unitary approaches with human beings.

Newman explicitly expresses a belief in the unitary nature of human beings, yet she also discusses the human being as a "system" made up of physiological structures and functions, such as the immune system and the genetic code, reflecting a natural science orientation. The unity of the human "system," for Newman, is predicated on the idea that "mind and matter are made of the same basic stuff" (1986a, p. 37). It is apparently quite appropriate within Newman's model to discuss the physiological, psychological, and emotional processes of the "human system" in conventional terms, so long as one remembers that everything, from the atom to the human being and beyond, is a manifestation of the implicate order, or "absolute consciousness" (pp. 33–37). Similarly, Watson (1985) maintains that the person is conceptualized as an irreducible whole, yet she repeatedly refers to body, mind, spirit and soul, and physical, emotional, and spiritual spheres. Her definitions of health and illness are dependent on the harmony or disharmony within these aspects. Watson also refers to several selves; the "real self," the "inner self," and the "ideal self" are presented as distinct entities. She refers to the "I" and the "Me" of the person and the potential disharmony of these aspects. It is not consistent to maintain that a person is a unitary whole and then to define the person according to these separate parts or spheres. Dilthey (1977a) maintained that "we continually experience a sense of connectedness and totality in ourselves" (p. 53). The authors' struggles to incorporate the concept of the unitary human being into nursing theory and practice parallel a long and complex tradition of discourse in the human sciences.

Intentional Free-Willed Beings

Human science conceptualizes human beings as intentional and inherently free willed; therefore the nurse would seek no more fundamental reference than the lived experience of the person. Paterson and Zderad (1988) address the nurse's intention and free will to commit authentically to another. The authors also regard the human being as free willed, yet they suggest, "The nurse is alert to opportunities for the patient to exercise his [sic] freedom of choice within the limits of safe and sound practice" (p. 17). The nurse is guided to monitor the patient's choices and to determine if they are responsible ones. To carry out this monitoring, the nurse would have to rely on some schema of normative standards or beliefs in order to judge what is "responsible," which is an inconsistent practice if the nurse wishes to respect the human science belief that the individual is an intentional being possessing free will.

Newman's (1986a) conceptualization of freedom describes an arc-like progression as consciousness expands. Human beings first lose freedom as they "come into being," are "bound in time" and "find . . . identity in space," until they reach a stage in which choice is engendered through movement (p. 46). "Restriction of movement forces one into a realm beyond space and time" (p. 62). Thereafter one throws off self-concerns, recognizes one's own "boundarylessness" and "timelessness" and gains the freedom of returning to "absolute consciousness" (p. 46). It is essentially the movement toward spirituality that imbues the human being with freedom, which is relative to the extent that consciousness is expanded.

The notion that human freedom underpins human science is quite different, in that freedom is never "lost," and there is no requisite for expanding consciousness to "gain" it. Human beings are believed to be free to choose meaning and direction because they make such choices continuously in living everyday life (Dilthey, 1988). "It is true," writes Dilthey (1988), "that the will depends on intellect, but the will can choose or not choose what the intellect understands. . . . In fact the will is free precisely inasmuch as in it the search for a reason ends" (p. 270). Newman's (1986b) proposal for "the diagnosis of pattern" would appear to be hinged on her notion of freedom as relative to expanded consciousness. She states, "The role of the nurse within a paradigm of pattern is to help clients recognize their own patterns," a process in which a "burst of insight" occurs that "opens up" a "pathway of action" (pp. 55–56). From a human science perspective, in contrast, the pathway of action is always open.

Watson (1985) says that human beings are free to self-determine and free to choose. Nurses are guided to hold nonpaternalistic values, which respect human autonomy and freedom. Yet this belief is violated in two ways. First, there are references to the nurse's helping, integrating, and "correcting" the patient's condition to increase harmony and to try to find meaning in the situation. Second, Watson maintains that

"ideally, a person should have the opportunity for self-determination of the meaning of a health-illness experience before professionals make decisions about treatments and interventions" (1985, p. 66). Human science philosophy abdicates the position of science as the arbiter of truth; the human scientist is a seeker of truth, a seeker rather than a dispenser of wisdom. Dilthey maintained that "understanding constitutes the goal of the human studies in the way that explanation defines the natural sciences" (cited in Makkreel, 1977, p. 7). Knowledge is not used or applied to the person, but rather knowledge enhances understanding for participating with the person in the process of becoming. Dilthey (1976) proposed, "In everything there is the same limitation of possibilities and yet freedom to choose between them, and the beautiful feeling of being able to move forward and to realize new potentialities in one's own existence" (p. 245).

The Nature of Reality

In a human science ontology, human beings and their worlds as experienced cannot be separated. Human science does not distinguish between subjective and objective realities because the focus of scientific activities is the humanly lived experience of the world, in which subjectivity is primal. Paterson and Zderad suggest that "nurses are drawn toward two realities—the reality of the objective scientific world and the reality of the subjective–objective world" (p. 36). The authors' endorsement of the traditional nursing process automatically places the person in the position of object and the nurse in the role of arbiter of truth. Again, this reflects the conflicting views proposed with respect to the nurse–patient relationship.

Newman's (1986a) view of the nature of reality draws on Bohm's (1980) theory of the implicate order. All humanly experienced phenomena comprising the explicate order are posited as manifestations of an unseen, unknowable implicate order which comprises the unity of all that is. According to this view, patterns of human experience are reflective of this underlying primary reality. Newman writes, "We need to remind ourselves that our manifest reality is a small portion of the total enfoldment of the pattern in time–space" (1986a, p. 15). Her model theoretically eliminates the subject–object duality, according to its ontology. However, Newman's (1986a, 1986b) view is that neither objectivity nor subjectivity has any validity, as the perspective adapted from Bohm says there are no boundaries to (physical) reality. From a human science perspective, this is still essentially an objectivist reality, founded on the basis of the speculations of physical scientists that the nature of reality is a complex, multidimensional whole. The human being in such a model is defined by what physical science says about matter and energy. In contrast, human science directly asserts that human reality as lived is itself a complex multidimensional whole (Dilthey, 1977a).

The preeminence of the human experience is ostensibly highly valued in Watson's theory. She speaks of developing knowledge about the lived world of human experience and contends that the phenomenological research method is most congruent with her theoretical perspective. However, Watson distinguishes the person's experience of the world (phenomenal field) from the world as it actually is. For example, she proposes that nurses "help integrate the person's subjective experience and emotions with the objective external view of the situation" (Watson, 1985, p. 65). Watson also suggests that there can be incongruencies between the person and nature (world). For example, she states, "If a person does not feel congruent with mind, body, and soul . . . or rejects the self . . . or is obsessed with an ideal self, the person will be dissatisfied and maladjusted" (p. 57). These distinctions reveal a belief in an objective reality separate from the person's experience of it. This essentially dichotomous view is inconsistent with human science philosophy, in which being human means participating in the creation of reality. Human consciousness already is the unity of the person's subjective–objective relationship with the world; it is not something to be aspired to (Dilthey, 1977a). The use of the conventional subjective–objective constructs speaks to the exigencies of traditional science but is inconsistent with the understanding of humanly lived reality that underpins human science.

Extending Essential Beliefs

In several instances within the frameworks examined, departures from the human science tradition were noted in areas where some congruence might be expected based on the overall presentation and central concepts.

Paterson and Zderad (1988) move from focusing on the human being's lived experience to focusing on nurses' lived experiences and their descriptions of human beings. Both Newman (1986a) and Watson (1985) go well beyond the lived experience as the primal foundation of human knowledge by assigning higher order importance to metaphysical concepts.

It is clear that the basic empirical datum in Paterson and Zderad's humanistic nursing is the nurse's experience, "the between" of existentially experienced nursing situations. The authors address the importance of meanings, patterns, values, and themes, but it is not clear whose experiences are paramount, the nurse's or the patient's. Paterson and Zderad contend that nursing must be described phenomenologically, that nurses' descriptions of nursing situations with patients will build the knowledge and "make explicit a science of nursing" (1988, p. 3). This is a description of the practice of nursing, however, not of a nursing science based on the health experience of human beings. Giorgi (1985) proposed that a discipline is not ready-made in the world and simply viewed and studied. Rather, it is created by a unique knowledge base that is housed within its theories. Thus, to study the nursing act phenomenologically as Paterson and Zderad suggest is to study the particular nurse's view of nursing. It is suggested in this article that nursing science focuses on the concepts of human–environment and health, not the nurse's views of the between. To be consistent with the human science approach nurses must rely on the person's description as it is given, and not on what that experience

is assumed to be. Paterson and Zderad's focus on the practitioner's experience reflects a serious departure from beliefs related to the practice of a human science, which investigates lived experiences and life expressions of human beings.

Human consciousness is an important concept in human science; it is the origin of all knowledge about lived experience (Dilthey, 1988). The ontology of Newman's theory is largely metaphysical, in that the key concept of "absolute consciousness" is beyond the realm of lived experience. Newman (1986a) ascribes consciousness to atoms, rocks, plants, animals, and unspecified "astral" and "spiritual" entities (pp. 33–37). In human science philosophy there is no way of knowing a more fundamental ground behind or beyond the lived experience of the person. One wonders why Newman (1986a), whose central thesis is "health as expanding consciousness," has completely ignored continental European philosophy and theory on consciousness throughout her work. Instead, Newman cites works of speculative physics as underpinning her theory, even when addressing human experience. Dilthey (1977a) maintained that "consciousness cannot go behind itself" (p. 75). It is the structure of consciousness that sheds light on the coherent unity of human life.

In human science, humanly lived experiences elaborated in thinking, feeling, and willing are the complex whole of reality. Watson emphasizes the significance of human experience as it is lived. However, her emphasis on the metaphysical, spiritual realm clouds the issue of the primacy of lived experience. Watson (1985) states that "the human soul is more than physical, mental, emotional existence. . . . The soul exists for something larger than physical life" (p. 45). She maintains, "The soul, inner self, spiritual self is tied to a higher degree of consciousness . . . that transcends time and space" (p. 46). This soul, which "may be underdeveloped and in need of reawakening" (p. 45), reflects a reality beyond that which is directly experienced by human beings and is in conflict with the purported human science origins of Watson's theory.

Watson explicitly presents her framework as emerging from the human science paradigm. Paterson and Zderad refer to their work as humanistic, a related term but not synonymous with human science. Although the concepts Newman uses are abundantly addressed in human science, the ontology underpinning her theory is derived instead from speculative physics The selective extraction of inconsistencies with the human science paradigm in these authors' works is not intended to suggest a failing on their part but is intended to foster greater conceptual clarity and is offered in the spirit of scholarly questioning and debate. The purpose of this analysis was to determine to what extent the values and beliefs of the human science paradigm were currently evident in nursing's extant knowledge base. The authors conclude that the human science tradition is present to varying degrees in nursing science.

Of the four theories explored here, Parse's (1981, 1987, 1990a) theory of human becoming remained consistent with the fundamental ontology and epistemology of the human science tradition. The theory can be seen to have expanded and clarified major ideas of the human science tradition. Parse's (1981) work was the first publication in nursing to specify nursing as a human science in Dilthey's traditional sense. Parse's theory is analyzed here with regard to both its adherence to and expansion of the human science tradition.

Parse's Theory of Human Becoming

Parse's first chapter begins, "To posit the idea of nursing rooted in the human sciences is to make explicit an alternative to the traditional practice of nursing as a medical model grounded in the natural sciences" (1981, p. 3). Parse describes nursing as a human science focusing on the unitary human being's experience of living and creating health, and she cites Dilthey in her explication of the concepts of her theory. She states that the methodologies of human sciences focus on "uncovering the meaning of phenomena as humanly experienced" and "on understanding the connectedness of life itself" (1981, p. 11). Dilthey (1977b) suggested that explicating human interrelatedness connects that which is universally human with that which is individual.

Parse (1981) synthesized concepts from Rogers' (1970) science of unitary human beings and tenets of contemporary existential phenomenology in such a way that the fundamental notion of human science proposed by Dilthey was brought to fruition for nursing science in the theory of human becoming. The tenets of human subjectivity and intentionality, and the concepts of human coexistence, co-constitution, and situated freedom, drawn from existential phenomenology, reflect the development of ideas germinated by Dilthey and others in the philosophy of human science. The synthesis of concepts from Rogers' work with concepts from existential phenomenology to form a unique, coherent theory of nursing underscores the compelling fit between human science philosophy and nursing as a unique and autonomous discipline. Parse (1987) avoided conceptual inconsistencies by inventing nursing practice and research methodologies that flow directly from the ontological and epistemological foundations of her theory. In this way there is no need to reconcile human science beliefs with biomedical traditions. Parse's theory and her practice and research methodologies express and structure the beliefs that underpin human science in a new way specifically for nursing science.

Parse's (1981, 1987, 1990a) theory of human becoming has three central themes: meaning, rhythmicity, and cotranscendence. Her explication of these themes moves her theory beyond human science as described by Dilthey (1961). Parse describes the human being as an open unity who freely chooses meaning in situations, bears responsibility for choices, and co-constitutes with the environment rhythmical patterns of relating in the process of co-transcending with emerging possibilities. Health is described as a "process of becoming, a co-created process of living

value priorities" (1981, p. 31). Health is the day-to-day living of rhythmical patterns reflecting the person's unfolding and co-transcending with the possibles (the moving onward in life in a chosen way) (Parse, 1981).

The goal of practice in Parse's theory is the quality of life from the person's perspective (1987). Nurses in true presence with people live the practice method, which revolves around the all-at-once of illuminating meaning through "explicating," synchronizing rhythms through "dwelling with," and mobilizing transcendence through "moving beyond" (1987, p. 167). Parse's research method is rooted in phenomenology and is structured to be congruent with the assumptions and principles of the human becoming theory. It focuses on uncovering the structures of universal lived experiences in the human–universe–health interrelationship. The goal of the method is to enhance understanding of lived experiences of health.

Critique of the Theory of Human Becoming

Parse presents her theory as emerging from the human science paradigm, and she remains congruent with those philosophical underpinnings throughout her work. The human being is viewed as unitary, mutually interrelating with environment, and there is no reference to human beings other than as living unities. The person's lived experience is clearly regarded as the preeminent ground of human health. The researcher explores universal lived experiences of health, with the goal of enhancing understanding. This is consistent with Dilthey's concern "to understand life as it is lived by man" (Ermath, 1978, p. 17). Both the research and practice methods focus on the lived experience of human beings. There is no subject–object dichotomy; reality is viewed as cocreated with the universe and others while experienced uniquely by the person. Nursing is seen as a scientific discipline in which the concepts of unitary human beings, mutual unfolding, human coexistence, intentionality, free will, and intersubjective sharing of meaning may at last be fully elaborated and incorporated in praxis. Dilthey consistently maintained that all theory was theory for praxis (Ermath, 1978).

Parse suggests that persons "unfold with contemporaries the ideas of predecessors . . . in a continuity that connects past with future" (1981, p. 26). The "way the person lives in interrelationship with others reflects chosen meanings and reveals cherished values" (1981, p. 48). Individuals freely choose the meaning of situations and freely live personal values by choosing ways of being/becoming from among possibilities. Again, this is consistent with Dilthey's (1961) view of human interconnectedness, yet it goes beyond his view.

Guided by Parse's theory, the nurse in true presence with the person focuses on the individual's own meaning without judging, labeling, or trying to change the person. The nurse goes with the person as he or she explores options, imagines consequences of choices, and plans to live hopes and dreams. In the true presence of the nurse, the individual clarifies the meaning of the situation and new meanings are uncovered; new insights generate new possibles, the understanding of opportunities and limitations in light of what is truly valued. The nurse coparticipates with the person in the process of moving beyond the now moment, guided by the theory to understand that the person chooses his or her own way (Parse, 1987). Parse maintains that individuals know their own way, reflectively and prereflectively. The nurse in true presence bears witness to the person's unfolding and becoming (Parse, 1990b). In creating the theory of human becoming, Parse has uncovered the intrinsic relevance of the human science perspective, which is centrally concerned with what it means to be human for the discipline of nursing.

In Parse's (1987) research methodology, the researcher "lives" dialogical engagements with participants. This is described as "an intersubjective being with, in which the researcher and participant live the I–Thou process as they move through an unstructured discussion about the lived experience" (1987, p. 176). The researcher views the participant as the expert on the lived experience being explored and remains focused on the phenomenon as it is revealed by the person. The researcher participates in generating enhanced understanding of the phenomenon by creatively abstracting the structure of the lived experience in the language of science.

In summary, Parse's theory, intentionally structured as a human science theory of nursing, accurately reflects the ontology and epistemology of human science philosophy. Parse's theory lays a foundation for a nursing science that is grounded in the meaning of lived experiences in the human–universe process. The theory focuses on the lived experience of unitary human beings in continuous interrelationship with their worlds. Reality as perceived by the person is not compared to an "objective" reality but is respected, as is the free will of the person, in choosing ways of becoming. Parse's theory is thus congruent with yet goes beyond the ontology and epistemology of human science as posited in this article and is an emergent, a newly created theory for praxis that uncompromisingly incorporates the beliefs of human science into nursing research and practice.

Conclusion

Nursing science is currently undergoing change as new views emerge that challenge the traditional methods of natural science-based, biomedical nursing. The human science paradigm is one such view. This perspective is surfacing in nursing at a time when nurse scholars are questioning the precepts of the natural science paradigm and, in doing so, are expressing many of the concerns that led Dilthey to propose a different approach to human science over a hundred years ago. It has been suggested in this article that the human science tradition is not merely any study of human beings, but a particular way of studying human life that values the lived experience of unitary persons and seeks to understand life in all its interwoven patterns of meanings and values.

Nurse scientists are defining boundaries and seeking knowledge that is unique to nursing. This knowledge is currently organized in conceptual and theoretical frameworks, some of which reflect the values and beliefs of the human science paradigm. Of the four frameworks explored here, one, Parse's theory of human becoming, was found not only to be congruent with but to go beyond the human science perspective. The other three frameworks, Paterson and Zderad's humanistic nursing, Newman's model of expanding consciousness, and Watson's human science and human care, demonstrated both consistencies and inconsistencies with the philosophy of human science. Continued explication of the assumptions, values, and beliefs that underpin different theoretical approaches is needed so that nurses can understand with depth and clarity the foundations of the unique knowledge base of nursing. Only through contemplative consideration of the philosophical basis of the extant body of theory and through open critique and discourse can nurses choose which paths to follow in the quest for knowledge.

References

Bohm, D. (1980). *Wholeness and the implicate order.* London: Routledge.

Connors, D. (1988). A continuum of researcher–participant relationships: An analysis and critique. *Advances in Nursing Science, 10*(4), 32–42.

Dilthey, W. (1961). Pattern and meaning in history: Thoughts on history and society (H. P. Rickman, Ed. and Trans.). New York: Harper & Row.

Dilthey, W. (1976). Selected writings (H. P. Rickman, Trans.). Cambridge: Cambridge University Press.

Dilthey, W. (1977a). Ideas concerning a descriptive and analytic psychology. (Original work published 1894.) In R. M. Zaner & K. L. Heiges (Trans.), Descriptive psychology and historical understanding (pp. 23–120). The Hague, Netherlands: Nijhoff.

Dilthey, W. (1977b). The understanding of other persons and their expressions of life. (Original work published 1927.) In R. M. Zaner & K. L. Heiges (Trans.), Descriptive psychology and historical understanding (pp. 123–144). The Hague, Netherlands: Nijhoff.

Dilthey, W. (1988). Introduction to the human sciences (R. J. Betanzos, Trans.). Detroit: Wayne State University Press. (Original work published 1883.)

Ermath, M. (1978). Wilhelm Dilthey: The critique of historical reason. Chicago: University of Chicago Press.

Gadamer, H. G. (1976). Philosophical hermeneutics (D. E. Linge, Trans.). Berkeley: University of California Press.

Geertz, C. (1973). The interpretation of cultures. New York: Basic Books.

Giorgi, A. (1970). Psychology as a human science. New York: Harper & Row.

Giorgi, A. (1971). Phenomenology and experimental psychology: II. In A. Giorgi, W. Fischer, & R. von Eckartsberg (Eds.). Duquesne studies in phenomenological psychology (vol. l, pp. 3–29). Pittsburgh, PA: Duquesne University Press.

Giorgi, A. (1985). Sketch of a psychological phenomenological method. In W. Fischer, & R. von Eckartsberg (Eds.). Phenomenology and psychological research (pp. 8–22). Pittsburgh, PA: Duquesne University Press.

Gortner, S. R., & Schultz, P. R. (1988). Approaches to nursing science methods. Image: Journal of Nursing Scholarship, 20, 22–24.

Heidegger, M. (1962). Being and time (J. Macquarrie & E. Robinson, Trans.). New York: Harper & Row.

Makkreel, R. A. (1977). Introduction. In R. M. Zaner & K. L. Heiges (Trans.), Descriptive psychology and historical understanding (pp. 1–20). The Hague, Netherlands. Nijhoff.

Meleis, A. (1990, September). Directions for nursing theory development. Paper presented at the National Nursing Theory Conference, Los Angeles, CA.

Munhall, P. (1989). Philosophical ponderings on qualitative research methods in nursing. Nursing Science Quarterly, 2, 20–28.

Newman, M. (1986a). Health as expanding consciousness. St. Louis: Mosby.

Newman, M. (1986b). Nursing's emerging paradigm: The diagnosis of pattern. In A. M. McLane (Ed.), Classification of nursing diagnoses: Proceedings of the seventh conference. St. Louis: Mosby.

Newman, M. (1990). Newman's theory of health as praxis. Nursing Science Quarterly, 3, 37–41.

Parse, R. R. (1981). Man–living–health: A theory of nursing. New York: Wiley.

Parse, R. R. (1987). Nursing science: Major paradigms, theories and critiques. Philadelphia: Saunders.

Parse, R. R. (1990a, September). [Speaker on] Panel of nursing theorists. National Nursing Theory Conference, Los Angeles, CA.

Parse, R. R. (1990b). Health: A personal commitment. Nursing Science Quarterly, 3, 136–140.

Paterson, J. G., & Zderad, L. T. (1988). Humanistic nursing. New York: National League for Nursing.

Polkinghorne, D. (1983). Methodology for the human sciences: Systems of inquiry. Albany: State University of New York Press.

Ricoeur, P. (1974). The conflict of interpretations: Essays in hermeneutics (W. Domingo et al., Trans.). Evanston, IL: Northwestern University Press.

Rogers, M. E. (1970). An introduction to the theoretical basis of nursing. Philadelphia: Davis.

Schutz, A. (1967). The phenomenology of the social world (G. Walsh & F. Lehnert, Trans.). Evanston, IL: Northwestern University Press.

Watson, J. (1985). Nursing: Human science and human care. Norwalk, CT: Appleton-Century-Crofts.

Webster's ninth new collegiate dictionary. (1985). Springfield, MA: Merriam-Webster.

Winch, P. (1958). The idea of a social science and its relation to philosophy. London: Routledge & Kegan Paul.

CHAPTER 20

Professionalism and the Evolution of Nursing as a Discipline: A Feminist Perspective

Judith Wuest, RN, MN

The evolution of nursing knowledge and nursing as a practice discipline has been stunted by the quest for professionalism. Liberal and socialist feminist theory clarifies the hazards inherent in the masculine institution of professionalism for a predominately female discipline. Socialist feminist theoretical perspectives facilitate a vision of nursing that includes altering social structure such that caring is valued.

The development of nursing as a discipline has been dominated by the hegemony of the patriarchal institutions of professionalism. Feminism can broadly be defined as seeking to end the domination of women (Jaggar, 1983). Nursing, historically a women's occupation, has been a vehicle of both liberation and oppression. The lens of liberal and socialist feminist theory provides a perspective for examining the evolution of nursing as a discipline. Professionalism has played a key role in marginalizing nursing and in constraining knowledge development. Feminism with its emphasis on praxis illuminates possible future directions in knowledge development for nursing as a practice discipline.

Feminist Theoretical Perspectives

Feminist theories have defined the causes of women's oppression and offer a means for

---

Source: Wuest, J. (1994). Professionalism and the evolution of nursing as a discipline: A feminist perspective. Journal of Professional Nursing, 10(6): 357–367. Reprinted with permission from W.B. Saunders. Copyright © 1994.

eliminating it (MacPherson, 1991). Alison Jaggar (1983) clearly distinguished between liberal and socialist feminism.

Liberal Feminist Theory

"Liberal feminism rests on a conception of human nature that is radically individualistic" (Jaggar, 1983, p. 355). Impartiality is a key tenet of liberal feminism. Thus, all individuals should be treated equally, and women should receive no special privileges. The focus of liberal feminism is on eliminating oppression by seeking equal opportunity for women, not on determining the factors that lead to women's oppression (MacPherson, 1991). The major approach to knowledge development is logical positivism, a legacy of Cartesian dualism. Adequacy of scientific theory is based on objectivity, scientific method, and value-free criterion. Within the liberal tradition, judgments must be impartial to the perspective of a particular group or individual.

Socialist Feminist Theory

Socialist feminism adopts the Marxist view that individual existence requires interaction with other humans and the nonhuman world. Knowledge development occurs in the process of human activity that is influenced by society. Knowledge is not value free and is always shaped by the perspective of the class from which the knowledge emerges. In contrast to the Marxist view that the perspective of the working class is most adequate, socialist feminism asserts that the standpoint of women is most valid because women's social position gives them access to a reality not accessible to men and because women have no vested interest in maintaining the status quo of a patriarchal society. Although this is a similar position to that of radical feminists, the difference lies in how the knowledge is acquired. Socialist feminists do not accept that the standpoint of women is expressed in "women's naive and unreflective worldview" (Jaggar, 1983, p. 371) because this is distorted by male-dominated structure and ideology. Instead, women's standpoint is continually evolving through scientific and political struggle. Jaggar acknowledged that individual women's standpoints may differ especially by race and class but suggested that this diversity contributes to a representation of reality that is continuously unfolding. Women's standpoint evolves in a matrix operation in which women's distinctive social experience guides the pattern of research in a particular discipline and the outcomes of the research are then tested within the social reality of women. Knowledge is deemed useful if it helps to reconstruct a world in which women's interests are not subordinate to those of men.

Feminism, Professionalism, and Nursing

Until recently, nursing links with feminism have been tenuous. A brief historical look at both the women's movement and the growth of professionalism in North America will shed light on the development of the discipline of nursing. From a socialist feminist perspective, examining historical context is essential; however, this examination reveals that any links between nursing and feminism have largely been in the liberal feminist tradition of seeking equality.

Early Women's Movement

Cott (1987) identified three foci in the women's movement of the 19th century: service and social action performed by charitable, altruistic women who felt their gender gave them a special mandate and who found new strength in their collectivity and self-assertion; women's rights action performed by individually motivated women who wanted "rights equivalent to those men enjoyed on legal, political, economic, and civic grounds" (p. 16); and action for self-determination through "emancipation from structures, conventions and attitudes enforced by law and custom" (p. 16). Regardless of specific beliefs, "the spectrum of ideology in the women's movement had a see-saw quality" (Cott, 1987, p. 19). At one end were elimination of limitations and the attainment of equal rights, a liberalist perspective. At the other was the desire to value the unique qualities and abilities that women had to offer society. This valuing resulted either in acceptance of the unique but subservient status of women's existing social order or in adoption of a socialist feminist approach to change the existing social order to one that valued women in different ways. "No collective resolution of these tensions occurred and seldom even did individuals resolve them in their own minds" (Cott, 1987, p. 20).

Nursing's Early Development in North America

The three positions of maintaining the status quo, seeking equality, and seeking to change the social order can be seen in nursing's development. "Nursing's identity has been inextricably bound to the very word and notion of nurturance as well as to the myth that women exist to be mothers" (Church, 1990, p. 7). Initially, nursing was simply one of the many domestic roles that women were expected to fulfill on the basis of love and obligation (Reverby, 1987). "To practice it [nursing] at home was to fulfill the true calling of womanhood" (O'Brien, 1986, p. 14). By the mid 1800s in North America, despite the desire of middle class women to be ladies, many found themselves economically in need of work. The affluent could afford to hire others to take on many of their domestic responsibilities. Hence, the emergence of the professed nurse.

> They brought to the bedside only the authority their personalities and community stature could command. Neither credentials nor a professional identity gave weight to their efforts. Their womanhood and the experience it gave them, defined their authority and taught them to nurse (Reverby, 1987, p. 6).

In contrast to factory work, "the nature of nursing with its roots deep in the domestic world of the family, muted the dramatic shift in self-perception that women in factory work experienced" (O'Brien, 1986, p. 13).

Reverby (1987) noted that within the hospital setting, working class women attempted to exert control on working conditions and relationships with physicians, despite their lack of formal training and subservient class position.

The sense of rights of working class womanhood gave them authority to press their demands. The necessity to care and their perception of its importance to patient outcome also structured their belief that demanding the right to be relatively autonomous was possible (Reverby, 1987, pp. 6–7).

Nevertheless, these women were unsuccessful largely because of class differences between nurses and hospital administrators, paternalism, and very demanding work.

Few nurses at this time were engaged in trying to change the social order. Lavinia Dock was a pioneer in nursing history who was labeled a suffragist, a pacifist, and a Marxist. Her overriding concern was self-determination for women, nurses, and nursing (Church, 1990). Throughout her life, she challenged nurses to fight against male dominance but was considered by the majority of nurses as deviant. Dock urged nursing leaders to involve public and political activism (Ashley, 1976). A more widely known nurse feminist was Margaret Sanger, birth control agitator, who championed women's rights to control their sexuality regardless of church or state (Cott, 1987). These nurses made a significant contribution to the development of nursing but were representative of a minority view within nursing.

During this time period, Nightingale's philosophy of nursing education, legitimated by her successes in the Crimea, was developing a following in North America. Her intentions were to establish autonomous schools of nursing, under the control of nurses who would ultimately share power with physicians in the health care setting. Although this approach was admirable from the liberalist feminist perspective, her intended hierarchy within the nursing school eliminated the possibility of equality among nurses (Reverby, 1987). Nightingale's vision was distorted in its implementation by the physicians and hospital superintendents in North America who viewed schools of nursing as vehicles for obtaining cheap labor. They supported the establishment of apprenticeship schools and in doing so gained control over nurse's labor (Melosh, 1982). Nightingale indicated that nurses were prepared by developing womanly virtue. Thus, she legitimized paid work by embodying in it 19th century social values and needs (O'Brien, 1986). From a socialist feminist perspective, nursing is an example of household work shifted to the outside world of production. Because this work was not valued when it took place within the home, it similarly received little economic or status reward when practiced publicly (Miller, 1991). Coburn (1987) noted that despite the desire of upper-class Nightingale nurses to attract refined women to nursing, the difficult working conditions and unpleasant work deterred many. The majority of recruits were working-class women whose only other option was factory work.

The school's emphasis on high moral character constituted an imposition of upper-class values on working-class women. The socialization process during training rested largely in the hands of middle- and upper-class nursing educators—women whose financial and social position allowed them to receive the necessary qualifications to teach (Coburn, 1987, p. 447).

This was the beginning of a class system within nursing: the elite educators and administrators versus the bedside practicing nurses. From a socialist feminist perspective, many of the decisions made from this point forward ensured the continuation of this division.

Ashley (1976) suggested that the apprenticeship system of nursing educations entrenched the domination of nurses by physicians and hospital administrators.

> Convinced of their inferiority and of the need for their subordination to the medical profession, many nurses identified with the system that oppressed them and worked to support its continuing existence. Nurses learned to believe in the virtues of hospital training. Early conditioning within these institutions intensified the capacity of women to aid the cause of their oppressors (Ashley, 1976, p. 32).

Nursing training was rigid, orderly, and disciplined and students were overworked. Nevertheless, standards of care were established, nurses developed pride in their skills, had their idealism nurtured, and felt empowered to care (Reverby, 1987).

> … nurses have emphasized perceived womanly qualities and differences

from men by stressing a role complementary to that performed by men. This position, often labelled anti-feminist, has led present-day feminists to disregard nursing because it tends to epitomize a set of characteristics and problems from which women are attempting to distance themselves (Kirkwood, 1991, p. 53).

In this sense, nursing embodies the dilemma of early (and present day) feminists who, by seeking equality, deny the very uniqueness of their contribution to society, but nursing was being controlled by forces beyond simply their desire to care.

> … caring was shaped not simply by women's psychological identity but by the social and political context in which nursing developed. It was a duty to care directed by a male medical hierarchy, not an ethic of care in which nurses would be able to make more autonomous judgments about the kind of care patients should receive (Baines, 1991, p. 63).

Nurses and Physicians

At the turn of the century, the medical profession was not well established in North America and was open to competition from nurses, pharmacists, and other allied occupations (Torrance, 1987). Medical students had no internship and nursing students in training schools had greater opportunity to observe and to care for the sick. Although the training system had established physicians as dominant, their position was not secure. In 1904 through 1905, Abraham Flexner, a sociologist, visited and assessed Canadian and American medical schools. His report, published in 1910, was highly critical of schools that lacked the facilities to teach laboratory-based scientific medicine and resulted in the closure or reorganization of 92 medical schools. "The Flexner Report . . . helped to consolidate the dominance of the allopathic practitioners and to establish laboratory-based scientific medical education and practice. This mechanistic-individualistic conception is currently pervasive in medical practice and research" (Bolaria, 1988, p. 3). The alliance of medicine with science and the subsequent entrenchment of medical education in the university resulted in the definition and domination of the health care field by the physicians. Flexner's study led also to a definition of "profession" and that had significant implications for the future of nursing.

Professionalism

In 1915, Flexner presented a paper that identified the criteria for characterizing professions from an analysis of the universally acknowledged professions of law, medicine, and clergy (Parsons, 1986).

> Professions involve essentially intellectual operations; they derive their raw materials from science and learning; this material they work up into a practical and definite end; they possess an educationally

communicable technique; they tend to self-organization; they are becoming increasingly altruistic in motivation (Flexner, 1915, p. 904).

This definition stressed rationalism, scientific standards, and objectivity, all characteristics that embodied the masculine ethos. His masculine, sociological view was never questioned and the criteria became the sociological standard for distinguishing professions (Parsons, 1986). Professions were dominated by men and "a culture developed that affirmed male-centered values of order, efficiency, and hierarchical division of labour" (Baines, 1991). Flexner's paper also suggested that occupations could alter their status and become professions by developing the traits that were lacking.

Professions, reinforced by their scientific credibility, became sources of power and prestige. Professionalization offered white, middle-class men a means of carving out new roles and obtaining monopoly on their services (Baines, 1991). Women who entered women-dominated professions were more motivated by an ethic of service or care than by a desire for power (Baines, 1991). "The bases for women's special expertise and place within the professions continued to rest on an ideology of service that lionized caring as a virtue particular to women" (Baines, p. 55). The norm of professionalism is historically and socially unacceptable to women because of their exclusion from its conception (Parsons, 1986). Cott (1987) noted that although women professionals were seen as leaders before obtaining the vote, once the vote was attained, the bond that held them together was gone. A barrier developed between women professionals and nonprofessionals. To progress within the professions, and hold the tenets of non-bias, objectivity, and impersonality, women were required to abandon allegiance to feminism and create a community of interest with professional men rather than non-professional women (Cott, 1987). Glazer and Slater (1987) noted that professionals scorned nurturant, expressive, and familial interaction, valuing expertise and monopoly over an ethic of service.

Nursing and Professionalism

"Prior to Flexner, American nurses . . . were secure in their identity as professionals" (Parsons, 1986, p. 273). However, nursing did not measure up to Flexner's criteria. By 1936, there were articles in nursing journals that indicated nursing was a developing profession (Parsons, 1986). Nursing had a limited body of scientific knowledge defined as nursing and exclusive of other disciplines. Because the phenomena unique to nursing had not been articulated and studied, nursing lacked control over practice and was subordinate to the medical profession (Lyon, 1990). Varying levels of educational preparation resulted in the absence of pervasive ideology and monopoly over work. Roberts (1984) asserted that nurses, once autonomous, became oppressed through societal forces and now exhibit the characteristics of an oppressed group. "Nurses have also accepted the fact that if they could only attain the characteristics of the powerful, or

professional status, they too would be powerful" (Roberts, 1984, p. 26).

In the early 20th century, women who wanted recognition for nurses as significant health care providers readily accepted Flexner's assertion that an occupation could become a profession. Acceptance of professional ideology can be viewed as a strength from a liberal feminist perspective. It pushed nurses to sever the link with domestic labor and establish standards of paid work, to refuse the limitations of gender in their own lives and in goals for nursing profession, and to challenge the traditional constraints on women in the workforce (Melosh, 1982). Because nursing was a women's profession, women had the potential monopoly and power to effect change. What nurses and other women striving for more traditional professions failed to recognize was that the criteria that they were trying to meet were established by men. The rightness of these criteria was not questioned. In fact, by accepting these criteria, and striving to meet them, nursing was supporting the existing patriarchal order. This decision resulted in securing privileges for few nurses at the expense of many (Melosh, 1982).

Knowledge Development

Professionalism and Knowledge Development

When nursing leaders decided to respond to the Flexner report by seeking to meet his criteria of profession, they recognized that nursing had to establish a scientific knowledge base. Because professionals had to be scientific, and the only academic preparation for nurses at that time was at the Columbia Teacher's College, most study and research related to education and administration and not to clinical practice (Baer, 1987). Thus, academically prepared nurses were further divided from those practicing at the bedside, and there was much debate about whose work was the most meaningful. This divisiveness is characteristic of the horizontal violence of oppressed groups. Roberts (1984) noted that whether nurses were in the hospital or the academic setting they were (and are) rewarded for being marginal and taking on the characteristics of the dominant groups. As nursing programs opened up in universities in Canada and the United States, nurses struggled to have their knowledge and experience validated as scholarship. "A knowledge base for nursing stemming from women's private, domestic sphere was suspect within the male-dominated culture of the university, which took pride in intellectual scientific achievements" (Kirkwood, 1991, p. 54).

World War II opened opportunities for nurses to expand their practice roles and to have advanced university study in post-war years; however, Baer (1987) noted that all nurses were not enthusiastic about these openings. Nurses seeking professionalization were anxious to upgrade their educational preparation, but this was very threatening to nurses who had trained under the hospital system. Hospital educators, anxious to support apprenticeship, failed to grasp post-war opportunities for upgrading. This further developed the class system in nursing.

Research became an issue for nurses as they attempted to establish a scientific knowledge base. Nurses ignored gender issues and moved away from its domestic heritage. "Nurses believed that, if they met university demands to demonstrate nursing was a scholarly discipline with a unique scientific base, nurses would be accorded the same professional respect as others in the university" (Kirkwood, 1991, p. 61). Hughes (1990, p. 31) noted that the development of nursing as a discipline is often equated with its evolution as a profession, but history "suggests that professional status is not likely to evolve passively from nursing's recognition as a scholarly discipline." However, it is significant that "by successfully developing and maintaining university nursing education, nurses have to some extent undermined the patriarchal structure of the university by locating work, traditionally assigned to women in the public sphere of higher education dominated by men" (Kirkwood, 1991, p. 62).

In November 1951, the American Journal of Nursing announced the publication of Nursing Research, noting that research was essential for knowledge development in nursing (Baer, 1987). It was 1976 before over half the articles published focused on clinical practice rather than education because most of the researchers were nursing faculty whose higher education had been in education. Whereas their institutions required that they participate in scholarly activity to meet criteria for tenure and promotion, service agencies and hospitals did not encourage such activity from practicing nurses (Baer, 1987). Hence, the gap widened with practitioners viewing educators as more and more removed from the real world of nursing.

> Nursing's major goal in fostering research was to achieve recognition of its professional status. Some individual nurses certainly saw research as a means, a method through which they could answer questions and expand their ideas, but for most nurses, it was an end, a criterion of professionalism they yearned to attain (Baer, 1987, p. 24).

Research and Theory Development

Early approaches to research followed the reductionistic methods of the biomedical model as the surest way to be credible as scientists (Nagle & Mitchell, 1991). Nursing adopted the empirical ethic of science through a research tradition "that concentrates on objectivity, facts, measurement of smaller and smaller parts, and issues of instrumentality, reliability, validity, and operationalization to the point that nursing is in danger of exhausting the meaning, relevance, and understanding of the values, goals, and actions that it espouses in its heritage and ideals" (Watson, 1988, p. 17). Researchers have only recently begun to recognize that the scientific method is insufficient for addressing many of nursing's concerns and are beginning to embrace more diverse, qualitative approaches to research.

Concern for nursing's lack of theory base developed in the 1960s when nurses began to study at a doctoral level in other disciplines. The embryonic nursing science was attached to other sciences and fed on their theories, methods, and instruments (Stainton, 1982). Much debate developed surrounding such issues as whether nursing theory should be borrowed from other disciplines, single versus multiple theories, and whether theories should influence or be influenced by practice.

At early nursing theory conferences, the views of theory development expressed by such leaders as Dickoff and James and Abdellah supported the logical empiricist tradition for the development of nursing science (Silva & Rothbart, 1983). "Early nurse theorists such as Roy and Orem maintained the status quo of objective reductionism by focusing on problems and defining health according to medical and/or societal norms" (Nagle & Mitchell, 1991, p. 18). Although nurses were strongly supporting this approach, the philosophers of science from where this tradition stemmed were seriously questioning the limitations of this approach (Silva & Rothbart, 1983; Webster & Jacox, 1985). Nurse researchers and theorists recognized the limitations of the received view in theorizing about people's experiences with health and illness; however, the drive for professionalism and scientific legitimacy resulted in nursing, as an emerging discipline, holding on to this respectable approach.

> In the 1960s, the unity and political and academic power of the received view theorists were sufficiently great that lip service had to be paid to their basic beliefs. Now we are free to choose among the insights of the received view and select only

those that we find useful and sound for our purposes in constructing nursing theory (Webster & Jacox, 1985, p. 27).

These authors suggest that nursing is free to develop its own philosophy of science. Evidence of changing views about the philosophy of science is in the works of such theorists as Watson (1988) and Parse (1981).

Theory and Nursing Practice Theory is argued to be important in the establishment of the unique body of knowledge essential for nursing to be recognized as a profession and as a means of fostering communication and improving patient care. Theory development through creative conceptualization expanded nursing knowledge. However, the language of theory is frequently abstract and there is much discussion among theorists and those attempting to understand and apply nursing theories to practice. "There are serious credibility gaps between the ideal prescriptive theory that is taught and the practical knowledge used by practitioners" (Aydelotte, 1990, p. 10).

> Resultant debates have tended to develop into a vicious circle, with theorists berating practitioners for their lack of concern with the conceptual basis for their actions, whilst practitioners bemoan theoretical approaches which are seen as having little or no relevance to their daily work (Nolan & Grant, 1992).

Fawcett (1992) asserted the existence of a reciprocal relationship between conceptual models and nursing practice, but she was adamant that the models come first and are tested for their credibility and refined in the field of clinical practice. This position fails to consider the fact that many practitioners find the conceptual model too obscure to enter into that reciprocity.

Nagle and Mitchell (1991) noted that nursing is being driven by professional licensing bodies and accreditation bodies to adopt a single theory as a base for practice within their agency. They suggested that this is a paternalistic action that denies nurses the autonomy of choosing their own theoretic base for practice consistent with their unique worldview. This suggestion assumes that most practicing nurses have articulated a worldview and is further evidence of the rift between practitioners and those nurses with advanced education. This imposition may give practicing nurses a means for voicing what they do and do not like about practicing within a specific, theoretical framework. This may be the key to Fawcett's reciprocity.

Feminism: Looking to the Future for Nursing

The acceptance of patriarchal professionalism has resulted in nursing adopting liberalist traditions for the development of research and practice. "Feminism, in its liberal form, appears to give nursing a political language that argues for equality and rights within the given order of things" (Reverby, 1987, p. 10). Nurses have often been criticized for rejecting liberal feminism.

From a feminist perspective, the individualism and autonomy promised by this rights framework often fails to acknowledge collective social need, to provide a way for adjudicating conflict over rights, or to address the reasons for the devaluing of female activity (MacPherson, 1991, p. 30).

Reverby (1987) suggested that nursing will have to create the social climate that values caring. This implies the need for a socialist feminist approach in which nursing takes a more active role in altering social structure.

Professionalization has objectified those for whom nurses care. "A feminist ethos of professionalism needs to be based on an ideology that integrates an ethic of care and forms a more equal partnership with the cared for" (Baines, 1991, p. 67). Feminism offers some revolutionary ideas for nursing (Chinn, 1987). "Feminism values and endorses women, critiques male thinking, challenges patriarchal systems, and focuses on creating self-love and respect for all others and all forms of life" (Chinn, 1987, p. 23).

Knowledge Development

Dorothy Smith (1990) addressed the impact that hegemony has on knowledge development by influencing the issues that are valued and by dictating an approach to those issues based on the conceptual view of those institutions rather than the lived experiences of the people involved. As people are educated to take up roles within institutions, they are exposed to a "conceptual imperialism" (Smith, 1990, p. 15) that ensures a perpetuation of the worldview of the institution under the guise of objectivity. People have two ways of knowing, experiencing and doing: one on a local, immediate, bodily level, and one that is at an objective, conceptual level. The objective account, giving the appearance of neutrality and impartiality, in fact conceals class, gender, and race and puts forward the ideology of the governing groups. The objectified text has power because of the way it organizes social relations. People read the objectified text as fact and repress their own lived experience. Thus, people begin to see things the same way. "Objectified knowledge, as we engage with it, subdues, discounts, and disqualifies our various interests, perspectives, angles, and experience, and what we might have to say speaking from them" (Smith, 1990, p. 80).

Smith's account sheds some light on the current division that exists between nursing theory and practice. Nursing theory has been developed by the elite and educated, the nurses who have wielded power in the development of nursing as a profession. The separation of these nurses from those at the bedside has been well documented. These nurses identified a professional route for the development of nursing knowledge and endorsed the patriarchal structure. Hence, the approaches to nursing theory reflect the dominant culture rather than the lived experience of nurses at the bedside.

Smith (1990) argued that women must create a reflexive critique through investigation that is grounded in the lives of women and people. This requires an exploration of women's everyday experience with socially organized practices and an examination of how women's practices contribute to and are articulated with the relations that rule our lives. This emphasis on praxis is most consistent for the development of nursing knowledge that reflects the human experience of nursing. However, a major barrier exists. Many nurses who wield educational and administrative power within nursing have a vested interest in maintaining their current positions of power and this is readily accomplished through Smith's "conceptual imperialism." For a significant change to occur nurse leaders and educators must be conscious of this oppression.

There is evidence that nursing is beginning to consider some more revolutionary approaches to knowledge development. Critical scholarship, a pattern of thought and action that challenges institutionalized power relations in the social reality of nursing has been suggested by Thompson (1987) as one means of addressing the issues that nursing faces. She urged nurses to question the assumption that underlie our liberal undergraduate education such as the logical positivist approach to science, the functionalist framework of the social world, and professional ideology because these assumptions foster acceptance of the status quo. "Critical scholarship in nursing can speak about the process of reweaving, regaining confidence in new reality, regaining a commitment to new definitions of nursing practice, and feeling grounded in new value orientations" (Thompson, 1987, p. 37). Anderson (1991, p. 2) noted that feminism and poststructuralist perspectives

> challenge us to extend our analysis of phenomena relating to the lives of clients or patients beyond the micro level of analysis to an examination of the broader social processes that influence health and illness behaviour. This has the potential for the development of nursing science that will be inclusive of the complex socioeconomic, historical, and political nexus in which human experience is embedded.

Silva and Rothbart (1983), drawing on the work of Laudan, suggested that nursing theory development is currently in a state of transition, that it will never result in a static set of truths but will always be evolving.

> Data for nursing theory development and testing will include the common practices of nurse clinicians, the social and psychological factors affecting the profession of nursing, the widely held beliefs of the community of nurses, and the reasoning patterns of individual nurse theorists. A result of integrating these data will be a nursing theory that more explicitly addresses the human dimension of nursing (Silva & Rothbart, 1983, p. 11).

The test for adequacy of theory will be more focused on solution of nursing care problems than on truth and error. This is very consistent with socialist feminist theory for which the criteria of adequacy is usefulness. These approaches hold promise for future development of nursing research and theory development.

Feminist Epistemology and Research Methodology

Jaggar and Bordo (1989, p. 4) indicated that feminist epistemology shares the critique of many philosophers that "the Cartesian framework is fundamentally inadequate, an obsolete and self-deluded world view badly in need of reconstruction and revisioning" borrowing from other traditions such as Marxist historicism, psychoanalytic theory, literary theory, and sociology of knowledge to support its claim. Contemporary feminism's arguments differ from others in the assertion that the Cartesian framework is not gender neutral. Feminist epistemology is not about women being able to conduct science in its current form as well as men can. "Rather its position is that women who have come to recognize and accept feminist assumptions about the world will practice science differently in a world that legitimates these assumptions. . ." (Farganis, 1989, p. 208). Belenky, Clinchy, Goldberger, and Tarule (1986) have identified that the epistemological perspectives that influence how women see and know the world are different from those of men.

Farganis (1989) suggested that feminism acknowledges that each person has a different position from which they view the world but does not accept that each view is equally good. Feminism has a moral dimension that opposes normative relativism. Because of their experiences as marginal persons and their experiences of care and concern, "women can offer an epistemically sounder and politically and morally better position" (p. 217). Rose (1988) supported this view urging that knowledge gained through the practice of caring be a base for a science that values people. Harding (1986) went one step further and suggested that the hierarchy of positivism should be reversed with studies directed by such moral emancipatory interests as the elimination of sexist, racist, and classist understandings of social life being most valued.

In the health care field, patriarchal standards have reigned and the personal experience of professional caregiving has been devalued. "Feminist ideology holds that marginal persons in society are those whose roles threaten those in power" (Miller, 1991, p. 49). Nursing can be considered marginal and this results in "the development of care modalities that are unspoken, unrecognized, and unappreciated by the dominant groups and, therefore, by society at large" (Miller, 1991, p. 49). Feminist approaches to science support the development of a nursing science based on the knowledge that nurses have gained through practice.

A further contribution that feminism makes to nursing knowledge development is direction for research. Fonow and Cook (1991) distilled four common, interdisciplinary themes of feminist epistemology and methodology that are helpful for nursing research.

Reflexivity This is the practice of reflecting on, examining critically, and exploring analytically the research process and using it to understand the underlying assumptions about gender relations. Consciousness raising is one method of reflexivity that is reflected in the increased consciousness of the researcher of the effects of the research process on the researcher's identity, the impact of the research on the subjects, and finally as a feminist research method. Collaboration between women researchers is another focus of reflexivity:

> . . . there is also the expectation among some scholars that feminist collaboration will bring about a deeper intellectual analysis, an original approach to framing questions, with a mind-set of innovation to deal with the gendered context of research (Fonow & Cook, 1991, p. 5).

Action Orientation The orientation of feminist research is toward social change. This can be accomplished by participating with people in an examination of positions and options, by historically analyzing the past for the purpose of future social change, or by focusing on the policy implications of research findings. "A personal commitment to feminism and to caring as a standard for professional nursing practice can only lead to the demand for major changes in the structure and provision of health care service to all human beings" (Gaut, 1991, p. 6). This change

can be accomplished by attention to research with an action orientation.

Attention to the Affective Components of the Research Act Feminist research recognizes the affective dimension and sees emotion as a source of insight. This can be connected to the notion of reciprocity between researcher and the researched manifested either in friendship or in negative interactions.

Use of the Situation at Hand This use of everyday, existing situations is particularly important for nursing research because nursing's major interest is the experiences of people in health and illness situations.

Conclusion

Professionalism has failed to bring nursing the power and prestige that were anticipated by nursing's early leaders. Professionalism is a patriarchal invention and by its very nature is alienating to women. By accepting the liberal tradition of knowledge development embodied in professionalism, nurses have not appreciated their own knowledge acquired through their caring experience. Rather than joining with other women to change the dominant social order to one that values women's unique differences, nurses have focused primarily on attaining professional status. Only recently have nurses begun to recognize that the received view of knowledge development is not sufficient for addressing the complex concerns of nursing as a human science. This realization has resulted in nursing seeking alternate approaches.

Feminism offers much to nursing through its focus on praxis. The liberalist feminist tradition of seeking equality is not sufficient to meet the challenges facing nursing. The socialist feminist perspective offers more direction. It suggests that nursing knowledge development should be directed toward creating a social order in which women are not subordinate to men. This means that our efforts should not be geared to maintaining the status quo within our field of practice but rather should be focusing on ways to alter public policy. Socialist feminism suggests that women as a social group have the more valid perspective because they have no vested interest in maintaining the status quo in society. Applying this view to nursing, nurses in practice have a more legitimate perspective of nursing than nurse leaders and educators. Thus, the distinctive experience of nursing practice should guide nursing research and the outcomes of research should be tested within the reality of practicing nurses because that reality may be quite different to that of the nurse researcher. The actual process of research should itself be dialectical, thus effecting some change in those participating. This approach may help to reduce the current chasm between nursing practice and research. Jean Watson urged nursing to "question its old dogmas, transcend its existing paradigms, and refocus its scientific attention to human phenomena that are consistent with the nature of nursing and preservation of humanity" (1988, p. 22). Feminism, particularly socialist feminism, has the potential to help nurses to meet this challenge and to make a significant contribution to changing the existing social order of health care and gender relations.

References

Anderson, J. (1991). Current directions in nursing research: Toward a poststructuralist and feminist epistemology. The Canadian Journal of Nursing Research, 23(3), 1–3.

Ashley, J. (1976). Hospitals, paternalism, and the role of the nurse. New York: Teachers College Press.

Aydelotte, M. (1990). The evolving profession: The role of the professional organization. In N. Chaska (Ed.), The nursing profession: Turning points (pp. 9–15). St. Louis: Mosby.

Baer, E. (1987). 'A cooperative venture' in pursuit of professional nursing status: A research journal for nursing. Nursing Research, 36, 18–25.

Baines, C. (1991). The professions and the ethic of care. In C. Baines, P. Evans, and S. Neysmith (Eds.), Women's caring: Feminist perspectives on social Welfare (pp. 36–72). Toronto, Canada: McClelland & Stewart.

Belenky, M., Clinchy, B., Goldberger, N., & Tarule, J. (1986). Women's ways of knowing. New York: Basic Books.

Bolaria, B. S. (1988). Sociology, medicine, health, and illness: An overview. In B. S. Bolaria & H. Dickinson (Eds.). Sociology of health care in Canada (pp. 1–14). Toronto, Canada: Harcourt Brace Jovanovich.

Chinn, P. (1987). Response: Revision and passion. Scholarly Inquiry for Nursing Practice, 1(1), 21–24.

Church, O. (1990). Nursing's history: What it was and what it was not. In N. Chaska (Ed.), The nursing profession: Turning points (pp. 3–8). St. Louis: Mosby.

Coburn, J. (1987). I see and am silent. In D. Coburn, C. D'Arcy, G. Torrance, & P. New (Eds.), Health care and Canadian society: Sociological perspectives (pp. 441–462). Markham: Fitzhenry and Whiteside.

Cott, N. (1987). The grounding of modern feminism. New Haven, CT: Yale University Press.

Farganis, S. (1989). Feminism and the reconstruction of social science. In A. Jaggar & S. Bordo (Eds.), Gender/Body/Knowledge: Feminist reconstructions of being and knowing (pp. 207–223). New Brunswick, NJ: Rutgers.

Fawcett, J. (1992). Conceptual models and nursing practice: The reciprocal relationship. Journal of Advanced Nursing, 17, 224–228.

Flexner, A. (1915). Is social work a profession? School Soc, 1, 901–911.

Fonow, M., & Cook, J. (1991). Back to the future: A look at the second wave of feminist epistemology and methodology. In M. Fonow & J. Cook (Eds.), Beyond method: Feminist scholarship as lived research (pp. 1–15). Bloomington: Indiana University Press.

Gaut, D. (1991). Caring and nursing: Explorations in feminist perspectives—Introductory remarks. In R. Neil & R. Watts (Eds.), Caring and nursing: Explorations in feminist perspectives (pp. 5–8). New York: National League of Nursing.

Glazer, P., & Slater, M. (1987). Unequal colleagues. New Brunswick, NJ: Rutgers.

Harding, S. (1986). The science question in feminism. Ithaca, NY: Cornell University Press.

Hughes, L. (1990). Professionalizing domesticity: A selected synthesis of nursing historiography. Advances in Nursing Science, 12(4), 25–31.

Jaggar, A. (1983). Feminist politics and human nature. Totowa, NJ: Rowman & Allenhead.

Jaggar, A., & Bordo, S. (1989). Gender/body/knowledge: Feminist reconstructions of being and knowing. New Brunswick, NJ: Rutgers.

Kirkwood, R. (1991). Discipline discrimination and gender discrimination: The case of nursing in Canadian universities, 1920–1950. Atlantis, 16(2), 52–63.

Lyon, B. (1990). Getting back on track: Nursing's autonomous scope of practice. In N. Chaska (Ed.), The nursing profession: Turning points (pp. 267–274). St. Louis: Mosby.

MacPherson, K. (1991). Looking at caring and nursing through a feminist lens. In R. Neil & R. Watts (Eds.), Caring and nursing: Explorations in feminist perspectives (pp. 25–43). New York: NLN.

Melosh, B. (1982). The physician's hand: Work culture and conflict in American nursing. Philadelphia: Temple University Press.

Miller, K. (1991). A study of nursing's feminist ideology. In R. Neil & R. Watts (Eds.), Caring and nursing: Explorations in feminist perspectives (pp. 43–56). New York: NLN.

Nagle, L., & Mitchell, G. (1991). Paradigmatic issues in research and practice. Advances in Nursing Science, 14(1), 17–25.

Nolan, M., & Grant, G. (1992). Mid-range theory building and the nursing theory-practice gap: A respite care case study. Journal of Advanced Nursing, 17, 217–223.

O'Brien, P. (1986). 'All a woman's life can bring': The domestic roots of nursing in Philadelphia, 1830–1885. Nursing Research, 36, 12–17.

Parse, R. (1981). Man-living-health: A theory of nursing. New York: Wiley.

Parsons, M. (1986). The profession in a class by itself. Nursing Outlook, 34, 270–275.

Reverby, S. (1987). A caring dilemma: Womanhood and nursing in historical perspective. Nursing Research, 36, 5–11.

Roberts, S. J. (1984). Oppressed group behavior: Implications for nursing. Advances in Nursing Science, 5(4), 21–30.

Rose, H. (1988). Beyond masculine realities. In R. Bleier (Ed.), Feminist approaches to science (pp. 57–76). New York: Pergammon.

Silva, M. C., & Rothbart, D. (1983). An analysis of changing trends in philosophies of science on nursing theory development and testing. Advances in Nursing Science, 6(3), 1–13.

Smith, D. (1990). The conceptual practices of power: A feminist sociology of knowledge. Toronto, Canada: University of Toronto Press.

Stainton, M. C. (1982). The birth of nursing science. Canadian Nurse, 78, 24–28.

Thompson, J. (1987). Critical scholarship: The critique of domination in nursing. Advances in Nursing Science, 10(1), 27–38.

Torrance, G. (1987). Socio-historical overview. In D. Coburn, C. D'Archy, G. Torrance, & P. New (Eds.), Health care and Canadian society: Sociological perspectives (pp. 6–32). Markham: Fitzhenry and Whiteside.

Watson, J. (1988). Nursing: Human science and human care: A theory of nursing. National League of Nursing.

Webster, G., & Jacox, A. (1985). The liberation of nursing theory. In J. McCloskey & H. Grace (Eds.), Current issues in nursing (pp. 20–29). Boston, MA: Blackwell.

CHAPTER 21

Rapture and Suffering with Technology in Nursing

Rozzano C. Locsin, RN, PhD, FAAN

Marguerite J. Purnell, RN, PhD, AHN-BC

Technology has shaped human life. As technology has become increasingly sophisticated, philosophers, such as Heidegger, have pondered the worth of its influence on the quality and duration of life. Concerns about technology encompass the experiences of persons whose lives depend on technologies and the experiences of those persons who care for them. Accompanying the rapture of technologies in nursing is the consequent suffering or the price of advancing dependency with technologies that critically influence contemporary human lives. With increased use of technologies and ensuing technological dependency experienced by recipients of care, the imperative is to provide technological competency as caring in nursing, guided by a formalized practice model such as the technological competency as caring in nursing theory.

Key words: *caring, intentionality, standing-reserve, technology.*

"I think people are often afraid that technology is making us less human."

—C. Brazeal (2001)

Technological advancements have shaped human life. As technology becomes increasingly sophisticated, philosophers carefully ponder the worth of its influence on the quality and duration of life. In health care, issues of the good, utility, and cost are foiled by the often fatal attraction of a glamorous drug or "technoluxe" cosmetic procedure (Frank, 2003) that promises rapture but instead delivers horror and suffering. From a Heideggerian philosophical view concerning technology and its "revealing" and complemented by Locsin's (1995) theory of technological competency as caring in nursing as framework, this chapter accentuates and discusses the effects of modern technology on

Source: Courtesy of the International Association for Human Caring

health care and focuses its influences primarily on nursing. The beneficial effects of technology are traced integral to health care, not only for nurses in professional practice but also for other professional caregivers who are faced with the burden of caring for persons in high-tech settings, including the home.

Over 50 years ago, well before the burgeoning of modern health care and specialized healthcare technology, the philosopher Martin Heidegger (1993) prophetically spoke of the danger of uncritical acceptance of technology and of disregard for its "ambiguous" (p. 338) essence. In dry, meaningful language he described how technology may not appear to be what it really is—coercive and consuming—and how human beings are simultaneously needed, both to bring order to or be ordered or used by technology. In describing the ways that modern technology is revealed, Heidegger observed, "The energy concealed in nature is unlocked, what is unlocked is transformed, what is transformed is stored up, what is stored up is in turn distributed, and what is distributed is switched about ever anew" (p. 322).

Heidegger's (1993) central concern was that future generations would not realize that this technological metamorphosis will create a "standing-reserve" (p. 322) that waits solely on and for the technology. Not only is nature in this standing-reserve but human beings both as sources and resources. For example, as Heidegger witnessed so many years ago, the "supply of patients for a clinic" (p. 323) was a standing-reserve. It is precisely the idea of human beings in this duality, influencing and

being influenced by healthcare technology, its iterations and various metamorphoses, and the challenges experienced in nursing caring in a technological environment that form the justification for this chapter.

The tension between the technological assessing of persons as objects, despite anthropomorphic "user friendly" external appearances, and the caring intention of nurses to know the person as whole and complete in the moment, obliquely pay homage to Heidegger's (1993) conception of the ambiguity (p. 338) of the essence of technology. Can this tension be ameliorated or reconciled?

Person or Object of Care?

The focus of nursing ought to be the understanding of patients as participants in their care rather than as objects of care. Often, the perspective of wholeness of person denotes the appreciation of the whole person as composite or derived from the understanding of an object-self. The object body is understood as that which can be known by an observer, a material entity, whereas the subject-self is the phenomenological body, "the body known from the inside, the body that is experienced, the lived body, the body as 'me'" (Sakalys, 2006, p.17). The conception of person as whole is predicated on the various understandings of this distinctive term.

The fundamental differences among knowing the composition of the person stem from the philosophical perspectives through which these terms are viewed. Commensurate with technology, from a positivist philosophical perspective, persons are appreciated through their component parts, recognizing the completeness of the person from a "lens" that depends on human sensory perception. The person is a whole being because the sensory (visual, hearing, touch, smell) data obtained by the observer, which are able to be machine replicated, reflect a "complete" person with physical composites and human physiological functioning.

Consider the subject of Shelley's (1919/1969) novel, *Frankenstein.* Frankenstein was a composite being and known for committing gruesome crimes. Created from several human body parts that were, in turn, obtained from as many different human beings, Frankenstein was put together, completed, made whole, and then brought to life. This human replica that was put together using various human parts was created biologically and humanly complete and eventually, when brought to life, appeared "more" human. Frankenstein came to be regarded as a human, albeit grossly distorted as a monster with characteristics "inherited" from the multiple donors of organ and limb to his life.

When viewing persons as participants in their care, instead of objects of care, biological wholeness and completeness as sensory evidence are not primary sources of knowledge. Rather, it is the relationship with others and the understanding of the value placed on life that allows nurses to know persons fully as "being cared for."

Influence of Technology on Practice

Such a concept, that a person is a person, may seem rhetorical. However, in nursing, views of persons range from the view of persons as whole in the moment to notions of persons as made up of parts. This latter understanding illustrates nursing practice as "fixing" persons to make them whole again and does not serve nursing well as a discipline of knowledge and practice profession. Rather, it perpetuates the understanding of nursing as a practice technique with a recipe to follow as guide to produce an outcome of care. Yet, the Heideggerian (1993) notion of "enframing" (p. 324), the coercive perpetuation of technology, forces nurses to objectify persons to care for them and challenges understandings of persons who are participating within the shared experience of a nursing situation. A glimpse of the influence of contemporary technology, with its extraordinary hold over human care and ethics, and the potential for nursing practice may be well perceived within the influences of social-political factors. Such a concern may happen to a person in custodial care and is in a "questionable" vegetative state. Is this person a living human being? Should the concern be that this person is only "like a human being" rather than "is a human being?"

In such a situation, when can a person cease to be a "real" human being? How often do similar objectifications and characterizations of persons not recognized as real human beings occur? In contrast, distinct and apart from this view of person as object dwells the particular idea of persons who are fully human, despite suffering endured and ensured by dependency on technological advances.

Punctuating this discussion of wholeness is a poignant story of an infant born in 1995 to migrant farmers working in the fields of South Florida. The infant was beautiful and healthy but was born without any arms or legs. It was totally dependent, then and now, on being cared for to supply every want and need. Yet, the infant is a whole person regardless of the missing parts. The customary technological resources used in assessing the health of persons created a distinct and limiting realization that with appendages missing, those vital "parts" around which the technologies were designed, for example, blood pressure cuffs, rendered the technologies deficient and immaterial. Physicians and nurses were concerned about how they could perform the usual but necessary technological care such as performing laboratory tests and the use of contraptions that traditionally require access through the limbs.

This situation emphasized Sandelowski's (1993) concern about the practice of nursing and the advent of technological dependency. Although the existence of modern, sophisticated, and advanced technologies were critical to modern nursing and health care, none of these technologies was up to the challenge of a person requiring unusual healthcare technological demands. "Knowing" the infant is a living and functioning human being, a person who is whole and complete in the moment regardless of the missing parts, was a reality, and coping with this reality was another challenge.

The focus of nursing is to know persons (Locsin, 2005). Ways of knowing persons are manifold and include empirical, ethical, aesthetic, and personal (Carper, 1978), as well as the symbolic and integrative ways of knowing (Phenix, 1964). In knowing persons the imperative is for nurses to focus on the "objective" composite of persons and, more important, on the "subjective" nature of being human. In a nursing encounter this particular view includes the moral imperative to know "who" is the person rather than the objectifying "what" is a person.

Coming to know the person is critical to nursing. Competently using technologies to achieve this goal is essential to appreciate nursing practice more fully as an integral aspect of human health care.

Human–Technology Interface in Nursing: Source or Resource?

The paradoxical enchantment/disenchantment of society with technology continues to spur the tension between subject and object, person and technology, source or resource, and the need for unified and integral care of the whole person. This disenchantment ripples from consumer to manufacturer to investor and is ultimately reflected in decreasing financial gains, far removed from the plight of the person experiencing the technology. In a report to over

700 investors, reporters, and entrepreneurs, Shipley (2006) stated the following:

> Making realistic robots is going to polarize the market, if you will. . . . You will have some people who love it and some people who will really be disturbed. . . . Individuals are becoming overwhelmed and worse, I believe that this state of being overwhelmed has moved the personal computing market to the point of diminishing returns.

The question arises of whether the disenchantment emanates from the view of technology as mere technology or is it something far deeper and primal? Is the acceptance of technology in various forms assisted by creating "user friendly" anthropomorphic attributes and human look-a-likes or, as this excerpt below recounts, a human feel-alike? Hogan (2004) stated as follows:

> After more than 2½ years of physical therapy and electronic stimulation, stroke victim Mike Marin still couldn't open a door with his left hand. Now, thanks to a robot, Marin can open a door. His atrophied left arm isn't completely useless anymore. Marin is at the forefront of what may seem an unlikely use for robots: providing the caring human touch.

This suggestion that robots and robotics-based technologies are designed to "provide the caring human touch" is intriguing. Although the goal is to provide the best quality of life for a person lacking the essential composites of a fully functioning human being, emulating a human through a provision of a robotic "caring human touch," although a technological advancement, seems to be a paradoxical answer to the challenges of human–computer interaction. Nevertheless, Hogan (2004) claimed the ability to show consistently improved therapy outcomes after using robots versus humans providing conventional, standard care. This is a far cry toward achieving even minimal "care" for persons who are technology challenged.

"Nursebot," a robot that alternately can assume the male and female personalities of Earl and Pearl by changing the voice gender, was tested among elderly patients. Despite the stereotype of older people being "technology phobic," the seniors accepted the robots. Their major concern was that the robots would not be able to do enough to provide adequate help for them. However, although robotic assistants are better suited for repetitive tasks, such as escorting persons to restrooms or reminding them to take medications, these same functions are now accomplished more cheaply by watches, radios, and the ubiquitous walker frame with tennis ball "gliders" on the legs.

The answer of society to the traditional ontological question, "What is nursing?", does not adequately reflect both the growth and development of nursing as a discipline of knowledge or as an expert, complex, practice profession. The need to continuously raise this question can be ascribed to the perennial use of the word "nurse" as narrowly referring to the routine performer of tasks and, as a consequence, to the image of nursing practice in all its complexity persisting as merely the performing of tasks. The creation of the robo-nurse—a complex piece of machinery that, in human fashion, is made to perform technical nurse activities such as taking a person's temperature (Gutierrez, 2000)—perpetuates this image. The robo-nurse simply facilitates completion of tasks for people, as does the nursebot described above. The persistent image of nursing as accomplishing tasks undeniably makes the nurse appear to be an automaton (Locsin, 2001). The essence of technology, whether enframed (Heidegger, 1993, p. 324) in complex anthropomorphic machinery or in graphic "live" viewing of functioning internal body parts, coerces and challenges caring as the essence of nursing in the expression of nursing practice.

Much can be said about technology in nursing, from its fascinating essence allowing greater dimensions of efficient and competent practice to the creation of phenomenal opportunities for persons to live more fully. From the appreciation of care practices as the skillful performance of activities for making persons well or healthy to the use of instruments and tools for promoting health and preventing illness, technology in nursing is critical to fostering health and wellness in contemporary times. The results of these technologies, however, also increase opportunities for care and cure activities, to the extent that contemporary health care appears to exist only because of the advantages of technological advances. Although technology captures our fascination with visions of an idyllic life, living out a life that

depends on technology can, likewise, lead to deep suffering. In doing so, understanding the ambiguity of the essence of technology and the consequences it evokes are befitting the revealing or poiesis (p. 317) of which Heidegger (1993) wrote. With increasing persistence for technological advancements and the dependency these technologies create for recipients and the users of the technologies, the imperative is to recognize and provide prospects for nursing guided by a framework of practice such as technological competency as caring (Locsin, 2005).

Two foci dictate the significance of technologies in nursing: *technological nursing*, described as the nursing of persons with lives that depend on technology, and *knowing persons*, described as the process through which nurses come to practice nursing using technological competency as caring in nursing to know persons more fully (Locsin, 2005). In each of these foci nursing provides the essential recognition of the influences of technology in nursing and health care. These essentials are directed toward the understanding of persons who experience life fully as human beings, regardless of depending on technologies.

Theory-Based Practice

Unraveling and acknowledging the allure of technology and the suffering occurring as a consequence of technology and its use are essential to nursing and its critical practice nature. *Technological Competency as Caring in Nursing* (Locsin, 2005) is a practice framework that allows for knowing the other as person and for providing self and the other opportunities to come to know through appreciating, affirming, and celebrating each other as person.

Practice of Nursing as Knowing Persons

How will the practice of nursing as knowing persons engage future human beings through caring, while simultaneously recognizing the often limited physical and psychological form and function of being human? How is competency with technology expressed in knowing persons as whole in the moment? The ultimate purpose of technological competency is to acknowledge persons as whole. Such acknowledgment compels the redesigning of processes of nursing—ways of expressing, celebrating, and appreciating the practice of nursing as continuously knowing persons as whole from moment to moment. In this practice of nursing, technology is used not to answer the question "What is a person?" but rather to come to know "Who is a person?" Although the former question alludes to the notion of persons as objects, the latter addresses the uniqueness and individuality of persons as human beings.

The advent of medical technology and its domination as a major influence in health care places nursing in an awkward position; being dependent on competencies for these technologies to engage in practice. The practice of nursing as technological competency—an expression of caring in nursing—is the achievement of knowing persons as whole moment to moment. It is the authentic, intentional, knowledgeable, and efficient use of technologies of nursing. These technologies influence the recognition of nursing as integral to health care. As such, this practice recognizes the role technology has on the practice of nursing. Technological competency allows the nurse to participate in the process of knowing persons as whole in the moment, the ultimate purpose of which is to continuously acknowledge persons as whole.

Nonetheless, in such a contemporary environment there is the possibility and likelihood that the nurse will be able to predict and prescribe for the one nursed. When this occurs, these situations forcibly lead nurses to appreciate persons more as objects than as persons. Such a situation can only occur when the nurse has assumed to "have known" the one nursed. Although it can be assumed that with the process of "knowing persons as whole in the moment," opportunities to continuously know the other become limitless. There is also a much greater likelihood that having "already known" the one nursed, the nurse will predict and prescribe activities or ways for the one nursed, and objectification of person ultimately occurs. This is the coercive yet elastic tension between the essence of technology and caring as the essence of nursing: Both are mediated by the thoughtful, technologically competent, and caring nurse. Although it is necessary to understand the operation of machine devices to understand the functioning human beings, the use of these technologies should not consign persons to be regarded as objects. The objectification of persons becomes an ordinary occurrence in situations wherein the practice of nursing is merely understood as achievement of tasks.

Technological competency as caring involves intentionality (Purnell, 2003) with compassion, confidence, commitment, and conscience as requisites to caring in nursing. Intentionality, in which are embedded patterns of values, ideals, and unique professional knowledge, which distinguish nursing, is active in shaping, guiding, and directing practice (Purnell, 2006). This is where the process of nursing takes on a focus different from the traditional series of problem-solving actions. By donning the lens of nursing as caring (Boykin & Schoenhofer, 2001), technological competency as caring in nursing is acknowledged. Through this lens, nursing is expressed as the simultaneous, momentary interconnectedness between the nurse and the nursed (Locsin, 1995). The nurse relies on the patient for calls for nursing. These calls are specific mechanisms that patients use, and they provide the opportunity for the nurse to respond with the authentic intention to know the other fully as whole person. Calls for nursing may be expressed as hopes, dreams, and aspirations. As uniquely as these nursing situations are expressed, the nurse is challenged to hear these calls for nursing and to respond authentically and intentionally in nurturance. These appropriate responses may be communicated as patterns of relating information, such as those derived from machineries like the electrocardiogram monitor, to know the physiological status of the person in the moment or to administer

life-saving medications, institute transfers, or to refer patients to other healthcare professionals as advocate for the patient in the moment.

The challenge of nursing is expressing technological competency as caring, ably focusing on the other as caring person, whole and complete in the moment, and growing in caring from moment to moment. Every human being uniquely responds to personal conditions in the moment. The nurse understands that the process of nursing occurs without preconceived views that categorize persons as needing to be fixed, like fitting the individuals into boxes of predicted conditions. By allowing the patient to unfold as a person and to live fully as a human being, the nurse facilitates the goal of nursing in the "caring between" and enhances personhood (Boykin & Schoenhofer, 2001) of both the nursed and the nurse.

Nursing practitioners long for a practice of nursing that is based on the authentic desire to know persons fully as human beings rather than as objects. Through this authentic intention and desire, nurses are challenged to use every creative, imaginative, and innovative way possible to appreciate and celebrate the person's intentions to live more fully and grow as a human being. Only with expertise with technologies of nursing can technological competence as an expression of caring in nursing be realized. The nurse as artist overcomes the essence of the technology with its continuing influence on the object or part and reveals what Heidegger (1993) called *physis* (p. 317)—a higher essence of poeisis, the unfolding of something into what it is, such as a blossom opening, or a call to a more primal truth (p. 333). In nursing, this primal truth is coming to know the one nursed through intention to care for wholeness of person, and for the whole person (Purnell, 2003), where in authentic presence the nurse brings all that he or she is to the nursing situation and attends to what matters.

It is evident from this description that describing nursing practice as the completion of tasks does not address the unfolding fullness of nursing. Nurses are urged to value technological competency as an expression of caring in nursing and as integral to health care. Otherwise, the image of the robo-nurse, simply facilitating completion of tasks for people, will render the nurse an automaton. The nurse will have fulfilled Heidegger's (1993) depictions of persons as standing-reserves, standing ready in endless cycles to serve the technology through a task-oriented practice.

Artificial Emotions and Evocative Objects

How will nursing be practiced in the future when human beings are partly machines? Turkle (2004) tapped into a side of technological dependence that is seldom addressed: that of emotional attachment:

> What has become increasingly clear is that, counter-intuitively, [human beings] become attached to sophisticated machines not for their smarts but their emotional reach. They seduce [human beings] by asking for human nurturance, not

intelligence. [Humans] are suckers not for realism but for relationships.

The advent of technological marvels in sustaining human lives, viewed from the ideals of persons as whole and the many ways nursing practice is grounded in caring perspectives, underscores nursing as a caring discipline. Nursing theories vicariously view human beings as whole and complete in the moment, as nursing transpiring between the nurse and the one nursed, and the appreciation of health as quality of life. The appreciation of these concepts dictates the understanding of how nursing is recognized, how it is practiced, and how nursing is integral to health care.

Reconciliation or Rift-Technology and Caring in Nursing

The focus of nursing is the person. However, technological advances, especially in modern medical and nursing practice, continue to challenge definitions of person. Through the lens of nursing as caring, all persons are understood as caring by the virtue of their humanness (Boykin & Schoenhofer, 2001). Persons are held to be whole in the moment with health as quality of life understood by the person being cared for. As human beings move closer toward the posthuman (Hayles, 2000), caring nursing theories must be flexible enough to accommodate new understandings of person. Traditionally, the central focus of nursing care has dealt with the human being as person. However, as modern and future advances in technology push toward our technological evolution, depending on our perspective, we will see partly human beings or partly human machines—cybernetic organisms (cyborgs) and other technosapiens as recipients of nursing. What will this nursing be like? How will nursing be experienced by the nurse and the one nursed? Will caring as the essence of nursing hold sway over technology? Heidegger (1993) said it best: "The closer we come to the danger, the more brightly do the ways unto the saving power begin to shine and the more questioning we become. For questioning is the piety of thought" (p. 341).

References

Brazeal, C. (2001). A sociable machine, *USA Today.*

Boykin, A., & Schoenhofer, S.O. (2001). *Nursing as caring: A model for practice.* Sudbury, MA: Jones and Bartlett.

Carper, B.A. (1978). Fundamental patterns of knowing in nursing. *Advances in Nursing Science,* 1(1), 13–23.

Frank, A.W. (2003). Connecting body parts: Technoluxe, surgical shapings, and bioethics. Paper presented at the "Vital Politics" conference, London School of Economics, September.

Gutierrez, L. (2000, March 1). Robo nurse? *The Palm Beach Post,* 3D.

Hayles, K. (2000). Visualizing the posthuman. *Art Journal,* 59(3), 50–54.

Heidegger, M. (1993). In D. F. Krell (Ed.), *Martin Heidegger: Basic writings.* San Francisco: Harper Collins.

Hogan, C. (2004). *The Boston Globe,* February 29.

Locsin, R.C. (1995). Machine technologies and caring in nursing. *Image: Journal of Nursing Scholarship,* 3(27), 201–203.

Locsin, R.C. (2001). *Advancing technology, caring, and nursing.* Westport, CT: Auburn House.

Locsin, R.C. (2005). *Technological competency as caring in nursing, a model for practice.* Indianapolis, IN: Sigma Theta Tau International Honor Society of Nursing.

Phenix, P.H. (1964). *Realms of meaning.* New York: McGraw Hill.

Purnell, M.J. (2003). Intentionality in nursing: A foundational inquiry. *Dissertation Abstracts International,* 64, 639.

Purnell, M.J. (2006). Development of a model of nursing education grounded in caring and application to online nursing education. *International Journal for Human Caring,* 10(3), 8–16.

Sakalys, J.S. (2006). Bringing bodies back in: Embodiment and caring science. *International Journal for Human Caring,* 10(3), 17–21.

Sandelowski, M. (1993). Toward a theory of technological dependency. *Nursing Outlook,* 41(1), 36–42.

Shelley, M. (1919/1969). *Frankenstein: Or the modern Prometheus.* New York: Oxford University Press.

Shipley, C. (2006). *Washington Post.* Retrieved February 8, 2006, from http://www.washingtonpost.com/wp/dyn/content/article/2006/02/08/AR200602080 2239.html

Turkle, S. (2004). A published interview by S. Allis. *The Boston Globe,* February 29.

CHAPTER 22

Exploring an Alternative Metaphor for Nursing: Relinquishing Military Images and Language

Gail J. Mitchell, RN, PhD

Mary Ferguson-Paré, RN, PhD, CHE

Joy Richards, RN, PhD

The language used to describe nursing practice and nursing leadership has a profound influence on what nurses believe about themselves, their work relationships, and indeed the very essence of their reason for being. Language often includes metaphor to help capture the complexities and layers of meaning that establish contexts for action. Nurses and others have relied on various metaphors to describe nursing work. However, one metaphor, more than any other, has shaped the context of nursing work and formed the images and the meanings that nurses have of themselves and their purposes in practice. The privileged one is the military metaphor. This chapter explores the notion of metaphor and its usefulness and potential to help nurses change their work patterns. The traditions and history of the military metaphor are examined and an alternative notion of the "frontier" is proposed to enhance understanding of the potential for change.

Key words: *metaphor, military model, hierarchy, nurse–client relationship.*

The use of language in nursing is a matter of longstanding interest and concern for the current authors. Discussions about language and the meanings and images used to describe nursing practice and nursing leadership have a profound influence on how nurses think about themselves, their work

Source: Mitchell, Ferguson-Paré, Richards. Exploring an Alternative Metaphor for Nursing: Relinquishing Military Images and Language. Nursing Leadership, 16(1) 2003: 48-60. Reprinted with permission from Longwoods Publishing Corporation.

relationships, and, indeed, the very essence of their reason for being. Language shapes how nurses define the nature of their presence with clients and families. Before that, it is language that houses one's reasons for being a nurse. Language reveals meaning in a public way. Language and attitude, together, show clearly how nurses think about their work and their relationships with clients, families, and colleagues. Belenky et al. (1986) proposed that women prefer to work toward a morality of responsibility and care for others that is informed by context and by the exchange of meaning through language and dialogue that enhances understanding and respect for multiple perspectives.

The choice of language used by women (and all persons) often includes metaphor to capture the complexities and layers of meaning that establish contexts for action. Nurses and others have relied on various metaphors to describe nursing work. However, the military metaphor, more than any other, has shaped the context of nursing work and formed the images and the meanings that nurses have of themselves and their purposes in practice.

The purpose of this chapter is to explore the notion of metaphor and its usefulness and potential to help nurses change their work patterns and their understanding of professional self in relation to other health professionals. To begin, we examine the traditions and history of nursing with the military metaphor to enhance understanding of the potential for change.

There is no question that part of our heritage flows from the reality of the military and the work that nurses performed during wars. Most notable is our greatest hero in nursing, Florence Nightingale, who achieved true greatness in her time and who continues to inspire nurses today. Nightingale served during the Crimean War, in which she ministered to sick, injured, and dying soldiers. Women of her time were expected to be obedient and subservient to hierarchies of power and authority. Belenky et al. (1986) proposed that women did not always develop language in ways that best represented their experiences and that many women clung to blind obedience to authorities for their very survival. Unquestioned authority continued to be the norm during development of the commodity- and manufacturing-based economies that have swept the globe. Chains of command and centralized centers of control have helped to solidify the military model deep in nursing's culture—deep into our language and beliefs about who we are and what our work is about. Although change in location may have occurred, we suggest here that centralized centers of control still dominate—even in organizations that claim to be decentralized.

We are proposing here that the military metaphor has served its purpose and has only limited, if any, usefulness for guiding nursing thought and work in today's complex healthcare settings. Today, nurses are expected to create meaningful relationships with clients and to individualize care and service with moral intent. It is our belief that nurses want to live compassionate and caring expressions that help clients heal, recover, and achieve quality of life or die with dignity. Nurse leaders are expected to inspire change, promote quality, and enhance retention of staff.

Today, nursing is about using knowledge for caring and being present in ways that promote, enhance, enable, and nurture health and quality of life. Nurses rely on nursing knowledge and discovery within the nurse–client relationship to know how to practice. Traditional images of unquestioned obedience to the dictates of other health professionals' knowledge and power are inadequate, restrictive, and increasingly offensive to professional nursing. The metaphor of battle and trenches, where survival is a triumph, does not help nurses attend to and abide with persons while they live experiences of health and illness. The military metaphor is no longer viable for achieving and sustaining meaningful nursing practices. It is our belief that future practitioners of nursing, and the clients they engage, will benefit from a different metaphor and a different way of thinking and working that is aligned with new images, new layers of meaning, and the potential for discovery and innovation.

Current and future leaders in nursing bear responsibility to lead the transformation of metaphoric thinking in the profession. We believe that nursing leaders at all levels have opportunities to explore meanings embedded in nursing work and nurse–client relationships and to explore different ways of thinking that support and enhance those relationships (Ferguson-Paré et al. 2002). Nursing leaders also have an obligation to advance nursing theories and processes of care and exploration so that the knowledge that serves nurses in their work is extended and advanced. Nursing theories define nurse–client processes and specify the reason for nurses being present and providing care that benefits individuals as they experience living and dying. We do not believe that references to the practice environment as a war zone or to the caring professional as a general duty nurse capture the important and unique nature or contributions of nurses in practice. For those of us in administrative positions, speaking about professional practitioners of nursing as frontline staff can imply that nurses are little more than cannon fodder in the pursuit of diagnoses and the treatment and management of problems defined by other disciplines.

The time is ripe for nurses to reflect seriously on the use of military language in their healthcare environments and to consider making the commitment to a different image of nursing work. Moving away from the military model is a difficult thing to do because it is ingrained in nurses educated in the 20th century from the beginning of our studies and experiences in nursing practice— especially in hospital settings. The military model, though pervasive and deeply engrained, is now showing cracks that are filled with possibility for new language and new kinds of practice. Inspired by recent discussions with colleagues in the Academy of Canadian Executive Nurses, many of whom revealed they share the concerns expressed above, we have undertaken the challenge to describe an alternative to the military metaphor, one that we believe is more fitting for nursing work. Our alternative is about presence, community, discovery, knowledge, and possibility. Before describing the alternative metaphor, we delve into the depths of the military metaphor and its ubiquitous presence in nursing life.

Military Metaphor and Its Integration in Nursing

In the not-so-distant past women were banned from universities, and medical experts proposed that too much learning would impair a woman's reproductive function (Rasmussen et al. 1976). We have witnessed resistance against baccalaureate entry for nurses; some physicians have denounced nurses as knowledge workers. Fearful that too much knowledge might interfere with nurses' willingness to follow medical orders, some physicians clearly prefer nurses who do not question authority. The submissive role of women fits with the military metaphor. Perhaps that is why contemporary nurses have not developed their own knowledge base and why many nurses in practice have opted for androgynous scrub suits, complete with sneakers, to present who they are to colleagues and the public. Modern nurses dress in uniforms fit for work in the trenches. Like Florence Nightingale, nurses today prepare themselves for battle and combat on the frontlines. But whom do they battle?

The standard of care expected of today's nurses was not developed in the 19th century. Nightingale had to create not only a structure for professional nursing but also a culture to support that structure. It was her mission to establish the concept of women nurses in

the military—women with excellent clinical skills and high moral character and a desire to serve others. Using the military structure as her prototype, she tried to introduce the role of nurse superintendent, a role with the mandate to follow all the rules and procedures set forth by the medical department and to develop consistent, measurable patient outcomes (Montgomery Dossey 1999). Against this backdrop we find the metaphor of the military, intricately woven as threads in a tapestry, holding this frail new discipline of nursing together. Over time, military language and context has been both assimilated and embedded into nursing structure and culture to a point that today, we propose, nurses are not fully aware of its power and influence.

Metaphor is, for most people, a device of poetic imagination and rhetorical flourish—a matter of extraordinary, rather than ordinary, language. Moreover, metaphor is typically viewed as characteristic of language alone, a matter of words rather than thought or action (Lakoff and Johnson 1980). Yet metaphor is pervasive in everyday life. Our conceptual system, in terms of which we both think and act, is fundamentally metaphorical in nature. For instance, Morgan (1997) portrays metaphor as the device through which we know, see, and express our everyday realities. He draws attention to the limitations of metaphor, to the biases they can create, and to the distortions that, if taken too literally, can become absurd. He offers the example of the metaphor of machines as a framework for organizations and notes that although somewhat useful, the machine model cannot address the human and political aspects that also have powerful impacts on organizational culture.

As noted by Morgan (1997) and others, the concepts that govern our thoughts are not just matters of intellect. Our thinking shapes and directs our choices and actions down to the most mundane details. Every person has a unique world view that structures what we think about, how we get along in the world, and how we relate with other people. Our conceptual systems or world views play a central role in defining our everyday realities, even when we are not fully aware of how this happens. In most things we do every day, we think and act more or less automatically along certain lines and in keeping with our unique patterns of living. It can be an enlightening process to examine our perspectives, and one place to begin looking is within our language. Our language tells others who we are. The language we choose also shows our thoughts, our cherished beliefs, our truths, and what we hope to realize (Parse 1998). Language is an important source of understanding, and it can disclose and illuminate hidden beliefs (Lakoff and Johnson 1980).

Military Language and Beliefs in Nursing

Initial introduction and orientation into military life is referred to as basic training, and many nurses also refer to their education as training. New military recruits are sent to boot camp, where the first goal is to break the new recruit's ego as well as to teach the basic skills needed to survive as a soldier. This process diminishes one's desire to think independently and individually. The hopeful outcome for all new recruits is to align them with authoritarian goals. Officers use rigid, humiliating, and punitive drills to train soldiers and to help them lose their sense of self. Loss of self is believed to be essential for effective teams and combat. Newly trained recruits know their place in the military hierarchy and will not question orders. They learn to respond by rote memory and impassive compliance. Military education is based on rules of conduct, policies and procedures, regulations and rules. Soldiers often refer to this as "earning their stripes."

Nurses new to the profession often describe experiences very similar to those of new soldiers earning their stripes. Senior nurses sometimes intimidate the young, yell at them, and belittle their novice knowledge. A rather distasteful metaphor is that "nurses eat their young." Senior nurses feel the need to "toughen up" new grads, and the more experienced believe they have earned the right to treat junior staff in a denigrating way. Many nursing schools, even those in universities, seem to structure experiences that leave nursing students feeling as though they must obey and comply with expectations defined by teaching authorities. In practice, nurses comply with team members' directives about how to treat patients; often, the directives are also punitive and regimented. Nurses who do not follow team directives can be viewed as poor team players. Not infrequently, these rebel nurses are ridiculed or punished by other nurses and team members.

Regimented military life has purpose; it promotes standardization and rote memory. These processes are devised to create personal safety, command routine, and promote the same level of ability among soldiers. Regimentation ensures sameness and control, both essential to the military culture. Based on the 24-hour clock, nursing has historically regimented and standardized the tasks and operations delegated to staff nurses. Regimented care—such as bowel routines, shower days, routine weights, and vital signs—is often performed in rigid ways according to schedules devised by the authorities. The work of nursing is executed through the use of standardized procedures, policies, rules, regulations, routines, and protocols. Most nurses have been trained to make beds in the military style, with sharply tucked corners and sheets stretched so tight a quarter could bounce a good 3 feet when dropped by a supervisor. Dress codes helped student nurses know they should be crisp and clean for inspection. Most nurses know how to follow prescriptive rules, even if they do not make sense, and most nurses also know that compliance, order, efficiency, and productivity are most important in the military culture. Even the term "orderlies" for unit workers speaks to the priority of keeping order. There is still talk of inspections within health care and the belief that order and compliance must prevail.

Soldiers in the military know their duties and the boundaries of roles and charges. Clear expectations and boundaries support parameters of responsibility. Consistent with military language, nurses use similar terms to describe their work. We have tours of duty, on/off duty, change of shift, and night duty. When away from work, nurses talk of lieu time, on call, leave of absence, time off, breaks, coverage, and replacements. Many nurses still work from master schedules or rotations of duties. Nurses at one time lived in nursing residences or quarters, similar to army barracks, and there were clear, paternalistic rules about how to act.

The tradition of the military is based on a model of hierarchical power, command, and control. Power is valued and feared, and respect is equated to rank. Subordination is an accepted and expected way of life—insubordination is not tolerated. Soldiers abide by orders, and a punitive stance is taken if they operate outside established rules and regulations and their rank. Punishment and humiliation are used as examples of how not to behave. Nurses too fear power and punishment, and fear may explain why some nurses are reluctant to report errors and near misses.

Hierarchy is not new to nursing, and even in today's flattened organizational structures we see the military influence on our roles. Nursing has a chain of command that starts with the chief nursing officer/director/head nurse/unit manager/clinical nurse specialist/charge nurse/team leader, down the rank and file to the resource nurse/general duty nurse/staff nurse. One way hierarchy is maintained is through uniforms. Uniforms in the military are used to create rank, and nursing and patient uniforms reinforce the notion that certain people dress in ways consistent with their rank. Along with rank, there are expectations of self-sacrifice, courage, bravery, and honor—for glory and heroism, which permeate military life.

Nursing work is typically generated from physician orders or medical/team directives, and the notion of nurses having their own knowledge base is foreign and unwelcome to some. Nursing theory and research still struggle within all ranks to rise above the oppression and anti-intellectualism that permeates nursing. Many hospital units still have charge nurses who accompany physicians on rounds, where many remain silent in the presence of doctors or wait to answer specific questions posed by the medical team. The silence is a throwback to the military rule not to question authority; and if nurses have no unique knowledge or practice, there is certainly no need for them to speak unless spoken to. Nurses, upon earning their stripes in the trenches, sometimes get promoted up the ranks, where they get special privileges, such as not having to work nights or weekends. And the military metaphor is alive and well in senior management discourse also.

One text about power and politics in nursing administration offers advice about how to swim with the sharks (Del Bueno and Freund 1986). In this text one can find phrases about treating strangers like the enemy, countering aggression with retaliation, surprising your adversary, diverting an attack, exciting enemies to fight among themselves, and trying not to bleed in front of others. Is it any wonder, then, that some nurses and nurse leaders choose isolation rather than community, control rather than collaboration, and punishment rather than development?

To summarize, nurses and soldiers work in the trenches where they are often in the line of fire. Both need to win the battles they fight and obey commands without question. Frontline activity is dangerous and violent; abuse is a common experience for nurses in the workplace. Both nurses and soldiers require well-defined roles and responsibilities that minimize innovation, discovery, reflection, and thought. Both groups must allocate scarce resources and develop procedures for dealing with casualties. Expression of feelings, unique thought, or objections are discouraged at best or ignored and ridiculed. Both nurses and soldiers know whom it is safe to talk to and when they will get in trouble. Members of each group know about reports and briefings; both know how to speak with as little personal disclosure as possible. The military metaphor embedded in nursing is masculine, power-based, patriotic, paternalistic, and violent: It is based on command and control and the principles of conquest and conflict. We assert that the metaphor has outlived its usefulness, and we call on our colleagues to declare its demise. It is our belief that the military model is a barrier to modern nursing concepts of client-centered care, personhood, participation, freedom, innovation, and potential. It is now time for the exploration of an alternative metaphor that may have the depth and richness to replace the military imagery and language.

Exploring the Frontier: A New Metaphor for Nursing

Consider for a moment that the nurse–client relationship may be embraced as the new frontier, one that awaits discovery and engagement and that holds promise for community and the co-creation of health and quality of life. It is our belief that even though human beings have charted the land-mass of the earth and ventured into space, they have not yet figured out how to relate to one another in ways that build respect, community, compassion, and quality of life. This is especially true in healthcare relation-ships. It may be that a new metaphor, such as the frontier, could change how nurses think and act so they are better prepared to con-tribute to the quality of lived experience for humankind. Morgan (1997) suggests an art to using metaphor in ways that can enliven and refresh thinking. The metaphor of fron-tier has been successfully used to describe how nurses can engage the process of change in complex healthcare settings (Liggett 1997). We suggest that the metaphor of frontier requires additional attention to explore its usefulness for conceptualizing not only the environment but also the nurse–client pro-cess and how nurses think about clients and themselves as scholars and practitioners.

We see the frontier as an open space full of promise, possibility, and discovery. Getting to the frontier is an adventure that requires courage bolstered by commitment to a dream. The frontier invites exploration. Life on the frontier involves excitement, danger, hope, struggle, joy, hardship, and growth. Nurses do not know what they will encounter when they go to be with clients and families. We believe that if nurses anticipate potential, promise, and mystery when working with others, they will think and act very differently in relationships with patients and families. If nurses were prepared in their educational programs to explore and innovate, instead

of being prepared to comply and standard-ize, they would rely on a distinct language to plan for such an adventure. Language would describe what nurses know as well as what they discover with clients and their lived experiences of health. Descriptions about possibilities with others would most likely be quite different from descriptions used to describe the problems and diagnoses encoun-tered in the military model.

Working on the frontier requires strength, maturity, courage, and a willingness to learn and to change continuously. Rasmussen et al. (1976) noted that during the early years, work on the frontier also meant times of intense loneliness and hardship. Let us emphasize also that women on the fron-tier were treated like property and denied education to increase the chances that they would stay at home, bear children, and take care of the farm (Rasmussen et al. 1976). As women ourselves, we find it impossible to escape our history. But, living on the frontier also required commitment to the activity of building, nurturing, gardening, sharing, and helping others. In the late 1800s women were largely responsible for finding ways to en-sure that families and communities flour-ished and thrived (Rasmussen et al. 1976). Today, in many healthcare settings nurses too are responsible for finding ways to ensure that patients and families thrive and live, despite the hostility of their surroundings.

The military model diminishes individu-ality to strengthen teamwork; in it, not only are nurses' uniqueness cloaked in procedure, but patient uniqueness can be ignored to achieve team goals set not by persons but by the "experts." One need only read patient accounts of care delivered within the military model to understand that the approach does not meet the needs of modern human beings (see, for example, Baier 1996; Gerteis et al. 1991). Teamwork may be the best way to do common work in some situations, such as war, but it does not necessarily build community—and it is community that establishes respect, collaboration, altruism, and the desire to be and work together.

This sense of community as a network of relationships that enliven and enhance mutual benefit is seriously threatened in nursing today. Nurses in one forum described how their sense of community and caring and working with others has been diminished by delivery models and role descriptions that define individual nurses working with patients/clients in a particular geographical area with little affiliation with patients/clients or nurses in other areas (Ferguson-Paré and Mitchell 2001). The metaphor of frontier may inspire different notions of how nursing work could be organized despite the challenges and struggles of modern healthcare settings. Perhaps, instead of units of nurses, we could create communities of nurses where respect and cooperation predominate.

People on the frontier had a profound respect for what they encountered there. The mysteries of weather, wild animals, and other peoples all represented enough strangeness and risk to warrant an attitude of respectful coexistence. Sharing lessons and respecting others who shared one's values and vision of life generated kinship and compassion, especially among women. Women were proud of their work and contributions, and they knew how to be creative and cooperative (Kirkpatrick 2001). It is our belief that nurses need to be supported with practices that help them innovate and to show profound respect for each other and for the people they encounter in their work.

Nursing work today may be as misunderstood as frontier work was for women 150 years ago. The similarities in the stories of frontier women and nurses are sometimes striking. Nursing is the fabric of modern health care, but it now needs to redefine itself in ways that promote nursing work and scholarship. Perhaps the metaphor of the frontier is too embedded itself in oppressive history. If so, let us ponder and ruminate until we find new images and metaphors that truly honor nursing relationships with patients and the work that nurses do to contribute to the betterment of humankind.

At this time we propose that the metaphor of frontier as an open place of exploration and discovery can be an alternative to the militaristic frontline trench. We need new ways of thinking about the place where nurse–client processes and relationships grow and contribute to human quality of life. The military metaphor is too restrictive and violent to support nursing in the next century. The frontier may not be exactly consistent with what we believe to be true about nursing, but it at least helps to focus on important concepts that we do believe are essential for the discipline of nursing. Some of the more appealing concepts linked with the frontier metaphor are exploration, discovery, promise, possibility,

Table 22-1   Contrasting Concepts
Between Military and Frontier Metaphors

Military	Frontier
Constancy	Change
Standardization	Variation
Compliance	Innovation
Control	Freedom/restriction
Labeling	Description
Team	Community
Authority	Discovery
Control	Collaboration
Medals	Dream catchers
Disparate ranks	Connectivity
Reports/briefings	Stories/narratives

hardship, community, altruism, hope, joy, struggle, and growth. These concepts could provide nurses with a different view of themselves and their role in helping others to live quality of life.

As noted in Table 22-1, the frontier concepts, when considered in light of the more familiar military concepts, show how language shapes thinking and acting. We look to the next generations of nurses to choose their language and the concepts they want to represent the work of nursing. The community of nurses awaits.

References

Baier, S. 1996. "The View from Bed Number Ten." *Healthcare Forum Journal 39*(2): 60–67.

Belenky, M.P., B.M. Clinchy, N.R. Goldberger and J.M. Tarule. 1986. *Women's Ways of Knowing.* New York: Basic Books.

Del Bueno, D.J. and C.M. Freund. 1986. *Power and Politics in Nursing Administration: A Casebook.* Owings Mills, MD: National Health Publishing.

Ferguson-Paré, M. and G.J. Mitchell. 2001. "Let's Get Real—Destroying–Restoring Community in Nursing." *Canadian Journal of Nursing Leadership 14*(2):7–9.

Ferguson-Paré M., G.J. Mitchell, K. Perkin and L. Stevenson. 2002. "Academy of Canadian Executive Nurses (ACEN) Background Paper on Leadership." *Canadian Journal of Nursing Leadership 15*(3):4–8.

Gerteis, M., S. Edgman-Levitan, J. Daly and T.L. Delbanco, eds. 1993. *Through the Patient's Eyes.* San Francisco: Jossey-Bass.

Kirkpatrick, J. 2001. What Once We Loved: A Sisterhood of Friendship and Faith. Colorado Springs, CO: Waterbook.

Lakoff, G. and M. Johnson. 1980. *Metaphors We Live By.* Chicago: University of Chicago Press.

Montgomery Dossey, B. 1999. *Florence Nightingale: Mystic, Visionary, Healer.* Springhouse, PA: Springhouse Corporation.

Morgan, G. 1997. *Images of Organizations* (2nd ed.). Thousand Oaks, CA: Sage.

Parse, R.R. (1998). The Human Becoming School of Thought: A Perspective for Nurses and Other Health Professionals. Thousand Oaks, CA: Sage.

Rasmussen, L., L. Rasmussen, C. Savage and A. Wheeler. 1976. *A Harvest Yet to Reap.*

Toronto, Ontario, Canada: The Women's Press.

Susko, M.A., ed. 1991. *Cry of the Invisible.* Montreal, Quebec, Canada: Conservatory.

Commentary

Barbara Paterson, RN, PhD

The article written by Mitchell, Ferguson-Paré, and Richards reminds us of something that we as nurses often take for granted: that our roots in the military are enacted in our everyday practices. I appreciated the thoughtful way in which the authors led readers to reflect on the consequences of remaining unreflective about the impact of our early history as a profession. Until we are able to articulate the effect of such historical roots on how nurses shape their role identity and practice, the nursing profession is unlikely to fully achieve the goals of professionalism to which it aspires.

I was intrigued with the authors' question: "With whom do they battle?" As they indicate, in the current healthcare environment, nurses battle almost everyone. The public has become skeptical of healthcare professions. Defensiveness, and at times aggression, is more common among patients and their families than ever before. Nurses fight physicians and other members of the interdisciplinary team who fear an erosion of their traditional roles by nurses' expanding roles. They do battle with administrators who threaten to take away already-limited services and resources. They even battle service staff, such as cleaning personnel, whose contracts delimit their responsibilities in such a way that nurses are frequently adding duties to their roles, simply to make the environment clean and safe for patients and others.

Because the metaphor of the military battle fits so well with nurses' experience, it is often readily accepted within the profession. Another reason for the popularity and pervasiveness of this metaphor over time is that it reinforces significant components of nursing that provide direction and a sense of purpose for nurses. For example, adopting the "one for all and all for one" military attitude reinforces the need for teamwork and commitment among nurses. However, the military metaphor also promotes ideas and practices that are incongruent with nursing's professional ideals. The authors clearly identify a number of the negative outcomes of the unquestioning adoption of the military metaphor in nursing, such as the power relations that are maintained in such a system.

A caution in interpreting the article written by Mitchell and her colleagues is that considering the military metaphor as separated and decontextualized from coexisting metaphors "obscure[s] the complex moral reality of nursing practice" (Wurzbach 1999). Like any metaphor, the military metaphor in nursing has its limitations; it cannot be translated to all aspects of the nursing experience, and nursing encompasses many metaphors, not just a military one (Wurzbach 1999). One example is the metaphor that arises from nursing's roots in religious convents. Although relying on similar notions of hierarchy and subservience, the convent metaphor differs from that of the military because religious orders contributed a moral metaphor of caring that subsumes gender, class, and age (Ross 1993). The goals subsumed in each metaphor (that is, to do battle and to care) are often exclusive. The clashes of these metaphors explain some of the tensions that have arisen in nursing's history as it has struggled to define its practice and to obtain status. For example, the conflicting metaphors of the military and the convent may explain why many nurses respond to assault by patients, physicians, and others by remaining silent or directing anger at others (Smith et al. 1996). It may also explain why, contrary to the authors' statement that nursing has been influenced primarily by the patriarchy characteristic of any military system, there is evidence of the domination of matriarchy, as was common in the convent model of early nursing history, in Canadian nursing history. Care and his colleagues (1996) believe it was this that prevented male registered nurses from being employed and conferred officer status in the Canadian military until 1967.

I appreciate whenever authors cause me to reflect on my practice as a nurse, and this article certainly has provoked my reflection. As I write this I am sitting in my office on a medical unit in a tertiary care hospital. I hear nurses in the hallway talking about "chain of command," "the charge nurse," and "what the doctor ordered." I am reminded that some of this terminology betrays an allegiance to another world of nursing, one that we commonly espouse as outdated and not reflective of who we are as professionals. Because of this chapter I renew my commitment to a "new frontier for nursing," one whose language is congruent with my beliefs and values as a nurse.

References

Care, D., D. Gregory, J. English and P. Venkatesh. 1996. "A Struggle for Equality: Resistance to Commissioning of Male Nurses in the Canadian Military, 1952–1967. *Canadian Journal of Nursing Research 28*(1):103–117.

Ross, K.R. 1993. "Women Are Needed Here": Northern Protestant Women as Nurses During the Civil War, 1861–1865. Unpublished doctoral dissertation, Columbia University, New York.

Smith, M., P. Droppleman and S.P. Thomas. 1996. "Under Assault: The Experience of Work-Related Anger in Female Registered Nurses. Part 1." *Nursing Forum 31*(1): 22–33.

Wurzbach, M.E. 1999. "The Moral Metaphors of Nursing." *Journal of Advanced Nursing 30*(1):94–99.

CHAPTER 23

Nursing Science in the Global Community

Shaké Ketefian, RN, EdD, FAAN

Richard W. Redman, RN, PhD

Knowledge development and research are generally embedded in cultural values and perspectives. This article examines the development of knowledge in nursing in a global context and addresses the degree to which Western values and the social environment in the United States shape nursing theory development. Three perspectives illustrate the influence of U.S. values and contextual factors. Questions are raised about the relevance of knowledge to other cultural or national contexts. Recom-mendations are made for nursing inquiry that makes knowledge more applicable to the global community.

Key words: *knowledge development, international nursing.*

For many years, nurses from other countries have been enrolled in U.S. graduate programs. Colling and Liu (1995) report a 10% increase in international students attending U.S. graduate programs in nursing in the past decade. In their survey of international students, these authors identified 239 students from 49 countries. In many parts of the world, U.S. nursing appears to be highly regarded.

As the diversity and ethnic mix of the U.S. population has increased, global awareness has also increased. In the past decade, many institutions and nurses have become involved in international activities such as consultation, collaborative research, and exchange visitor arrangements.

Yet, despite the increase in international activities, the nature of nursing theory, research, education, and practice has not

Source: Ketefian, S., Redman, R. (1997). Nursing Science in the Global Community. Journal of Nursing Scholarship, 29(1):11–15. Reprinted with permission by Sigma Theta Tau International.

changed appreciably to be globally relevant. The degree to which parochialism may have played a role in explaining the slow pace of change in this regard has not been fully examined.

Boyacigiller and Adler (1991) examined the degree to which Western parochialism and ethnocentrism are embedded in the concepts of organizational theory. These authors reviewed the research literature in management science from three perspectives: (a) the influence of post World War II America and its environment on organizational theory development (b) the volume of international articles published in American management journals and (c) the degree to which American beliefs and values have shaped organizational theory development. Their assessment, overall, was that organizational theories are parochial and many do not acknowledge awareness of non-U.S. contexts, models, or values. Many Americans have shaped theories central to organizational and human behavior with the assumption that these beliefs have universal applicability. Free will (versus determinism) and individualism (versus collectivism) are just two examples of how Western values have shaped research and theory in organizational science. The authors call for the development of organizational sciences in which universal, intercultural theories are clearly explicit.

Following the approach taken by Boyacigiller and Adler (1991), we describe three perspectives in our examination: (a) contextual—the influence of the U.S. social environment on nursing theory development (b) quantitative—the rapid

expansion of U.S. doctoral programs in nursing, the shaping of nursing journals by U.S. nurse scientists, and the degree of international scientific representation in these journals and (c) qualitative—the degree to which U.S. values have shaped nursing theory development. The status of multicultural knowledge development in the United States is then presented followed by selected recommendations. Given the magnitude of the topic, no attempt is made to be comprehensive. Rather, the ideas presented represent select perspectives and observations of the authors who are educators in the United States, but who have had extensive international experience. The views presented here are intended to serve as catalysts for further discussion.

Perspectives

Contextual Perspective

The influence of social forces on American nursing can be examined from several perspectives. These include (a) social trends and values and how they shape nursing knowledge development, (b) the influence of technology and reimbursement systems on nomenclature in nursing, and (c) the development of nursing education and research infrastructures as social phenomena. Each is described briefly to illustrate the contextual influences.

Many recent U.S. social movements have had considerable effect on nursing theory. One example is the emphasis on health promotion and risk reduction. The social emphasis on behavior related to diet, exercise, and other types of health-promoting behaviors have influenced the shaping of public policy as well as the education of health professionals. To a considerable degree, they have also shaped the direction of nursing science and research. Another example is the way in which the emergence of the women's movement has shaped the thinking of a whole generation of women and has led to the development of new public policies in education, employment, health, and other domains. Recognition that women's health problems should be given priority has led to research by health professionals, including nurses, resulting in a body of scientific knowledge in this domain.

The Nursing Interventions Classification (NIC) work at Iowa (McCloskey & Bulechek, 1994) is another example of a social force influencing nursing knowledge development. NIC has been developed as a comprehensive classification of treatments that nurses perform in an attempt to create a standardized language of both nurse- and physician initiated nursing interventions. Interest in developing this taxonomy can be traced in part to the need for nurses to develop a universal language. Catalytic social forces such as the rapid technologic development of literature data bases, clinical information systems in practice settings, and the need for taxonomies that are compatible with reimbursement systems have resulted in the need for standardized nursing nomenclature. This development has profound implications for nursing practice and knowledge development internationally. The degree to which

U.S. nursing interventions are shaping the rapid development of "universal" taxonomies and languages that reflect nursing practice throughout the world is a pressing question. In addition, there is considerable interest in using taxonomies such as NIC to redefine nursing knowledge inductively. Again, the degree to which U.S. nursing interventions and practices reflect nursing practice in other countries is a question of critical importance internationally.

Social values and contextual influence also relate to the quality of nursing care. Definitions of nursing care quality vary, ranging from using the proper amount of resources to accomplish nursing goals to meeting patients' requirements. Assessing the quality of nursing care, whether focused on the appropriateness of a given intervention to a patient's needs or the selection of alternatives as a function of resources available illustrates how context-dependent quality can be. The expectations of a client, the socially defined role of the nurse, and the technology available can vary considerably. Furthermore, the importance of each of these variables in the quality equation can vary, depending on the context, and in turn drive the research questions and methodologies. Thus, the manner in which the pressing questions of the discipline are framed are very likely to reflect the values, philosophy, and practices of the culture and society in which they are asked.

Explorations of theory in nursing began in the 1960s. Since then, in an effort to define what is distinctive about nursing science and theory, nurse scholars and theorists have widely debated their ideas. Many of these ideas have been characterized as metatheories or conceptual frameworks. In the past decade, the nursing literature has reflected a shift in thinking. Now many investigators favor working with propositions and theories characterized as middle-range theories rather than with conceptual frameworks because middle-range theories provide the basis for generating testable hypotheses related to particular nursing phenomena and to particular patient populations.

Expansion of doctoral programs along with the magnitude and refinement of nursing research over the past several decades has been impressive. Thus, it can be argued that such advances in U.S. nursing have rightfully placed it in an enviable position vis-à-vis international peers.

The scope and orientation of much of nursing research is American without global characteristics. Frequently, research findings are presented and received by international colleagues as though the work is applicable to other national and cultural contexts. In addressing such issues, Zwanger (1987) states that American nurses are recognized as leaders in doctoral education in the world and that

> They are . . . the oracles of the international academic nursing community. As a consequence, in many instances, their ambiguous tendencies, unclarified ideas, and conceptions are accepted as bona fide facts. (pp. 33–34)

Zwanger draws on the Israeli experience in stating that some of those who complete their degree in the United States wish to transplant American ideas to their native land. She then describes the inappropriateness of doing so, which in some cases results in failure to function effectively in one's home settings. She makes a case for U.S. doctoral faculty to "pay attention to global content and international nursing issues," emphasize comparative studies, and assist international students to gear their doctoral research to problems in their own countries.

Quantitative Perspective

The International Council of Nurses now represents 110 national associations as members, with a total of 1 million nurses (Splane & Splane, 1994). Of 110 schools worldwide offering doctoral degrees in nursing, 62 are in the United States and 48 in all other countries combined. Moreover, according to anecdotal data, an indeterminate number of non-U.S. educational programs are programs where nurses have the opportunity to obtain doctoral degrees in fields other than nursing.

A limited number of international exchanges of students and faculty have occurred over the years (Fenton, 1994), although exchange has gained momentum recently, yet such opportunities are not made available to students by many institutions further, international exchanges typically occur during undergraduate study rather than graduate study. At the doctoral level, during the 1970s, many institutions either abandoned a second language requirement altogether or began accepting a computer language in its stead. A recent American Academy of Nursing publication (1995) identifies five graduate programs in nursing in the United States with a cross-cultural focus, some of which include international nursing. Thus, in most cases, doctoral students' exposure to the world beyond the United States might come when they have the opportunity to study with international students as peers.

Examination of the growth in journal publication and in doctoral education gives readers another perspective on the growth in nursing knowledge and science. The major journal for reporting research in nursing, Nursing Research, was established in 1952 by the American Journal of Nursing Company later it was followed by the publication of Research in Nursing and Health in 1977 and Advances in Nursing Science in 1978. Since that time, many journals have been established that report research in nursing, nursing theory, and nursing practice. As specialty organizations grew, so did journals concerned with the practice and research of their clinical area of practice. In the early days of Nursing Research, it was not uncommon to see papers authored by social scientists, reporting on studies concerned with nurses rather than with nursing.

Ketefian and Redman (1994) reported that the first doctoral programs in nursing were established in 1933 (Teachers College, Columbia University) and 1934 (New York University), both offering the Doctor of Education degree. In the next 25 years, only two more programs were established. Growth in doctoral programs since then has been exponential. Of the 62 institutions in the United States offering doctoral degrees in nursing, 75% offer the PhD, the remainder offers a DNS, DNSc, or EdD. As to the nature of these programs, Grace (1978) and Murphy (1981) have described the development of doctoral programs in three phases: Phase I (inception to 1959) is characterized by focusing on education for nurses for functional roles; Phase II (1960–69) is characterized by a focus on education for nurses in a second discipline, referred to as nurse scientist training; Phase III (1970 to the present) is characterized by a focus on education in and of nursing.

A review of the content of U.S. journals suggests that many report on international issues, some have articles co-authored by nurses from overseas, and others have a regular international column, however, the effect of these developments, although significant, is not major. Many libraries now subscribe to international journals yet class assignments do not often include readings from these journals. A few journals now have international representatives on their review boards.

Qualitative Perspective

The Code for Nurses (American Nurses Association, 1985) represents embodiment of the values of American Nursing. The preamble reads, in part,

When making clinical judgments, nurses base their decisions on consideration of consequences and of universal moral principles, both of which prescribe and justify nursing actions. The most fundamental of these principles is respect for persons. Other principles stemming from this basic principle are autonomy (self-determination), beneficence (doing good), nonmaleficence (avoiding harm), veracity (truth-telling), confidentiality (respecting privileged information), fidelity (keeping promises), and justice (treating people fairly). (p. i)

The values in the code, and others emanating from them, find expression in nursing theories and conceptual frameworks developed by U.S. scholars. Indeed, they permeate the nursing literature. These values are at times explicit and at other times implicit.

Why are value assumptions important? Values have important effects on people, communities, and societies the primary concern of nursing is people—individually or in the aggregate. An understanding of behavior and the values that underlie behavior becomes a critical starting point for designing and implementing nursing interventions. Value assumptions underlying U.S. nursing are profoundly influenced by American culture, social mores, and the biases of the people who produce this literature. Yet a reading of U.S. literature suggests that the ideas therein are claimed to be either acultural or universal.

Most nursing theories and nursing research are developed and implemented in the United States and, therefore, can be said to be influenced by the social and cultural context of this country. In the next section, we offer specific examples of the influence of culturally specific values and

assumptions—and present comparisons or contrasts gleaned from the literature.

Graduate and Higher Education in Nursing In the United States, it is assumed that academic study is "good" and necessary for nursing education and that higher education (at college and university level) is even better. However, in many countries these are not assumptions; the terms often have different meanings.

Hockey (1987) draws on her knowledge and experience in European countries, and states that in some countries "higher education" refers to academic study beyond that required for qualification for practice. In addition, she explains that typically with higher education come leadership positions, even though some nurses do not wish to assume such positions. Thus, she poses the dilemma in ethical terms: Is "higher education" necessary for nursing? In another poignant example from the Austrian experience, she reveals that nurse training begins at age 15 and notes that "nursing autonomy assumes a different meaning" under these circumstances (p. 77).

Another author from the same conference describes the experience of Norway and its dilemmas that highlight value conflicts and value differences of a significant magnitude for that country. The main dilemma posed by Haugen Bunch (1987) is whether Norwegian nurses should study in the United States or in Norway. Each choice is described as having significant consequences for Norwegian nursing. She describes the choices as (a) studying social and natural sciences, (b) developing nursing science, or (c) blending the two. At the University of Bergen (Norway), where an Institute of Caring Sciences was established in 1979, many believe that caring is not subject to scientific inquiry, that nursing cannot be both holistic and scientific, that science may compromise the nursing discipline, that nursing can use relevant scientific principles from other disciplines, and that there is no need for a separate nursing science. Thus, if nurses study in Norway, with its tutorial educational model, their role models will not be nurses and they will learn the traditions of other disciplines rather than of nursing. If, on the other hand, they study in the United States, they will be socialized in nursing's scientific tradition and will have nurse role models. Haugen Bunch warns that for those educated in the United States there will be the danger of bringing back to Norway "undigested American knowledge that is presented as 'Norwegian truisms'—forgetting the need for value clarification so that the knowledge will fit Norwegian culture and traditions" (p. 103). Throughout her presentation she emphasizes the importance of adapting and testing theories and concepts before, "being applied and integrated to the Norwegian culture" (p. 103).

Nursing Science and Japan According to a Japanese nurse who did graduate work in the United States, Japanese nurses have imported nursing knowledge and literature since the end of the 19th century. The works of many American authors and theorists have been translated into Japanese by exchange nurses and by those who came to the U.S. for master's and doctoral degrees (Minami, 1987). Minami claims that many of these nurses "were not aware of the differences between the Japanese and American cultures or social context" (p. 66) and claimed that nursing was universal. She describes fundamental differences in the cultural milieu of the two countries that make concepts developed in one country inapplicable or irrelevant in the other. She also describes dilemmas faced by American-educated Japanese nurses in functioning in their home settings. Communication differences, for example, exist in eight areas: physical proximity, self-disclosure, trust in words, boundary in human relationships, commitment, contract dependency, independence autonomy, independence, and confrontation (p. 70). She says that Americans communicate with language while Japanese communicate with empathy, and she provides examples. These differences are characterized by Boyacigiller and Adler (1991) as high-context or low-context cultures. The external environment, the situation, and nonverbal behavior determine communication in high-context cultures like the Japanese, and subtlety, facial expression, relationship, and timing are valued. In low-context cultures like the United States, meaning comes from the spoken word and legal contracts are valued.

Multicultural Knowledge Development in the United States

Rapid change in the demographic composition of the U.S. population has occurred within the past several decades. Some demographers estimate that by the 21st century, one third to one half of the population will be other than Euro-Caucasian. Thus, a reversal is anticipated whereby groups that were minorities will collectively become the majority. The importance of a change of such magnitude is immense. An appreciation for diversity and for the varying needs of people who are different—with regard to any number of characteristics—is needed. Nowhere is this appreciation more compelling than in health care and nursing.

A small group of nurse investigators has been developing research and theory that is culturally sensitive. In a recent American Academy of Nursing monograph (AAN, 1995), a group of authors define culturally competent care as that which "takes into account issues related to diversity, marginalization, and vulnerability due to culture, race, gender, and sexual orientation" (p. 4). In their assessment of the state of knowledge development in this area, the authors identify the dearth of principles to guide selection of culturally sensitive research questions and selection of culturally appropriate methodologies. Many nursing programs do not offer content relevant to this area and fewer still require doctoral students to enroll in seminars about cross-cultural nursing.

The authors of the AAN monograph (1995) identify two metatheories and studies based on them that have shown promise of generating knowledge that is culturally sensitive. One theory is Leininger's (1985), wherein she posits that care, as the essence of nursing, is universal across cultures, although its forms and expressions may vary. The authors cite a number of nursing studies in which Leininger's theory helped researchers generate knowledge related to cultural care.

The other metatheory cited is the "care deficit theory" (Orem, 1991). This theory enables study of self-care practices used by diverse social groups. Its relevance for populations in a number of European countries—as well as Mexico and Thailand—is being studied by a network of collaborators (AAN, 1995).

In addition to the two metatheories, others are being developed that are referred to as "situation-specific theories" (AAN, 1995). Examples are studies of Middle Eastern immigrants (Lipson, Reizian, & Meleis 1987; Meleis, 1981; Meleis & Jonsen, 1983), patterns of health-seeking behaviors among Arab children (May, 1985), and postpartum transition among Arab women (El Sayed, 1986). The authors contend that, collectively, such studies can be synthesized to provide conceptualizations of patterns of responses to health–illness transitions, thus enabling development of a situation-specific theory in a particular population (AAN, 1995, p. 10).

Methodological concerns in the conduct of research with ethnically and racially diverse groups have received increasing attention as well. The U.S. Department of Health and Human Services (1990) has recently stipulated that ethnically and racially different groups be included as research subjects. Porter and Villarruel (1993) provide a cogent analysis of research issues and propose a set of guidelines to be considered for the design of research. Consideration of appropriate sensitivity is reflected in conceptualizing and conducting research, including each step of the research process and investigator activities. It is implied that unless these design considerations are present and deliberatively addressed, the relevance and applicability of the outcome of the research to diverse populations would be questionable.

Other Knowledge Development Strategies Over the years, nurses in many countries have identified their inability to describe nursing practice, client populations, or geographic areas as a serious constraint (Clark, 1994). To meet this need and to contribute to knowledge development for nursing, various classification systems have been developed. The Nursing Minimum Data Set was developed by Werley in the late 1960s (Werley & Lang, 1988) and in turn spurred other developments.

In the early 1980s, a classification of nursing diagnoses was proposed by the North American Nursing Diagnosis Association, where the phenomenon of concern is patient status (McLane, 1987). More recently, the Nursing Interventions Classification (NIC) project was developed. The use of nursing diagnoses and NIC is becoming widespread in the United States and internationally. Such standardization has many advantages: it helps expand nursing's knowledge base, provides a common language to communicate the functions of nursing, provides shared understanding of nursing practice across national and cultural boundaries, and highlights the distinctive contribution nursing makes toward solving health problems. The International Council of Nurses currently has a project in progress with these goals in mind (Clark, 1994). Although we do not know how the different knowledge development

strategies will evolve, significant developments are providing the basis on which to build continuing work by nurse scholars in doctoral programs around the world.

Next Steps

Some authors discuss the urgent need to develop nursing knowledge relevant to the health of the global community (Meleis, 1993). A Western perspective generally pervades organizing concepts and frameworks in nursing and thus is a dominating influence in knowledge development and research. Meleis expressed concern that U.S. nursing doctoral programs may be producing nurse scientists who do not challenge Western perspectives, particularly in terms of definitions and assumptions related to nursing phenomena.

In 1997, we are at a critical juncture for American nursing science. Given the global society in which we live, nursing science now faces the challenge of moving to its next phase of development, which we call "becoming globally relevant." This movement entails a variety of activities and changes in the way we do science, a responsibility that should be shared by scientists in the U.S. and internationally. We need to test nursing models, propositions, and hypotheses in several countries, include relevant content in educational programs, provide opportunities for doctoral students to develop nursing research internships abroad, involve international scholars in editorial review boards, increase the representation of international authors in U.S. journals and vice versa, encourage international students to focus their dissertations on topics pertinent to their countries, integrate collaborative international research in the ongoing work of scientists in leading nursing institutions throughout the world, and expand the criteria for promotion and tenure to include such activity.

We hope the questions raised in this essay will be viewed as opportunities by the global nursing community. If future discussions result in recognition of the challenges facing nursing knowledge development and doctoral education throughout the world, then our purpose will have been served.

References

American Academy of Nursing. (1995). Diversity, marginalization, and culturally-competent health care: Issues in knowledge development. Washington, DC: Author.

American Nurses Association. (1985). Code for nurses with interpretive statements. Kansas City, MO: Author.

Boyacigiller, N. A., & Adler, N. J. (1991). The parochial dinosaur: Organizational science in a global context. Academy of Management Science, 16(2), 262–290.

Clark, J. (1994). The international classification of nursing. In J. McCloskey & H. K. Grace (Eds.). Current issues in nursing (4th ed.) (pp. 143–147). St. Louis: Mosby-Year Book.

Colling, J. C., & Liu, Y. C. (1995). International nurses' experiences seeking graduate education in the United States. Journal of Nursing Education, 34(4), 162–166.

El Sayed, Y. A. (1986). The successive-unsettled transitions of migration and their impact on postpartum concerns of Arab immigrant women. Unpublished doctoral dissertation, University of California, San Francisco.

Fenton, M. V. (1994). Development of models of international exchange to upgrade nursing education. In J. McCloskey & H. K. Grace (Eds.). Current issues in nursing (4th ed.) (pp. 202–206). St. Louis: Mosby-Year Book.

Grace, H. (1978). The development of doctoral education in nursing: An historical perspective. Journal of Nursing Education, 17(4), 17–27.

Haugen Bunch, E. (1987). International perspectives and implications for doctoral education in nursing: Norwegian perspective. In International perspectives and implications for doctoral education in nursing (pp. 97–105). Portland, OR: Oregon Health Sciences University School of Nursing.

Hockey, L. (1987). Ethical issues in higher education in nursing. In International perspectives and implications for doctoral education in nursing (pp. 75–85). Portland, OR: Oregon Health Sciences University School of Nursing.

Ketefian, S., & Redman, R. W. (1994). The changing face of graduate education. In J. McCloskey & H. K. Grace (Eds.). Current issues in nursing (4th ed.) (pp. 188–195). St. Louis: Mosby-Year Book.

Leininger, M. M. (1985). Ethnography and ethnonursing: Models and modes of qualitative data analysis. In M. M. Leininger

(Ed.). Qualitative methods in nursing. New York: Grune & Stratton.

Lipson, J. G., Reizian, A., & Meleis, A. I. (1987). Arab-American patients: A medical record review. Social Science and Medicine, 24(2), 101–107.

May, K. M. (1985). Arab-American immigrant parents' social networks and health care of children. Unpublished doctoral dissertation, University of California, San Francisco.

McCloskey, J. C., & Bulechek, G. M. (1994). Standardizing the language for nursing treatments: An overview of the issues. Nursing Outlook, 42(2), 45–63.

McLane, A. M. (1987). Classification of nursing diagnoses: Proceedings of the seventh conference. St. Louis: Mosby-Year Book.

Meleis, A. I. (1981). The Arab-American in the Western health care system. American Journal of Nursing, 6, 1180–1183.

Meleis, A. I. (1993). A passion for substance revisited: Global transitions and international commitments. In Proceedings of the 1993 Annual forum on doctoral nursing education (pp. 5–22). St. Paul, MN: University of Minnesota School of Nursing.

Meleis, A. I., & Jonsen, A. (1983). Ethical crises and cultural differences. Western Journal of Medicine, 138(6), 889–893.

Minami, H. (1987). Reflections of the cultural and social milieu on the development of nursing science in Japan. In International perspectives and implications for doctoral education in nursing (pp. 63–74). Portland, OR: Oregon Health Sciences University School of Nursing.

Murphy, J. F. (1981). Doctoral education in, of, and for nursing: An historical analysis. Nursing Outlook, 29(11), 645–649.

Orem, D. E. (1991). Nursing: Concepts of practice (4th ed.). New York: McGraw-Hill.

Porter, C. P., & Villarruel, A. M. (1993). Nursing research with African American and Hispanic people: Guidelines for action. Nursing Outlook, 41(2), 59–67.

Splane, V. H., & Splane, R. B. (1994). International nursing leaders. In J. McCloskey & H. K. Grace (Eds.). Current issues in nursing (4th ed.) (pp. 49–56). St. Louis: Mosby-Year Book.

U.S. Department of Health and Human Services. (1990). Healthy people 2000: National health promotion and disease prevention objectives. Superintendent of documents. Washington, DC: U.S. Government Printing Office.

Werley, H. H., & Lang, N. M. (Eds.). (1988). Identification of the nursing minimum data set. New York: Springer.

Zwanger, L. (1987). International perspectives and implications for doctoral education in nursing: The Israeli case. In International perspectives and implications for doctoral education in nursing (pp. 17–43). Portland, OR: Oregon Health Sciences University School of Nursing.

CHAPTER 24

Nursing Practice with Aboriginal Communities: Expanding World Views

Othmar F. Arnold, RN, BScN

Anne Bruce, RN, PhD

Through advances in interpretive inquiry, diverse ways of knowing and experiencing reality are increasingly made explicit in nursing literature. Nevertheless, the privileges of empiricism continue alongside a lack of language to consider other realms of reality. In this chapter aboriginal ways of constituting health and reality are explored. Morley's four categorizations of health belief systems provide a useful tool for understanding diverse world views. In contrast, Atleo drew on Nuu-chah-nulth origin stories to address the complexities and ambiguities of aboriginal health beliefs. Approaches for bridging cultural differences are explored with a view toward inclusive health care and nursing practice.

Key words: *aboriginal health, culture, health beliefs, world view.*

The traditional model of knowledge generation in nursing has been the analytic, empirical model of the natural sciences. This view of basic science and nursing has shifted in the past 20 years recognizing the necessity of humanistic, interpretive, and phenomenological approaches as aspects of scientific inquiry. Distinctions between epistemologies in understanding phenomena within diverse ontological domains are now made more explicit in nursing literature. However, the question of dominance remains. The concern is not that different ways of knowing exist or that different epistemologies are necessary in knowledge development; rather, the issue remains one of the privileged position of empiricism and a lack of language to consider other realms of reality and knowledge. The dominance of biomedical perspectives in health care poses challenges as nurses engage with people and communities who live and interpret their worlds otherwise. In this chapter we explore aboriginal world views and understandings of health, drawing particularly on the writings of E. R. Atleo (2004) of the Nuu-chah-nulth First Nations whose aboriginal lens guided his interpretations and actions.

Differing World Views

According to Uys and Smit (1994), a world view is a comprehensive framework of basic beliefs. Individuals and groups use their basic beliefs to guide their actions. People cannot be without a world view, yet more often than not the basic beliefs remain unarticulated (Edwards, 1997). World views guided by values, beliefs, and an intuitive understanding of reality are expressed in everyday life in responding spontaneously to concrete situations. Without inquisitiveness and understanding, differences in beliefs and world views can lead to frustration, domination, and oppression. For healthcare providers working in aboriginal communities, this is particularly relevant. To better understand the nature of these differences, aboriginal perspectives of health and implications within intercultural care are explored.

Aboriginal Health

"Individual beings are designed to help one another in order to fulfill the requirements of wholeness, balance and harmony, interconnection, and interrelationality. Therefore, to practice vanity as a lifestyle can be destructive."

—*E. R. Atleo (2004, p. 35)*

Aboriginal Views

In the Cree language of the Whapmagoostui, there is no word that translates directly into *health* (Adelson, 2000). As in any society or culture around the globe, there is no singular definition of health and no essential perspective among aboriginal communities. For many First Nations' people, today's understanding of health is influenced by traditional knowledge, colonial history, Western medical science, mass media, and the healthcare system as experienced in aboriginal communities (Atleo, 1997). Nevertheless, scholarly views on aboriginal health belief systems identify commonalities and similarities that include the concept of living in harmony with nature (Spector, 1996). Adelson (2000) described health based on Cree experience as a complex, dynamic process that has to do with social relations, land, and cultural identity, which are integrally linked to quality of life. E. R. Atleo (2004), whose Nuu-chah-nulth name is Umeek, did not mention health per se, but through using the traditional Nuu-chah-nulth origin stories he suggested that health cannot be isolated as a stand-alone concept from the unity of creation. Umeek's world view holds that life is an orderly whole, a continuum of harmony within the physical and metaphysical worlds: "the universe is unified, interconnected, and interrelated" (Atleo, 2004, p. xix).

Biomedical Representations of Aboriginal Health

Despite diverse and highly complex world views and beliefs, aboriginal health is mainly discussed in the literature in relation to incidence and prevalence of disease; deficits are emphasized from a Western medical science point of view supported with epidemiological data (Health Canada, 2003). Identified deficits form the rationale for program design and delivery. First Nations' people are identified as being disadvantaged in accessing health services due to remoteness, socioeconomic factors, or open, direct racism by healthcare providers (Browne & Fiske, 2001; Commission on the Future of Health in Canada, 2002). Yet despite these disparities and recent shifts toward capacity building through health-promotion strategies, it is difficult to find information on the inherent strengths and abilities of First Nations' populations for their own health and healing. Healthcare providers using the current literature as evidence see aboriginal health constituted primarily within a biomedical framework of disease, treatment, and prevention.

Aboriginal Health Belief Systems

Aboriginal and Western concepts of health hold divergent world views. The Nuu-chah-nulth First Nation is located on Vancouver Island, British Columbia, and has an oral tradition of stories that reflect the entire range of human experience. These tales provide an orientation to life and reality. The stories are implicit rather than explicit and are told through the fables of animals or beings that exist in both spirit and animal/human/material realms (Atleo, 2004). Although translated into and recorded in English, E. R. Atleo

cautioned that Nuu-chah-nulth language is more complex than English, that the stories are embedded within cultural assumptions and contexts that differ from those of other cultures.

To explore these differences a model proposed by Morley (1987) provided a useful perspective for Western-trained practitioners. Morley described four common categories of causation beliefs with various health belief systems: (1) immediate, (2) nonsupernatural, (3) ultimate, and (4) supernatural causes. These categories of beliefs about causation are illustrated using examples from a Western scientific point of view alongside Nuu-chah-nulth traditional stories. Morley's framework of causation beliefs clearly demonstrated the narrow dimensions within which traditional Western biomedicine is located.

The first category of *immediate causes* includes beliefs about direct influences resulting in imbalance or illness. In this perspective it is possible to link immediate causes with resultant effects. In health care this category includes physical injury. For example, with a fall the mechanism of injury is the cause, whereas the broken limb is the effect. In Nuu-chah-nulth stories immediate cause and effect is well represented and sometimes provides for very dramatic effects (Atleo, 2004, p. 44):

> The chief came forward and welcomed (Aint-tin-mit) and asked him to sit by the fire. Even while he was being seated, the fire was being built into a roaring inferno. Hotter and hotter it grew. When the fire

finally became unbearably hot, Aint-tin-mit took some of his medicine [barnacle] powder and threw it into the fire. Ho! The flames died down.

In this story the fire had the potential for serious injury and caused discomfort to the point where Aint-tin-mit needed to interfere to maintain his safety and comfort in the situation. Immediate cause and effect are shown between adding fuel to the fire and the increase of heat and also between the medicine powder and the immediate decrease in flames. In the first example Western minds accept the link between cause and effect because they know and accept the correlation of fuel and heat and can provide scientific evidence with understanding. The second example belongs, from a Western point of view, in the realms of storytelling and imagination. The sprinkles of barnacle powder have no scientific merit as a fire extinguisher. However, in the Nuu-chah-nulth view cause and effect in this case are immediate and real. This understanding is based on the implicit knowledge of a supernatural cause that transformed the attributes of the barnacle powder.

Linked to the immediate causes is the second category of *nonsupernatural causes*, which tries to explain why a particular situation occurred. It is also based on observable cause–effect relationships with the addition of explanatory reasoning that may not be immediately observable. For example, germ theory falls under this category. It can be established that with the help of technology there is a direct relationship between the presence of a pathogen and the resulting signs and symptoms of disease. In a nonmedical context the construction of a road with the resulting decline of certain game animals due to the disruption of their established migration patterns is considered a nonsupernatural cause. In Umeek's account of Nuu-chah-nulth origin stories, we find instances of teasing that can cause temporary imbalances based on an observable cause–effect relationship with reasoning (Atleo, 2004, p. 43):

> First he must see the two snail women. One was blind and the other almost blind. He went to their house and found them cooking. He decided to tease them good-naturedly. Very carefully and quietly, he took some food from the plate of one of the women. When she discovered the missing food, she turned to her friend and scolded her, "What are you doing?" "Eh!" the other said in surprise. "Why are you stealing my food?" the other replied indignantly. As the two old snail women quarreled, Aint-tin-mit interrupted them with a chuckle. "Hold on there," he said. "Here is your food. I was only teasing. I'm sorry if I upset you."

The teasing was not apparent for the main characters in the story; the listener of the story was able to know what was going on. Hiding food from a blind person is creating insecurity, which may result in conflict. The key is not in the direct action of cause and effect but in the reasoning of why a certain effect is created. The same act in a different context may not establish a comparable cause–effect relationship. The nonsupernatural causes are an expression of intersectionality of various concepts and ways of knowing.

The third category, *ultimate causes*, seeks to explain health states and diseases as based on nonobservable interactions between human beings, the environment, and properties beyond the physical realm. For example, smudging, or burning a particular plant or herb, is attributed to cleansing qualities that are used in conjunction with events where emotional, psychic, and spiritual purification is desired (Spector, 1996). Other examples include people living near industrial sites or high-voltage power lines experiencing unexplained signs and symptoms that have no observable or measurable cause. Despite the lack of empirical evidence they still claim the exposure to immeasurable or legally sanctioned levels of contamination of soil, water, air pollution, noise, or electromagnetic fields is the likely source of their illnesses. In the field of complementary and alternative medicine, ultimate causes are frequently used to make claims for healing properties that cannot necessarily be proven using Western scientific methods or theories.

In the Nuu-chah-nulth origin stories birthright and membership in the family, community, or nation are important factors in maintaining balance and harmony and are often based on nonobservable interactions between humans and properties beyond the physical realm. In opposition to factors that maintain balance and harmony, one also encounters disharmony and forces that obstruct or destroy life and creation. One such negative force is exemplified in Aulth-ma-quus, the Pitch Woman, who is a destroyer of interrelatedness and harmony. The archetypal Pitch Woman is seen as an enemy of family, wholeness, and interrelatedness. "She is an inverse of a *quus* (human) living in community" (Atleo, 2004, p. 34).

In the representation of Aulth-ma-quus, Atleo (2004) drew parallels to contemporary, individualistic society: "she is alienated, surrounded by people yet alone, and has a closer relationship with technology than with family" (p. 34). Aulth-ma-quus' evil spirit is defined by the negative relationships she forms with human beings that prevent her from acquiring rights and creative participation in the community. In contrast, Aint-tin-mit, Son of Mucus, is described as a more positive force because he was born into a particular community and he was meant to help. His birthright afforded him membership, responsibilities, and rights in the community that supported his ability for maintaining balance and harmony.

Aulth-ma-quus and Aint-tin-mit are both part of the physical world. The two characters represented by Pitch Woman and Son of Mucus have both spiritual dimensions and claim a place in the world of the Nuu-chah-nulth (Atleo, 2004). Their importance in health (balance and harmony) or disease (destruction) is associated with their characteristics of kindness, generosity, selfishness, and egotism respectively. These characteristics are not mentioned by normative standards but are determined by individual experiences in the context of communal experience. Membership is both an individual experience (personal belonging) and a communal experience (contributor to wholeness and beneficial reciprocity). Therefore, ultimate causes do not need scientific proof. They exist based on experience, they may be inconsistent and contradictory, and they may defy logical reasoning.

In the final category, *supernatural causes* are explanations that Western scholars categorize as spirit and demon intrusion and are generally considered scientifically irrelevant and associated with religious practices (Spector, 1996). A strong element of supernatural causes is their characteristic to explain fortune and misfortune. In the Nuu-chah-nulth origin stories we find many instances of transformations of people and objects. In Umeek's world view there are no exclusionary boundaries between the physical and the spiritual world. The design of creation is based on strong relationships between the two worlds; therefore, it is only natural that spiritual powers are associated with persons and objects in the physical world. The creative interaction between the two worlds requires strict observation of protocols, rituals, and spiritual contracts, an aspect that is closely linked to membership and initiation (Atleo, 2004). Umeek shared a whaling story from his great-grandfather Keesta that illustrated the union between the spiritual and physical world as well as the whaler's changing fortunes (Atleo, 2004, p. x):

> All of a sudden something went wrong . . . everyone in the whaling canoe remained true to the

protocols—cleansed, purified, and in harmony. Prayer songs intensified. Still, the great whale refused to turn toward the beach, heading straight off shore. Keesta and the paddlers had kept true to their agreements, and now there seemed nothing left to do except to cut the *atlu,* the rope attached to the whale. Keesta took his knife, and as he moved to cut the rope, Ah-up-wha-eek (Wren) landed on the whale and spoke to Keesta: "Tell the whale to go back where it was harpooned." Keesta spoke to the whale, and immediately the great whale turned according to the word of Wren.

In explanation, the excitement over the successful hunt led some family members ashore to prematurely break away from the ritual necessary for the whale hunt. Only a spiritual power, in the form of a little bird with the ability to communicate with humans, was able to intervene and restore the harmony required to finish the hunt and provide for the community.

The supernatural causes involve beliefs outside the usual inquiry in Western science, and, like the spiritual field, supernatural events are left to philosophical and religious interpretation. Supernatural influences are used to explain fortune and misfortune. They do not follow a cause–effect pattern and have esoteric qualities, which mean they are only accessible to the specifically initiated. Many ceremonial and healing traditions, such as the *syewen,* or winter dance in the Coast

Salish Longhouse, can only be understood with great difficulty by lay people (noninitiated, or without membership in the cultural community) by using an expanded vocabulary and world view (Denis, 1997).

In Western world views the first two categories of immediate and nonsupernatural causes are acknowledged as reality, but the ultimate and supernatural categories go unattended except as folklore or cultural mythology. In contrast, aboriginal inquiry as described by E. R. Atleo (2004) integrates all four categories into one paradigm that embraces the universe as a whole. Although Morley's (1987) model provided a useful tool for Western-trained practitioners to begin to expand their world views, its categorizations are less than adequate in addressing the complexities and ambiguities of aboriginal health beliefs. For example, by listening to or reading First Nations' stories, we begin to understand how the four categories are presented not as discrete units but all-at once as multidimensional and paradox. Similarly, the Society of Obstetricians and Gynaecologists of Canada (2001) presented an aboriginal framework that addresses the complexities of health beliefs using the medicine wheel as a circular paradigm with a three-dimensional overlay to illustrate the cyclical, holistic perspective of health in the life cycle. Atleo's (2004) approach drew from origin stories based in the First Nations' ontology and exposed readers to alternative understandings. Nurses wishing to work with aboriginal peoples and communities need to try to understand and explore diverse perspectives.

Bridging Intercultural Gaps

Although differences in world views exist, possibilities of inclusivity also arise. Biomedical approaches in aboriginal health can be appropriate for concerns located in the immediate and nonsupernatural categories. However, the ultimate category, which also includes consideration of social justice issues and the supernatural, can only be addressed through an expanded, progressive application of health care that goes beyond the first two categories alone. Holistic initiatives for aboriginal health remain absent or grossly underrepresented and necessitate the inclusion of aboriginal modes of inquiry in all categories of causation.

Health promotion from an aboriginal perspective is primarily an issue of ultimate and supernatural causes. Further, Denis (1997) suggested that until the demons of century-old oppression are tamed, a successful healing of the human being will not occur. Alcohol, drug prevention, and treatment programs that attend to broader notions of health must go hand in hand with restoring cultural identity and self-government initiatives to achieve long-term positive outcomes for aboriginal people and communities. In M. R. Atleo's (1997) words, there is a "gap between the concept of holistic health and machinations of bureaucracy" (p. 70) that prevents a culturally sensitive way of healing for aboriginal populations. Therefore, culturally responsive health services in aboriginal communities require the ability to operate within at least two different paradigms. Biomedical knowledge and other explanatory models and ways of knowing must be integrated within a holistic approach. Without such recognition of diversity, care providers will not be able to see the human being beyond the aboriginal patient and the ineffectiveness of prescribed cures will continue with considerable frustration to all involved.

The adoption of the human becoming theory (Parse, 1998) as a foundation for practice is one possible approach to bridging intercultural gaps with aboriginal communities. The phenomenon of concern in human becoming theory is the human–universe–health process that, as in aboriginal world views, acknowledges the interconnected and interrelated continuum of universe–health and beings. Within the human becoming theory, human beings are postulated as co-creating with the universe. In community practice the nurse–community process focuses on the community's intentions and is guided by community priorities. Nurses are with a community to initiate and unfold change (Parse, 2003). The emphasis of the healthcare provider's role in intercultural health services is no longer a paternalistic health expert but rather an ally (DiClemente, Crosby, & Kegler, 2002).

In New Zealand Maori nurse leaders have developed an educational strategy of cultural safety for healthcare providers. Their goal is for health providers to offer culturally safe care in intercultural environments, particularly in aboriginal communities, within a colonial context (Polaschek, 1998; Ramsden, 2002). The concept of cultural safety formally recognizes unequal power relations between healthcare providers and clients and its consequences, based on colonial history. It acknowledges the social, political, and economic factors that influence and shape individual and collective attitudes. Through exposing postcolonial ideologies, cultural safety emphasizes the limitations of the assumptions of the dominant cultural values that underlie health policies, research, and interactions. Awareness is drawn to the discrepancies in health delivery and health status among diverse groups based on the cultural, social, and political processes of healthcare systems (Smye & Browne, 2002). In examining the transferability of the cultural safety framework for use in other contexts, Anderson and colleagues (2003) suggested that adopting cultural safety principles in Western scholarship will change the way healthcare providers interact and will open a path to healing in many intercultural environments.

Current approaches within the existing healthcare system that seek to acknowledge diverse world views and aim to correct disparities in aboriginal health often remain located within the categories of immediate and non-supernatural causes. Even the adoption of Ramsden's (2002) cultural safety theory does not go beyond cause and effect understandings. Parse's (1998) human becoming school of thought, on the other hand, does not support any reductionistic causal interpretations on the part of nurse.

Efforts in nursing scholarship are shifting the discourse of aboriginal health to better appreciate the legacy of colonialism and oppression in the past. Another frequently overlooked domain that warrants further inquiry is the dimension of membership. Membership is constituted in the Nuu-chah-nulth world view through rights and responsibilities and includes dimensions that blur spiritual and physical boundaries. The sense of belonging as a personal and communal experience, creating an understanding of wholeness and wellness, is a central theme in Nuu-chah-nulth creation stories (Atleo, 2004). Based on Morley's (1987) model, the notion of membership holds promise for further understanding of the role and relationship of healthcare providers engaging with aboriginal communities with a view toward inclusion.

Conclusion

The significance of world views in providing nursing care cannot be overstated. In understanding aboriginal communities' values and experiences of health and healing, nurses must consider diverse perspectives in addition to the dominant world view of biomedical science. Diverse health beliefs are evident in the complexities and ambiguities of knowing the reality in aboriginal world views and can be explored through a framework such as Morley's (1987) categorizations of causation. If holistic care is to be fully enacted, diversity in the ways of knowing and being among healthcare providers and the aboriginal communities must be recognized.

References

Adelson, N. (2000). *Being alive well: Health and politics of Cree well-being.* Toronto, ON: University of Toronto Press.

Anderson, J., Perry, J. A., Blue, C., Browne, A., Henderson, A., Basu Khan, K., et al. (2003). "Rewriting" cultural safety within the postcolonial and postnational feminist project: Toward new epistemologies of healing. *Advances in Nursing Science, 26,* 196–214.

Atleo, E. R. (2004). *Tsawalk: A Nuu-Chah-Nulth worldview.* Vancouver, BC: University of British Columbia Press.

Atleo, M. R. (1997). First Nations healing: Dominance or health. *Canadian Journal for the Study of Adult Education, 11*(2), 63–77.

Browne, A. J., & Fiske, J. A. (2001). First Nations women's encounter with mainstream health care services. *Western Journal of Nursing Research 23,* 126–147.

Commission on the Future of Health in Canada. (2002). *Building on value: The future of health care in Canada.* Ottawa, ON: Author.

Denis, C. (1997). *We are not you: First Nations and Canadian modernity.* Peterborough, ON: Broadview Press.

DiClemente, R. J., Crosby, R. A., & Kegler, M. C. (Eds.). (2002). Emerging theories in health promotion practice and research: Strategies for improving public health. San Francisco: Jossey-Bass.

Edwards, S. D. (1997). What is philosophy of nursing? *Journal of Advanced Nursing, 25,* 1089–1093.

Health Canada. (2003). A statistical profile on the health of First Nations in Canada. Ottawa, ON: Author.

Morley, P. (1987). Culture and the cognitive world of traditional medical beliefs: Some preliminary considerations. In P. Morley & R. Wallis (Eds.), *Culture and curing: Anthropological perspectives on traditional medical beliefs and practices* (pp. 3–12). Pittsburgh, PA: University of Pittsburgh Press.

Parse, R. R. (1998). *The human becoming school of thought: A perspective for nurses and other health professionals.* Thousand Oaks, CA: Sage.

Parse, R. R. (2003). Human becoming community change concepts. In R. R. Parse (Ed.), *Community: A human becoming perspective* (pp. 23–47). Sudbury, MA: Jones & Bartlett.

Polaschek, N. R. (1998). Cultural safety: A new concept in nursing people of different ethnicities. *Journal of Advanced Nursing, 27,* 452–457.

Ramsden, I. M. (2002). *Cultural safety and nursing education in Aotearoa and Te Waipounamu.* Wellington, New Zealand: Victoria University.

Smye, V., & Browne, A. (2002). "Cultural safety" and the analysis of the health policy affecting aboriginal people. *Nurse Researcher, 9,* 42–57.

Society of Obstetricians and Gynaecologists of Canada. (2001, March). *Health issues affecting aboriginal peoples: A guide for health professionals working with aboriginal peoples* (SOGC Policy Statement No. 100). Retrieved April 11, 2005, from http://sogc .medical.org/sogcnet/sogc_docs/ common/guide/pdfs/ ps100_4.pdf

Spector, R. E. (1996). *Cultural diversity in health & illness* (4th ed.). Stamford, CT: Appleton & Lange.

Uys, L. R., & Smit, J. H. (1994). Writing a philosophy of nursing. *Journal of Advanced Nursing, 20,* 239–244.

Interrelationships Among Nursing Theory, Research, and Practice

The clarion call for evidence-based practice is but one among many contemporary influences that demand that the advanced practice nurse have a clear and expandable understanding of the interrelationships among nursing theory, research, and practice. In Part Four, these interconnections are explored in three chapters by a collection of nurse leaders, offering opportunities for reflection.

As established in Chapter 1 and carried on as a thread throughout this book, a useful distinction can be made between practice and care, although this distinction is rarely observed in the literature. The logic, coherence, and utility of construing practice as values based and practitioner driven and care as evidence based and consumer driven can

certainly be put to the test in this part of the book. The rubric of values-based practice and evidence-based care is offered here as a kind of organizing principle. Although the language of the chapters does not match the language of values-based practice and evidence-based care, it may be useful for the reader to evaluate this organizing principle as a means to reach a greater understanding of the issues at stake in identifying guides to practice.

In Chapter 25, Pipe discusses optimizing patient safety and outcomes by aligning the concepts of evidence-based practice and theory-driven care. In Chapter 26, five well-known and influential nurse scholars offer a view of nursing theories and evidence that seeks to expand the received view of scientific evidence to admit of philosophical, autobiographical, and aesthetic "evidence." Clearly, the case has been made many times over that the knowledge needed for nursing practice is far greater than scientific knowledge alone. For this author the question arises as to whether it is necessary or appropriate to expand the notion of evidence from its traditional science base or whether it may be preferable to speak of philosophical, auto-biographical, and aesthetic ways of knowing in altogether different ways arising from their different traditions. Does it confuse the issue to introduce notions of multiple kinds of evidence alongside the traditional view of scientific evidence? To those who are familiar with the processes through which the most objectively rigorous integrative reviews are conducted to evaluate evidence and construct standards of care, it is plain that discourses such as this are unlikely to alter the standards by which quantitative research studies are evaluated and counted as solid evidence. Why use the language of evidence for values, beliefs, and lived experiences when these phenomena have their own discursive traditions?

In Chapter 27, Mitchell offers a critique and alternative view of evidence-based practice. Mitchell asserts that "professional nursing practice requires the risk to embrace the inherent ambiguity of the moment and to be with others with explicit commitment, responsiveness, openness, compassion, and the intent to serve." She goes on to present four principles generated by a long-time patient, which include "I am the only legitimate decision-maker," and "I must have complete information." These assertions resonate harmoniously with the organizing rubric of values-based practice and evidence-based care as delineated in this book.

CHAPTER 25

Optimizing Nursing Care by Integrating Theory-Driven Evidence-Based Practice

Teri Britt Pipe, RN, PhD

An emerging challenge for nursing leadership is how to convey the importance of both evidence-based practice (EBP) and theory-driven care in ensuring patient safety and optimizing outcomes. This chapter describes a specific example of a leadership strategy based on Rosswurm and Larrabee's model for change to EBP, which was effective in aligning the processes of EBP and theory-driven care.

Key words: *evidence-based practice, Jean Watson's Theory of Human Caring, leadership, nursing theory, Rosswurm and Larrabee.*

A professional work environment that engages and optimizes the empirical and theoretical foundations of nursing can advance patient health and safety. Core beliefs in nursing include that care should be based on the best empirical evidence available, incorporate patient/family beliefs and preferences, and be guided by the strong theoretical foundations of our discipline. The recent emphasis on evidence-based practice (EBP) in nursing has moved the discipline forward in understanding the importance of the empirical underpinnings of practice. However, some have argued that the theoretical and aesthetic ways of knowing in nursing have been overshadowed by this emphasis on the empirical way of knowing. The purpose of this chapter is to describe the leadership strategy used in the implementation of an integrated emphasis on EBP that is guided by nursing theory. The chapter highlights the interplay of nursing theory and EBP to optimize patient outcomes.

A key challenge for nursing leadership is how to convey the importance of blending both EBP and theory-driven care in terms of ensuring patient safety and optimizing outcomes. Specifically, nursing leadership wanted

Source: Pipe, T. Optimizing Nursing Care by Integrating Theory-Driven Evidence-Based Practice, Journal of Nursing Care Quality. 22 (3): 234-238. © 2007 Lippincott Williams & Wilkins, Inc.

to engage nurses in the process of adopting a unifying nursing conceptual framework, highlighting the linkages between the theory and outcomes of caring behaviors, communication, and patient safety. Simultaneously, the organization was engaged in educating nurses about EBP and its importance to patient care outcomes. The same framework was used for both endeavors—Rosswurm and Larrabee's Model for Evidence-Based Practice.[1] The description of the work on EBP has been described elsewhere.[2] This chapter describes the application of Rosswurm and Larrabee's model as a leadership strategy that led to the adoption of Jean Watson's Theory of Human Caring.[3]

Setting

The hospital and clinic system described in this chapter has 208 licensed beds, 15 operating rooms, and a level II emergency department. The clinic system was in place before the opening of the hospital. The environment uses state-of-the art technological innovations, with an electronic medical record for nursing documentation and tracking of quality indicators. The hospital staff members are registered nurses assisted by patient care assistants. Staff participation in nursing committees is encouraged. Nursing roles include, but are not limited to, educators, nursing informatics specialists, a nursing quality coordinator, nurse practitioners, and specialty-based clinical nurse specialists. Participation in nursing and other clinical research is encouraged.

Application of the Rosswurm and Larrabee Model

Rosswurm and Larrabee[1] proposed a model for guiding nurses through a systematic process for the change to EBP. This model recognizes that to translate research into practice, there must be a solid grounding in change theory and the principles of research utilization and use of standardized nomenclature. The model has six steps: (1) assess the need for change in practice, (2) link the problem with interventions and outcomes, (3) synthesize the best evidence, (4) design a change in practice, (5) implement and evaluate the practice change, and (6) integrate and maintain the practice change. The model provides a pragmatic, theory-driven framework for empowering clinicians in the process of EBP. In this project the model was used as a leadership strategy to guide the transition to theory-driven practice.

Assess the Need for Change in Practice

The process of strategic planning during a leadership retreat revealed a need to revisit the conceptual model for nursing. The former conceptual framework fitted well during the time when most nursing service delivery was in the outpatient setting, but the organization had grown to include a hospital with multiple specialties and an emerging wide range of nursing roles. It was time to look for a unifying model that would accommodate the complexity and diversity of patient populations and nursing care roles that were now in place.

During this phase it was important to include key stakeholders and gather baseline data. Nursing leaders and staff nurses were the key stakeholders included in the discussion about the need for a nursing model that fit the vision for the Division of Nursing Services. A vital part of the process was collecting internal data about current practice and comparing it with external benchmarks. One of the outcome indicators identified was a specific item contained in a survey designed to monitor nurses' perceptions of the work environment. Nurses at the hospital and clinic were invited to participate in an online survey using the National Quality Forum measure of the Nursing Work Index.[4] One of the items pertained to the perception of nurses that there was "a clear philosophy of nursing that pervades the patient care environment." The survey responses to this specific item were favorable, indicating that a large majority (89%) agreed with this statement. It was important for nursing leadership to ensure continued strength in this area, so this metric will continue to be monitored, using our internal data as a benchmark.

Link the Problem with Interventions and Outcomes

The problem was defined as the need to identify a vital nursing theory that could guide, richly describe, and give life to the language of nursing care. The theory had to be directly linked with patient health and safety. It was a priority to find a theory that was patient centered. It was also important that the theory provide language that helped nurses delineate the distinct discipline of nursing and at the same time was useful in collaborative care within an interdisciplinary team. The theory would be required to "travel with the patient" across various settings and levels of care. For example, we wanted the language of caring to be used in nurse-to-nurse report when patients are transferred between units or levels of care. Another requirement was that the theory was flexible to encompass all patient populations and all stages of the lifespan. Another desirable attribute for the theory was that nurses in all roles could use it to guide practice. For example, we wanted a theory that would be useful in multiple roles such as nurse educators, advanced practice nurses, nursing quality coordinators, nursing administrators, and researchers.

In this phase we identified potential interventions and activities that would help match a theory with the desired attributes. Outcome indicators included the Nursing Work Index data element as described in phase 1, pertaining to nurses' awareness of a guiding philosophy of nursing. We also included more process-oriented outcomes such as gathering consensus approval during the theory selection process and identifying steps to raise awareness about the chosen theory among nurses across the organization. The overarching goal was that nurses would adopt the theory and that nursing care would be theory driven and evidence based and would result in positive patient outcomes.

Synthesize the Best Evidence

The framework for choosing a theory was to select one that would be practical and relevant to nurses and patients across the care continuum and that could be used to link nursing care with pragmatic clinical outcomes. Examples of pragmatic outcomes included patient-centered caring behaviors, communication, and patient safety. The first step in this phase was a literature review. The priority was to adopt a theory that was linked with patient safety. During a previous EBP endeavor,[2] a literature search revealed the critical link between knowing the patient and detection of early warning signs of patient health declines as well as positive clinical indicators.[5–9] The theory motivating these studies was Jean Watson's Theory of Human Caring.[3] The theory met all the requirements identified earlier in phase 2. Of primary importance was its usefulness in linking patient-centered caring behaviors, communication, and patient safety. An added benefit of the Theory of Human Caring was its beneficial way of focusing on the nurse as a developing professional.

During this phase the feasibility of implementing the theory was assessed. The facilitators included the already high standards of care and professionalism among nursing staff, the level of engagement and intellectual excitement, the value on creativity and innovation, and the congruency between the Theory of Human Caring and the mission and vision of nursing within the organization. Another facilitating factor was that many nurses are in graduate programs and actively learning about nursing theory. They were interested in serving as change agents, integrating theory in their practice settings.

In addition, there were several barriers. Some nurses were not interested in nursing theory and did not see the link between theory and practice, especially between theory and patient outcomes. The challenge was to provide practice-based scenarios depicting how the Theory of Human Caring could guide practice in reality and specifically how the caring behaviors depicted in the theory could be linked with patient safety outcomes.

Design Practice Change

The proposed change was to adopt the Theory of Human Caring as the model that guided nursing care and practice throughout the organization. The resources needed for this to happen included a mechanism for knowledge transfer across the Division of Nursing Services and the willingness of nurses to make the theory live within the context of their practice. The Nursing Research Subcommittee took on the responsibility of being the team to begin the diffusion of innovation. The team identified nurses working in a wide variety of practice settings who were then invited to teach in an educational series about the Theory of Human Caring. The nurses were committed to learning about the theory and providing an interactive, creative series based on clinical realities in nursing. The team developed a curriculum on the basis of our organizational model of practice, education, and research.

Implement and Evaluate the Change in Practice

A formal educational series was implemented, led by key members of the Nursing Research Subcommittee. The sessions were primarily taught by nurses engaged in clinical nursing practice. The series included four interactive sessions that focused on the theory's practical uses in patient care, education, and research. The sessions were conducted in the outpatient setting and in the hospital, and the participants were awarded nursing continuing education units. The series was taped and thus available to nurses who could not be present for the live presentations. In addition to the series, members of the Nursing Research Subcommittee were invited to unit meetings and educational offerings to present the theory in various settings. On some units nurses took the lead in learning about the theory themselves and presenting to their colleagues at staff meetings. Presentations were made available to unit educators to tailor to their clinical environments.

The outcomes of this phase were measured by tracking the large number of participants in the educational offerings and their high ratings of the sessions. The question-and-answer sessions were particularly lively, with nurses commenting on how empowering it was to adopt a theory that gave them a language of compassion to link with patient safety and high quality outcomes. Two small research studies were also conducted to measure "caring efficacy"[10,11] as an outcome of participation in the educational series. The decision was made to adopt Jean Watson's Theory of Human Caring as the unifying nursing conceptual model for the organization.

Integrate and Maintain the Change in Practice

The change in practice, the adoption of the theory, was communicated in several ways, including the nursing newsletter, through minutes of various nursing committee meetings, and informally by nurses talking to others about the theory. Key in these communication strategies was making the explicit link between the theory and the outcome of patient safety. The nursing strategic plan and related documents are being changed to reflect the incorporation of the Theory of Human Caring into practice across the Division of Nursing Services. Monitoring is in place to ensure the continued relevance of the theory for the state of nursing in our organization.

Using the Rosswurm and Larrabee model as a leadership strategy was an effective way to guide change and achieve the desired outcome. Although the model has been established for EBP, it was expanded in this case to motivate and inform a movement toward theory-driven care.

Lessons Learned

- Staff nurses were positive and enthusiastic about the systematic translation of theory into practice. It made sense to nurses that as they are simultaneously learning the processes related to EBP, integrating nursing theory is a fitting companion journey. Multiple nurses have given presentations on their units about the theory, and several have used the theory in work they are doing related to continuing education.
- Nurses appreciate having a theory-driven practice with a language that empowers them to speak about

what they do and who they are with patients. Nurses are particularly enthusiastic when the theory helps them link caring behaviors (in which they already engage) with patient outcomes. We continue to monitor nurse-sensitive patient safety outcomes (falls, medication errors, patient injuries, etc.) and discuss them within the context of Watson's theory. However, because there are multiple quality improvement strategies in place at any one time, a direct causal link between the adoption of the theory and specific outcomes is not possible.

- Nurses are able to give multiple anecdotal examples of times when caring behaviors such as intentional presence, listening, and developing empathy with patients had led to focused advocacy for patient health and safety. For example, the Division of Nursing Services has adopted new processes and procedures for patient advocacy and communication, particularly during transitions or handoffs in care. In addition, because we wanted to learn more about the patient's ability to detect nursing caring behaviors, a specific item was included in our Nursing Quality Clinical Scorecard that focuses on "understanding and caring by nurses" as reported through the Professional Research Consultants methodology. This item is benchmarked with more than 1,500 hospitals. Our results for the quarters since the theory was adopted have been

above the 90th percentile, indicating that patients are able to detect nurses' understanding and caring behaviors.

Conclusion

Rosswurm and Larrabee's framework for translating evidence into practice is versatile and relevant for other related leadership processes, such as translating nursing theory into practice. The ultimate goal of both processes is to improve patient outcomes by optimizing the level and quality of nursing care. The example provided in this article is meant to highlight the potential benefits to patients and to nurses when nursing practice is both theory driven and evidence based and that the discipline will be enriched when both processes occur simultaneously.

References

1. Rosswurm MA, Larrabee JH. A model for change to evidence-based practice. *Image J Nurs Scholarsh.* 1999;31:317–322.
2. Pipe TB, Wellik KE, Buchda VL, Hansen CM, Martyn DR. Implementing evidence-based nursing practice. *Med Surg Nurs.* 2005;14:179–184.
3. Watson J. *Postmodern Nursing and Beyond.* New York: Harcourt-Brace; 1999.
4. Lake ET. Development of the practice environment scale of the Nursing Work Index. *Res Nurs Health.* 2002;25:176–188.

5. Minick P, Harvey S. The early recognition of patient problems among medical-surgical nurses. *Med Surg Nurs.* 2003;12:291–297.

6. Minick P. The power of human caring: early recognition of patient problems. *Sch Inq Nurs Pract.* 1995;9:303–317, 319–321.

7. Erci B, Ayse S, Tortumluoglu G, Kilic K, Sahin O, Gungormus Z. Effectiveness of Watson's Caring Model on the quality of life and blood pressure of patients with hypertension. *J Adv Nurs.* 2003;41:130–139.

8. Smith MC, Kemp J, Hemphill L, Vojir CP. Outcomes of therapeutic massage for hospitalized cancer patients. *J Nurs Scholarsh.* 2002;34:257–262.

9. Smith M. Review of research related to Watson's Theory of Caring. *Nurs Sci Q.* 2004;17:13–25.

10. Watson J. Assessing and Measuring Caring in Nursing and Health Science. New York: Springer; 2002.

11. Coates CJ. The Caring Efficacy Scale: nurses' self-reports of caring in practice settings. *Adv Pract Nurs Q.* 1997;3:53–59.

CHAPTER 26

On Nursing Theories and Evidence

Jacqueline Fawcett, RN, PhD, FAAN

Jean Watson, PhD, FAAN

Betty Neuman, PhD, FAAN

Patricia Hinton Walker, PhD, FAAN

Joyce J. Fitzpatrick, PhD, FAAN

Purpose: To expand the understanding of what constitutes evidence for theory guided, evidence-based nursing practice from a narrow focus on empirics to a more comprehensive focus on diverse patterns of knowing.

Organizing construct: Carper's four fundamental patterns of knowing in nursing—empirical, ethical, personal, and aesthetic—are required for nursing practice. A different mode of inquiry is required to develop knowledge about and evidence for each pattern.

Conclusions: Theory, inquiry, and evidence are inextricably linked. Each pattern of knowing can be considered a type of theory, and the modes of inquiry appropriate to the generation and testing of each type of theory, provide diverse sources of data for evidence-based nursing practice. Different kinds of nursing theories provide different lenses for critiquing and interpreting the different kinds of evidence essential for theory-guided, evidence-based holistic nursing practice.

Key words: *nursing theory, patterns of knowing, evidence-based practice.*

Evidence-based practice is in the forefront of many contemporary discussions of nursing research and nursing practice. Indeed, the term "seems to be the up-and-coming

Source: Fawcett, J., Watson, J., Neuman, B., Walker, P.H., Fitzpatrick, J.J.; Journal of Nursing Scholarship Second Quarter. 2001; 33:2, 115–119 © 2001 Sigma Theta Tau International. Reprinted with permission by Blackwell Publishing, Ltd.

buzzword for the decade" (Ingersoll, 2000, p. 151). The current call for evidence-based nursing practice has set the debate in a conventional, atheoretical, medically dominated, empirical model of evidence, which threatens the foundation of nursing's disciplinary perspective on theory-guided practice (Walker & Redmond, 1999). More specifically, as Ingersoll (2000) pointed out, almost all discussions of evidence-based practice are focused on the primacy of the randomized clinical trail as the only legitimate source of evidence. Furthermore, most discussions of evidence-based practice treat evidence as a theoretical entity, which only widens the theory-practice gap (Upton, 1999). Moreover, although multiple patterns of knowing in nursing have been acknowledged at least since the publication of Carper's work in 1978, nurses have ignored this disciplinary perspective and reverted to a medical perspective of evidence when discussing evidence-based nursing practice.

The purpose of this paper is to invite readers to join in a dialogue about what constitutes the evidence for theory-guided, evidence-based nursing practice. We are initiating the dialogue by offering a comprehensive description of theoretical evidence that encompasses diverse patterns of knowing in nursing. We advance the argument that each pattern of knowing can be considered a type of theory and that the different forms of inquiry used to develop the diverse kinds of theories yield different kinds of evidence, all of which are needed for evidence-based nursing practice.

On Nursing Theories

Diverse patterns of knowing were identified by Carper (1978), who expanded the historical view of nursing as an art and a science in her classic paper, "Fundamental Patterns of Knowing in Nursing." She identified four ways or patterns of knowing in nursing: empirics, ethics, personal, and aesthetics. Carper's work is significant in that it "not only highlighted the centrality of empirically derived theoretical knowledge, but [also] recognized with equal importance and weight, knowledge gained through clinical practice" (Stein, Corte, Colling, & Whall, 1998, p. 43). Chinn and Kramer (1999) expanded Carper's work by identifying processes associated with each pattern of knowing. Their work has enhanced understanding of each pattern of knowing and has brought Carper's ideas to the attention of a wide audience of nurses.

The pattern of empirical knowing (**Table 26-1**) encompasses publicly verifiable, factual descriptions, explanations, and predictions based on subjective or objective group data. In other words, empirical knowing is about "averages." This pattern of knowing, which constitutes the science of nursing, is well established in nursing epistemology and methods. Empirical knowing is generated and tested by means of empirical research. The next section of this paper extends the common focus on empirics as the primary focus of evidence, and offers a new lens for considering theory-guided evidence and

Table 26-1 Patterns of Knowing: Types of Nursing Theories

	Description	Mode of Inquiry	Examples of Evidence
Empirics	Publicly verifiable, factual descriptions, explanations, or predictions based on subjective or objective group data; the science of nursing	Empirical research	Scientific data
Ethics	Descriptions of moral obligations, moral and nonmoral values, and desired ends; the ethics of nursing	Identification, analysis, and clarification of beliefs and values; dialogue about and justification of beliefs and values	Standards of practice, codes of ethics, philosophies of nursing
Personal	Expressions of the quality and authenticity of the interpersonal process between each nurse and each patient; the interpersonal relationships of nursing	Opening, centering, thinking, listening, and reflecting	Autobiographical stories
Aesthetics	Expressions of the nurse's perception of what is significant in an individual patient's behavior; the art and act of nursing	Envisioning possibilities, rehearsing nursing art and acts	Aesthetic criticism and works of art

diverse ways of knowing that can and should be integrated into nurses' evidence-based practice initiatives.

Diverse Patterns of Knowing

In contrast to empirics, the other patterns of knowing are less established, but they are of increasing interest for the discipline of nursing in particular and for science in general. Ethical knowing, personal knowing, and aesthetic knowing are required for moral, humane, and personalized nursing practice (Stein et al., 1998). The pattern of ethical knowing (Table 26-1) encompasses descriptions of moral obligations, moral and nonmoral values, and desired ends. Ethical knowing, which constitutes the ethics of nursing, is generated by means of ethical inquiries that are focused on identification and analysis of the beliefs and values held by individuals and groups and the clarification of those beliefs and values. Ethical knowing is tested by means of ethical inquiries that focus on dialogue about beliefs and values and establishing justification for those beliefs and values.

The pattern of personal knowing refers to the quality and authenticity of the interpersonal process between each nurse and each patient (Table 26-1). This pattern is concerned with the knowing, encountering, and actualizing of the authentic self; it is focused on how nurses come to know how to be authentic in relationships with patients and how nurses come to know how to express their concern and caring for other people. Personal knowing is not "knowing one's self" but rather knowing how to be authentic with others, knowing one's own "personal style" of "being with" another person. Personal knowing is what is meant by "therapeutic nurse-patient relationships." Personal knowing is developed by means of opening and centering the self to thinking about how one is or can be authentic, by listening to responses from others, and by reflecting on those thoughts and responses.

The pattern of aesthetic knowing shows the nurse's perception of what is significant in the individual patient's behavior (Table 26-1). Thus, this pattern is focused on particulars rather than universals. Aesthetic knowing also addresses the "artful" performance of manual and technical skills. Aesthetic knowing is developed by envisioning possibilities and rehearsing the art and acts of nursing, with emphasis on developing appreciation of aesthetic meanings in practice and inspiration for developing the art of nursing.

Carper (1978) and Chinn and Kramer (1999) pointed out that each pattern of knowing is an essential component of the integrated knowledge base for professional practice, and that no one pattern of knowing should be used in isolation from the others. Carper (1978) maintained that "Nursing . . . depends on the scientific knowledge of human behavior in health and in illness, the aesthetic perception of significant experience, a personal understanding of the unique individuality of the self and the capacity to make choices within concrete situations involving particular moral judgments" (p. 22). Elaborating, Chinn and Kramer (1999) pointed out the danger of using any one pattern exclusively. They said

> When knowledge within any one pattern is not critically examined and integrated with the whole of knowing, distortion instead of understanding is produced. Failure to develop knowledge integrated within all of the patterns of knowing leads to uncritical acceptance, narrow interpretation, and partial utilization of knowledge. We call this "the patterns gone wild." When this occurs, the patterns are used in isolation from one another, and the potential for synthesis of the whole is lost. (p. 12)

The current emphasis on empirical knowing as the only basis for evidence-based nursing practice is an outstanding example of a "pattern gone wild."

Patterns of Knowing as Theories

The question arises as to whether the multiple, diverse patterns of knowing can be considered sets of theories. The answer to that question depends, in part, on one's view of a pattern of knowing and a theory. A pattern of knowing can be thought of as a way of seeing a phenomenon. The English word "theory" comes from the Greek word theoria, which means "to see," that is, to reveal phenomena previously hidden from our awareness and attention (Watson, 1999). For the purposes of this paper, a theory is defined as a way of seeing through "a set of relatively concrete and specific concepts and the propositions that describe or link those concepts" (Fawcett, 1999, p. 4). Theories constitute much of the knowledge of a discipline. Moreover, theory and phenomena are the lenses through which inquiry is conducted. The results of inquiry constitute the evidence that determines whether the theory is adequate or must be refined.

Collectively, the diverse patterns of knowing constitute the ontological and epistemological foundations of the discipline of nursing. Inasmuch as both patterns of knowing and theories represent knowledge and are generated and tested by means of congruent, yet diverse processes of inquiry (Table 26-1), we maintain that each pattern of knowing may be regarded as a type of theory. These four types of theories are subject to different types of inquiry. Henceforth, then, we will refer to the patterns of knowing as empirical theories, ethical theories, personal theories, and aesthetic theories. Our decision to regard the patterns of knowing as types of theories is supported by Chinn and Kramer's (1999) reference to ethical theories and Chinn's (2001) articulation of a theory of the art of nursing. Other global perspectives

indicate the direction of diverse patterns of knowing as types of theories. For example, Scandinavia nurses view nursing within a caring science model, and they acknowledge personal knowing, personal characteristics, and moral and aesthetic knowing of caring practices as theoretical ways of knowing the elicit diverse forms of evidence (Dahlberg, 1995, Fagerstrom & Bergdom Engberg, 1998; Kyle, 1995; Snyder, Brandt, & Tseng, 2000; von Post & Eriksson, 2000).

Furthermore, we, like some of our international colleagues, maintain that the content of ethical, personal, and aesthetic theories can be formalized as sets of concepts and propositions, just as the content of many empirical theories has been so formalized (Fawcett, 1999; von Post & Eriksson, 2000). Moreover, regarding all four patterns of knowing as types of theories reintroduces the notions of uncertainty and tentativeness that typically are associated with empirical theories (Fagerstrom & Bergdom Engberg, 1998; Morse, 1996; Polit & Hungler, 1995).

The four types of theories constitute much, if not all, of the knowledge needed for nursing practice. A potentially informative analysis, which follows from the conclusion that the patterns of knowing can be regarded as sets of theories, is the examination of extant theories to determine in which pattern of knowing each is located. That analysis is, however, beyond the scope of this paper and will not be pursued here. Rather, we are attempting to make connections between the four types of theories, representing the four patterns of knowing, and what constitutes evidence for nursing practice.

On Evidence

These four types of theories underlie all methodological decisions, and they are the basis for generating multiple forms of evidence. The question of what constitutes evidence depends, in part, on what one regards as the basis of the evidence. We maintain that theory is the reason for and the value of the evidence. In other words, evidence itself refers to evidence about theories. Similarly, theory determines what counts as evidence. Thus, theory and evidence become inextricably linked, just as theory and inquiry are inextricably linked.

Any form of evidence has to be interpreted and critiqued by each person who is considering whether the theory can be applied in a particular practice situation. This view indicates acknowledgment of diverse forms of knowing as inherent in any global or cultural interpretation of knowledge or theory (Zoucha & Reeves, 1999). The four types of theories are diverse ontological and epistemological lenses through which evidence is both interpreted and critiqued. The current emphasis on the technical-rational model of empirical evidence denies or ignores the existence of a theory lens. In contrast, our theory-guided model of evidence requires and acknowledges interpretation and critique of diverse forms of evidence. As shown in Table 26-1, we regard the scientific data produced by empirical research as the evidence for empirical theories. We count as scientific both qualitative and quantitative data and we support the call for palliative outcome analysis (Kyle, 1995; Morse, Penrod, & Hupcey, 2000; Snyder et al., 2000). The evidence for

ethical theories is illustrated in formalized statements of nurses' values, such as standards of practice, codes of ethics, and philosophies of nursing. The evidence for personal theories is found in autobiographical stories about the genuine, authentic self. The evidence for aesthetic theories is manifested or expressed as aesthetic criticism of the art and act of nursing and through works of art, such as paintings, drawings, sculpture, poetry, fiction and nonfiction, dance, and others.

Our view of the reason for evidence differs from the prevailing discussion in the literature. In current literature, typically a procedure or intervention is presented in isolation from the theory that undergirds that procedure or intervention, and in isolation from the value of the evidence-hence the term "evidence-based practice." We maintain that the more appropriate term is "theory-guided, evidence-based practice" (Walker & Redmond, 1999). Given the diversity of kinds of theories needed for nursing practice (see Table 26-1), evidence must extend beyond the current emphasis on empirical research and randomized clinical trials, to the kinds of evidence also generated from ethical theories, personal theories, and aesthetic theories.

Our view of the diversity of types of theories and the type of evidence needed for each type of theory addresses, at least in part, current criticisms of the evidence-based practice movement. We agree with Mitchell (1999) that the "proponents of evidence-based practice have . . . grossly oversimplified and misrepresented the process of nursing" (p. 34). Mitchell was particularly concerned that "the notion of evidence-based practice is not only a barren possibility but also that evidence-based practice obstructs nursing process, human care, and professional accountability" (p. 30). We respond to Mitchell's concern by including evidence about personal theories, which include authenticity in nurse–patient interpersonal relationships. Moreover, Mitchell (1999) maintained that "Evidence-based practice does not support the shift to patient-centered care, and it is inconsistent with the values and interests of consumers" (p. 34). Here, we respond to Mitchell's concerns by including evidence about ethical theories, which include the values of nurses. Mitchell (1999) also was concerned that "evidence-based practice, if taken seriously, may restrain some nurses from defining the values and theories that guide the nurse–person process" (p. 31) and relationship. This point relates to our view that the art of nursing is expressed through the nurse–person process and the evidence derived from interpretations of tests of aesthetic theories and ethical theories.

Furthermore, our view of the diversity of types of theories and corresponding types of evidence needed for theory-guided, evidence-based nursing practice elaborates Ingersoll's (2000) definition of evidence-based nursing practice. Her definition is as follows: "Evidence-based nursing practice is the conscientious, explicit, and judicious use of theory-derived, research-based information in making decisions about care delivery to individuals or groups of patients and in consideration of individual needs and preferences" (p. 152). Our view makes explicit the multiple kinds of theories—ethical, personal,

aesthetic, and empirical—whereas Ingersoll's reference to theory could easily be construed to mean only empirical theory or, perhaps because of the reference to individual needs and preferences, to include empirical and aesthetic theories.

We maintain the appropriateness of recognizing and appreciating empirical, ethical, personal, and aesthetic theories and the corresponding critique and interpretation of the evidence about each kind of theory. Such critique and interpretation of evidence is crucial for nursing practice because it is embedded in the values and phenomena located within a broad array of nursing theories. Moreover, by recognizing the four types of theories, more nurses and other health professionals may appreciate and use theories. They may agree with us that theories and values are the starting point for the critique and interpretation of any evidence needed to support clinical practices that may enhance the quality of life of the public we serve.

Conclusions

We invite readers to expand the dialogue about theory-guided, evidence-based practice. We urge nurses everywhere to consider the implications and consequences of the current virtually exclusive emphasis on empirical theories and empirical evidence-based nursing practice. We urge our nurse colleagues throughout the world to join us and those who have accurately pointed to the limitations of viewing nursing as a strictly empirical endeavor (Bolton, 2000; Dahlberg,

1995; Fagerstrom & Bergdom Engberg, 1998; Hall, 1997; Zoucha & Reeves, 1999) to consider what might be gained by recognition and development of ethical, personal, and aesthetic theories and by formalization of those kinds of theories. Accordingly, we encourage all nurses to actualize their claim of a holistic approach to practice by adopting a more comprehensive description of evidence-based nursing practice, a descriptive that allows for critique and interpretation of evidence obtained from inquiry guided by ethical, personal, aesthetic, and empirical theories, as well as by any other kinds of theories that may emerge from new understandings of nursing as a human science and a professional practice discipline.

References

Bolton, S. C. (2000). Who cares? Offering emotional work as a "gift" in the nursing labor process. Journal of Advanced Nursing, 32, 580–586.

Carper, B. A. (1978). Fundamental patterns of knowing in nursing. Advances in Nursing Science, 1(1), 13–23.

Chinn, P. L. (2001). Toward a theory of nursing art. In N. L. Chaska (Ed.), The nursing profession: Tomorrow and beyond (pp. 287–297). Thousand Oaks, CA: Sage.

Chinn, P. L., & Kramer, M. K. (1999). Theory and nursing: Integrated knowledge development (5th ed.). St. Louis: Mosby.

Dahlberg, K. (1995). Qualitative methodology as Caring Science Methodology. Scandinavian Journal of Caring Science, 9, 187–191.

Fagerstrom, L., & Bergdom Engberg, L. (1998). Measuring the unmeasurable: A caring perspective on patient classification. Journal of Nursing Management, 6, 165–172.

Fawcett, J. (1999). The relationship of theory and research (3rd ed.), Philadelphia: F. A. Davis.

Hall, E. O. C. (1997). Four generations of nurse theorists in the U.S.: An overview of their questions and answers. Vard I Nordeu: Nursing Science and Research In the Nordic Countries, 17(2), 15–23.

Ingersoll, G. L. (2000). Evidence-based Nursing: What it is and what it isn't. Nursing Outlook, 48, 151–152.

Kyle, T. V. (1995). The concept of caring: A review of the literature. Journal of Advanced Nursing, 21, 506–514.

Mitchell, G. J. (1999). Evidence-based practice: Critique and alternative view. Nursing Science Quarterly, 12, 30–35.

Morse, J. M. (1996). Nursing scholarship: Sense and sensibility. Nursing Inquiry, 3, 74–82.

Morse, J. M., Penrod, J., & Hupcey, J. E. (2000). Qualitative outcome analysis: Evaluating nursing interventions for complex clinical phenomena. Journal of Nursing Scholarship, 32, 125–130.

Polit, D. F., & Hungler, B. P. (1995). Nursing research: Principles and methods (5th ed.). Philadelphia: Lippincott.

Snyder, M., Brandt, C. I., & Tseng, Y. (2000). Measuring intervention outcomes: Impact of nurse characteristics. International Journal of Human Caring, 5(3), 36–42.

Stein, K. F., Corte, C., Colling, K. B., & Whall, A. (1998). A theoretical analysis of Carper's ways of knowing using a model of social cognition. Scholarly Inquiry for Nursing Practice, 12, 43–60.

Upton, D. J. (1999). How can we achieve evidence-based practice if we have theory-practice gap in nursing today? Journal of Advanced Nursing, 29, 549–555.

Von Post, L., & Eriksson, K. (2000). The ideal and practice concepts of "Professional Nursing Care." International Journal for Human Caring, 5(3), 14–22.

Walker, P. H., & Redmond, R. (1999). Theory-guided, evidence-based reflective practice. Nursing Science Quarterly, 12, 298–303.

Watson, J. (1999). Postmodern nursing and beyond. New York: Churchill Livingstone.

Zoucha, R., & Reeves, J. (1999). A view of professional caring as personal for Mexican Americans. International Journal of Human Caring, 3(3), 14–20.

CHAPTER 27

Evidence-Based Practice: Critique and Alternative View

Gail J. Mitchell, RN, PhD

Recent calls to promote evidence-based practice in nursing raise serious concerns. It has been suggested that evidence should be the primary source of knowledge for nurses. The general literature supporting evidence-based practice indicates that evidence will take nurses away from tradition, intuition, and anecdote to factual, scientific practice. The suggestion is that evidence can provide nurses with directives about how to think and act with patients, families, and groups. However, I contend that the notion of evidence-based practice is not only a barren possibility but also that evidence-based practice obstructs nursing process, human care, and professional accountability.

Prior to presenting arguments against evidence as the guide for nursing practice, let me state up front that evidence, defined here as conclusive statements based on findings from randomized controlled trials, has two areas of relevance. First, evidence may provide direction for development of procedures, techniques, and protocols that nurses and others are asked to perform. Healthcare professionals and nonprofessionals require such knowledge to guide their performance of tasks, and large systems require protocols to coordinate hospital-based care. Naturally, people who require knowledge and skill in these areas value the most effective techniques for preventing complications or performing tasks such as delivering medication,

Source: Nursing Science Quarterly, Vol. 12, No. 1, January 1999. 30–35. Reprinted by permission of and copyright © (1999) Sage Publications, Inc.

for instance, but evidence about procedure or service delivery is different from knowledge that informs the nurse–person process. Nurses may use techniques and technologies, but the knowledge base of nursing is not technical.

Second, evidence may provide one more resource for clients and nurses to consider the latest developments in the diagnosis and treatment of illness and disease. This information is available to any person who has access to libraries or to the Internet. Television broadcasts regularly offer the latest developments about links between heart disease and smoking or drug trials and side effects, for example. Healthcare professionals no longer control access to health-related information, and the general public will have increasing opportunities to consider the latest developments and to weigh their relevance in light of personal life circumstances.

In a general way, evidence may well be useful to people for making decisions about how they wish to approach their care and what options are available. Pharmacological or medical information may be a launching pad for discussions with people as they figure things out—but evidence will not build a knowledge base for nursing practice. The usefulness of evidence has been wrongfully cast in the context of legitimizing nursing as a profession instead of describing evidence as one possible resource for supporting clients' processes of decision making.

Rather than legitimizing nursing, evidence-based practice entraps nurses in the role of medical extender or medical technician, but even in these roles, evidence will not provide a foundation for practice. The idea that nurses in practice can access the relevant literature, make the required judgments about credibility of findings, interpret the significance of the findings in light of the guiding theory, and implement changes in practice is inconsistent with current realities. For one thing, nurses are expected to follow procedures written by multidisciplinary groups that are responsible for updating clinical practice, in particular medical specialties. In the more technical practice contexts, nurses are rewarded for complying, message is that nurses are the experts who intervene (try to manage and control) to create change toward provider-defined goals.

The term evidence-based practice, rather than being restricted to its technical and medical context where it may have some relevance, is being applied to the nurse–person process as the primary mode of knowing for relating with patients and families. Nursing practice happens in the nurse–person process, and to suggest that this process can be directed by evidence is not a supportable position; it is actually inconsistent with professional ethical codes, with current philosophical thought, and with what people say they want from nurses. Once again, it is obvious that nurses require current knowledge and skill for guiding activities involved in the delivery of health care, especially in hospitals. However, the nurse–person process is not data based—it is human based and must be guided by values and theoretical principles.

Specific Issues of Concern

Specific issues, then, about evidence and its use for guiding nursing practice are as follows. First, there is no body of evidence that can justify nursing as an applied science; current evidence is contradictory, tentative, unethical, and in some instances absurd. Second, proponents of evidence-based practice do not sufficiently acknowledge that all evidence is value laden and theoretically driven. Third, evidence-based practice is inconsistent with nursing's societal mandate to serve others rather than nurses themselves. Fourth, proponents of evidence-based practice oversimplify and misrepresent the complexities of human relating and the realities of multiple competing values, including those of the client, in the nurse–person process. Each of these points deserves thoughtful and scholarly attention by the nursing community. The following is an attempt to initiate discussion about these four issues.

Where Is the Evidence?

Proponents of evidence-based practice suggest that there is a body of knowledge that, if accessed by nurses, could provide clear direction about how to benefit others. In reality, the evidence does not exist. What do exist are multiple calls for more research and multiple reports that offer generalized statements that in many instances merely confirm the obvious. For instance, research findings about crisis intervention have led to recommendations that nurses should listen to people experiencing crisis, or studies of quality of life have suggested that people with more resources have different health patterns than those who have no resources at all. This confirmation of the obvious is absurd. It should be a fundamental assumption that listening to all clients is essential in nursing practice—listening should be a core value of the nursing discipline. Directives for listening should be explicit in theories and standards that guide nursing practice. As a nurse leader, I prefer directing my time and energy to promoting practices that ensure that all persons experience being listened to by nurses so that the patient's reality provides the foundation for any care offered. If nurses began by listening, they would know how to be helpful and what actions and information might help people in light of their personal health experiences. The unsettling reality is that patients and families consistently report that many nurses, similar to other professionals, do not listen.

Most nursing philosophies specify nursing's commitment to treat all patients as unique human beings who define and live health differently; therefore, should not nurses already know and expect that all people have unique health patterns, not just those reported in research studies? Do we need evidence to know that some percentage of unemployed, single mothers with several children would benefit from more resources in the community? How will the evidence from these sorts of studies help nurses to practice with a particular mother and her children? Will nurses share with the mother that research evidence suggests that if she just had more money or more support she would be better off and her health patterns might improve? Nurses should be offended by the presentation of the obvious; it insults the knowing of both patients and nurses.

I am very concerned that nurses are being portrayed as empty (thoughtless) beings who must be directed when to speak, what to think, and when to listen—based on research evidence. The idea that nurses require evidence to know they should listen or be open to unique patterns of health, for instance, is a dangerous notion—if one can take it seriously at all. It is possible to imagine that evidence-based practice could propel nursing toward a purely technical vocation, which questions the need for professional nurses. Unregulated workers can certainly follow menu-driven directives based on evidence. I concur with White (1997), who suggests that evidence-based practice may represent one more example of how nurses embrace what they think will liberate them when, in reality, the initiative ensures their subservience to other interests and other disciplines.

Professional nursing practice requires the risk to embrace the inherent ambiguity of the moment and to be with others with explicit commitment, responsiveness, openness, compassion, and the intent to serve. Professional practice demands an engagement with the unknown in light of a broad knowledge base and understanding of lived experience and not the enforcement of predefined directives based on generalized and often meaningless statements of evidence. Beneficial outcomes for patients surface in genuine engagements with nurses—as persons (clients) themselves clarify meanings, ask questions, explore concerns, discover strengths, and make plans to change health and quality of life. Patients and families indicate that they want to be treated as human beings, and the essence of this kind of human relationship is unscripted engagement in which nurses live the commitment to be with clients and to listen, respect, provide, and be involved as directed by clients. Knowledge about how to be with others in ways that respect the client's power and direction can only be found in nursing theories, because theories direct the "how" of nursing in light of its human context. Unfortunately, evidence-based practice obscures the critical links among practice, theory, and the client's experience of nursing.

Obscuring the Theory–Practice Link

Contemporary scholars endorse the belief that all thinking is theoretical and value laden, yet many supporters of evidence-based practice fail to acknowledge that nursing practice requires thought and is therefore also guided by theory. All the thinking and acting that happens in nursing moments are already guided by theory. Moments with nurses help or hinder persons as they struggle and plan to change patterns of health. In evolving as a discipline, nursing has relied on theory from other disciplines to guide practice, but it is becoming increasingly obvious that nurses require nursing theories to fulfill their societal mandate to provide a service that enhances health and quality of life. Introducing evidence as the guide for practice obscures the linkages that already exist between practice and theory. This is a critical omission in the literature promoting evidence-based practice because the reality is that, despite evidence, some theories are not appropriate for professional nursing because of what people experience when the theory is used and because the goals of some theories are not consistent with nursing's ethic.

For instance, there may be research evidence to support the use of behavior modification to make patients comply with medical directives, but this evidence does not justify the nurse's choice to reward and punish patients in a paternalistic model of care. In this example, there are clear directives from the theory that shape the nurse–person process and the patient's experience of nursing. Behavior modification, a theory borrowed from psychology, does not uphold nurses' commitment to a dynamic (open and changing), nonjudgmental process that respects human freedom. I have heard nurses describe both the burden of policing patients and the harm to relationships that can accompany behavior modification. Any evidence that is unexamined in light of the guiding theory and uninformed about the client's experience is not consistent with nursing. One need only listen to patients describe what it is like to be on the receiving end of rewards and punishments to know that behavior modification is inconsistent with the mandate of nursing. In my opinion, it is essential

to question who is being served when punitive interventions are used by professionals to bring about desired change.

Self-Serving or Other Serving

I have heard claims that disciplines are merely self-serving. Much of this antidisciplinary sentiment emerged a decade ago in North America when it was discovered that disciplines created large departments and complex care processes that had questionable benefit to the persons being served. Many health disciplines wanted to ensure a holistic approach to care and so their members developed extensive multisystem assessments for problem identification. Meanwhile, patients were being subjected to multiple, redundant questions and interventions that may or may not have been relevant to their immediate concerns and interests. The question of whether disciplines are self-serving is legitimate, and nurses especially must question whose interests they serve in day-to-day practice.

For instance, some nurses perform assessments and use tools that may harm patients or that diminish their quality of living. Nurses may lose sight of the client's experience and focus more on collecting evidence than on satisfying or comforting patients. There are multiple examples of this self-serving phenomenon, but two that are particularly meaningful are linked with nurses doing routine Mini Mental State Examinations (MMSE) and pain scale ratings. The MMSE is a tool for detecting problems with orientation and memory. In some institutions, nurses routinely complete the MMSE daily or weekly to collect evidence of change. Fluctuations in scores, however, are not usually explainable even from a medical perspective, and there is no clear direction about what nurses should do in the nurse–person process in light of any particular score. Furthermore, many patients find the MMSE unsettling at best, and for some, it leads to crying and upset as they try to find the right answer to please the healthcare professional. Nurses must begin to question this routine collection of data that does not inform their practice and that often leads to embarrassment for clients.

Similarly, frustrations have been reported by patients who are asked to rate their pain on a scale of 1 to 10. I recently heard a very compelling story from a patient who was being pressured to rate his pain on a scale of 1 to 10 before staff would respond to his requests for medication. He expressed frustration and anger about being treated as if he were wrong and having to say the right things to get pain medication. The message being given to patients who prefer not to rate their pain on a scale of 1 to 10 is that their language does not count as credible evidence. If a patient prefers to use the word terrible to describe pain, and if the person can only say that the pain is "somewhat" or "mostly better," it should be enough for nurses. From my view, we are already bordering on negligence by forcing patients to comply with our tools so that we can collect numerical evidence instead of attending to patients' concerns and issues with compassion and respect for their choice of words

and descriptions. The previous examples about patient dissatisfaction lead one to the following question: Who are nurses serving in their day-to-day practice?

I support the belief that nursing practice should integrate particular values and principles to structure the nurse–person process. The only evidence that can help nurses understand the benefit of nursing will come from clients' personal descriptions of how health and quality of life change with nursing care. The notion of evidence-based practice should be clearly limited to the technical/procedural realm of clinical care so that nurses are not expected to relinquish their responsibility to live certain values and theoretical principles with all human beings. Nurses must begin to ask clients what difference nurses' attitudes, actions, and expressions make to their experiences of health and quality of life.

There are extensive reports from patients that indicate that they want to be accepted, listened to, involved, respected, and treated as unique human beings (see e.g., Gerteis, Edgman-Levitan, Daley, & Delbancho, 1993; Young-Mason, 1997). One man who spent a great deal of time with healthcare professionals developed his own principles that helped him deal with a medical belief system that consistently ensured staff had power and control (Macurdy, 1997). Macurdy's four principles, which are echoed in many stories from patients, are as follows:

1. As the person with the greatest stake in my healthcare, I make the decisions, and no health professional can overrule my preferences.

2. I am the only legitimate decision maker, and no one else is permitted to speak for me.
3. I must have complete information.
4. Health care is a means to a full and meaningful life; it is not an end in itself. I will not allow the medical agenda to rule my life. I choose to lead my life and accept the risks and consequences of a meaningful existence.

The knowledge base for ensuring that all patients have experiences that support their being listened to, involved, respected, and treated like human beings flows from guiding nursing theories rather than evidence. Theories guide how nurses think and act with individual persons and families as clients provide direction by identifying concerns, what is helpful, what information might be useful, what things mean, what is possible, and what choices are most important. The nurse–person process is very complex, and proponents of evidence-based practice have, in my view, grossly oversimplified and misrepresented the process of nursing.

The Misrepresentation of Evidence

To say nursing is evidence based misrepresents what is in reality a complex, intimate, and multidimensional process of interhuman relating. Despite claims that are in contrast (DiCenso et al., 1998), evidence-based practice does indeed promote a routinized process of care that is dehumanizing. Nurses want and need to know how to practice with people in open, nonjudgmental, participative relationships that enhance quality from the client's perspective. If nursing is to remain a human science concerned about quality of life and lived experience, then it is essential that nurses identify the specific values and theories that will guide the nurse–person process toward this goal. Proponents of evidence have not explicitly addressed the influence of values, assumptions, interpretations, intentions, and desired outcomes in practice.

It is also essential that nurse leaders acknowledge that there are higher values in the discipline of nursing (such as respect for self-determination, mutual process, and individual uniqueness). Any evidence or theory selected by nurses should be coherent with such values. The very term evidence flows from certain assumptions that are not consistent with nursing practices that honor situated freedom, human uniqueness, and client as leader. Nursing's responsibility should be first and foremost to develop and sustain knowledge that honors the client's meanings, realities, possibilities, wishes, and choices. The nurse–person process must be informed by values and theories that provide nurses with the knowledge to participate with human beings in changing health and quality of life as directed by people themselves.

Also underestimated by proponents of evidence-based practice are that hospitals, clinics, and other service-oriented centers already embrace some philosophy for practice that influences decisions made by frontline providers. Nurse leaders are responsible for creating settings that nurture specific values and beliefs about patient care. As a chief nursing officer, I want nurses to practice patient-focused standards that are consistent with the human becoming school of thought (Parse, 1998). The notion that individual nurses could or should practice in ways supported by any evidence is inconsistent with the expectation that nurses should represent specific values and principles when it comes to human care.

Research involving human beings is infinitely complex, open to interpretation, and value laden. If research expands and informs the guiding theory, then findings must be considered in light of the practice prescribed by the theory. The most challenging aspect of nursing is the reasoning and thinking required to be with others in open, participatory, nonjudgmental relationships in which multiple forces and struggles come into play. Therefore, nurses should be given opportunities to look at their practices in light of the values and beliefs of nursing philosophy and theory. Changes in practice happen through personal insights about the linkages among beliefs, values, and actions—not through presentation of data.

The responsibility of all nurses should be to continue to integrate and develop theories that assist practitioners to be helpful and to have meaningful relationships with clients. Evidence in the absence of values and theories about human care and participative

relationships is meaningless unless nursing is to be reduced to a purely technical, menu-driven enterprise. It is unfortunate that some nurses have failed to be guided by the concerns and wishes of those served by nursing—patients and families—because there are opportunities for professionals to create practices that enhance quality of life and consumer satisfaction. Some people are coming to hospitals with extensive knowledge and with a greater understanding of their health situations than many professionals. People want dialogue that is relevant to their personal lives. Evidence-based practice does not support the shift to patient-focused care, and it is inconsistent with the values and interests of consumers. This gap between what evidence-based practice promotes and what consumers want raises this question: To what end? This question may indeed hold the essential seed of controversy that is fueled by the evidence-based initiative.

Proponents of evidence-based nursing practice contend that the initiative is consistent with practices that are patient focused and with qualitative research methods. I respectfully disagree. The ultimate goal of evidence-based practice is control. No matter what patient-friendly words are picked up along the way and no matter what research methods are employed, the values and assumptions embedded in evidence-based practice lead to a particular place—prescriptive interventions aimed at managing patients. Nurses and other professionals have been trying to manage people for many decades, and people have indicated that the management approach is not wanted. It is folly to think that people will embrace professionals who judge them and who do not recognize their knowledge and their investment in the healthcare process.

It is my hope that nurses will seriously consider the complex issues surrounding the evidence-based initiative. Debate will continue to shed light on how nursing is evolving as a human science. There are alternative views and different roads that lie in nursing's path. The call issued here is for nurses to choose a path that ensures a value-specific, theory-guided knowledge base that clearly places the client as the expert about health and change—a path that places nurses as accountable to clients for the quality of nursing care.

References

DiCenso, A., Cullum, N., & Ciliska, D. (1998). Implementing evidence-based nursing: Some misconceptions. Evidence-Based Nursing, 1(2), 38–40.

Gerteis, M., Edgman-Levitan, S., Daley, J., & Delbancho, T. L. (Eds.). (1993). Through the patient's eyes. San Francisco: Jossey-Bass.

Macurdy, A. H. (1997). Mastery of life. In J. Young-Mason (Ed.), The patient's voice: Experiences of illness (pp. 9–15). Philadelphia: F. A. Davis.

Parse, R. R. (1998). The human becoming school of thought. Thousand Oaks, CA: Sage.

White, S. J. (1997). Evidence-based practice and nursing: The new panacea? British Journal of Nursing, 6(3), 175–178.

The Future of Advanced Nursing Practice

In Part Five, four chapters are presented that offer innovative ways of addressing the complexity of advanced nursing practice in the contemporary healthcare environment. In Chapter 28, the late Janet Kenney, sole editor of the first three editions of this book, discusses nursing theory-based advanced practice nursing. Kenney's discussion (left intact for this edition) is broad ranging and thorough, and it offers the reader the opportunity to synthesize all that has come before to construct a personal perspective on the alternative theoretical and philosophical perspectives available in the literature. In Chapter 29, Reeder focuses on the changing definition of evidence between eras and seeks to determine the kind of evidence to be pursued in the future and how it will be obtained.

As the future brings changes to advanced practice nursing curricula, four researchers in Chapter 30 examine the need to have a clear understanding of nursing's meta-theoretical space to ensure adoption of only those values truly nursing oriented. In Chapter 31, Bunkers delineates the portrait of the 21st century nurse scholar as committed to human freedom and choice, openness, meaning, and social justice; pursuing an understanding of health as process, community as process, and the nature of suffering; believing in the power of personal presence; and focused on ethics and quality of life while acknowledging the centrality of mystery and uncertainty in human experience. Bunkers's nurse scholar, a kind of renaissance person for the new millennium, would surely be well prepared to explore the depths of values-based practice and the intricacies of evidence-based care and is, therefore, an excellent role model for the reader of this book who is likely a graduate student or doctoral student in nursing.

CHAPTER 28

Theory-Based Advanced Nursing Practice

Janet W. Kenney, RN, PhD

All professional disciplines are based on their unique knowledge, which is expressed in models and theories that are applied in practice. The focus of nursing knowledge is on humans' health experiences within the context of their environment and the nurse–client relationship. Theory-based nursing practice is the application of various models, theories, and principles from nursing science and the biological, behavioral, medical, and sociocultural disciplines to clinical nursing practice. Conceptual models and theories provide a broad knowledge base to assist nurses in understanding and interpreting the client's complex health situation and in planning nursing actions to achieved desired client outcomes. "Explicit use of conceptual models of nursing and nursing theories to guide nursing practice is the hallmark of professional nursing"; it distinguishes nursing as an autonomous health profession (Fawcett, 1997, p. 212).

This chapter describes the value and relevance of theory-based nursing for advanced practice nurses and discusses some underlying concerns about applying theories in nursing practice. The structure of nursing knowledge and the transformative process for theory-based practice are explained, along with the importance of critical thinking. An overview of various models and theories of nursing, family, and other disciplines is provided. Finally, the process for selecting and applying appropriate models and theories in nursing practice is thoroughly described.

Relevance of Theory-Based Practice in Nursing

The value of theory-based nursing practice is well documented in numerous books and journal articles. Although many articles illustrate the application of a nursing model or theory to clients with a specific health problem, Alligood (1997b) recently reviewed the nursing literature and found that about 68% of the articles reflect a medical approach to nursing. She also noted that most nurses described their practice in terms of a specialty area, types of care or health problems, and nursing interventions.

All nurses use knowledge they acquired during their formal education and clinical experience to guide their practice. Some nurse practitioners consistently use models and theories to guide their practice, but most nurses are unaware of existing theories and models or do not know how to apply them. Many nurses are not aware of what knowledge they use or where they learned it; thus, their implicit knowledge tends to be fragmented, diffused, incomplete, and greatly influenced by the medical model (Fawcett, 1997). Although graduate nurse practitioner students learn about nursing models and theories, their education often emphasizes application of medical knowledge as the base for their nursing practice. Thus, the use of medical knowledge and policies of health care delivery systems has replaced nursing knowledge and influenced some nurses to become "junior doctors," instead of "senior nurses" (Meleis, 1993).

Theories and models from nursing and behavioral disciplines are used by advanced practice nurses to provide effective, high quality nursing care. Many nurses believe that use of nursing theories would improve the quality of nursing care but that they do not have sufficient information about them or the opportunity to use them (McKenna, 1997b). According to Meleis (1997), theories improve quality of care by clearly defining the boundaries and goals of nursing assessment, diagnosis, and interventions and by providing continuity and congruency of care. Theory also contributes to more efficient and effective nursing practice and enhances nurses' professional autonomy and accountability. Aggleton and Chalmers (1986) claim that providing nursing care without a theory base is like "practicing in the dark." Kenney (1996) reported that professional nurses can effectively use theories and models from nursing and behavioral disciplines to:

- collect, organize, and classify client data
- understand, analyze, and interpret client's health situations
- guide formulation of nursing diagnoses
- plan, implement, and evaluate nursing care
- explain nursing actions and interactions with clients
- describe, explain, and sometimes predict clients' responses
- demonstrate responsibility and accountability for nursing actions
- achieve desired outcomes for clients (p. 9)

As we enter the next millennium, the health care revolution requires that nurses demonstrate efficient, cost-effective, high-quality care within organized delivery systems. "Nursing theory-based practice offers an alternative to the dehumanizing, fragmented, and paternalistic approaches that plague current delivery systems" (Smith, 1994, p. 7). With changes in the current third-party reimbursement systems, nurses will be paid for effective theory-based practice that enhances clients' health and their quality of life. To accomplish this, nurse practitioners must use critical thinking skills combined with theory-based knowledge and clinical expertise to achieve desired client outcomes.

Issues Related to Theory-Based Nursing Practice

In recent years, the enthusiasm for using nursing models and theories in practice has waned due to criticisms about the "theory–practice gap" and the lack of relevance to clinical practice. Also, there are philosophical concerns about whether only nursing models should guide practice and whether models and theories of nursing and other disciplines may be integrated in practice. This section discusses some of these issues.

The "theory–practice gap" refers to the lack of use or inability of nurses to use nursing and other theories in clinical practice. McKenna (1997b) claims that theories are not being used in a systematic way to guide nursing practice, although using theories may improve the quality of care. He believes nurses do not use nursing theories because they do not know about them, understand them, believe in them, know how to apply them, or are not allowed to use them. Professional nursing practice more often reflects the medical or organizational model of care than application of relevant nursing models or theories.

According to Rogers (1989, p. 114), "Nursing knowledge . . . is often seen as being unscientific, intuitive, and highly subjective." Some nurses believe that conceptual models and theories are too abstract to apply in nursing practice: they do not provide sufficient information to guide nursing judgments, are subject to different interpretations, are incomplete, and lack adequate testing and refinement (Field, 1987; Firlet, 1985). Others argue that some nursing theories were never meant to be directly applied in nursing practice but were intentionally abstract to stimulate thinking, provide new insights, and develop creative ways of viewing nursing (McKenna, 1997b).

As a practice discipline, nursing models and theories should be useful in practice, or their value is questionable. When models and theories are logical and consistent with other validated theories, they may provide the rationale and consequences of nursing actions and lead to predictable client outcomes. There are numerous articles and chapters describing application of various models to clinical nursing practice. However, rigorous research studies on how nursing models and theories contribute to desirable nursing actions and client outcomes are lacking.

Another issue is whether only nursing models and theories are appropriate for the discipline, as nursing is an applied science. Most professional nurses are familiar with theories from other disciplines, such as systems theory, family theories, developmental theories, and others; in clinical practice, nurses often combine their nursing and medical knowledge with theories from other disciplines. Some nurse scholars argue that nursing practice must be based on nursing models and theories, as they are consistent with nursing's view of human science and provide the structure for explaining nursings' unique contribution to health care (Cody, 1996; Mitchell, 1992). Because nursing models or theories represent the theorist's unique beliefs about persons, health, and nursing and guide how nurses interact with clients, McKenna (1997b) believes that an eclectic approach, combining theories from nursing and other disciplines, may compromise nursing theories if the concepts are removed from their original context and interwoven with other theories.

In contrast, Meleis (1997) argues that because nurses study other disciplines, nursing theory tends to reflect a broad range of perspectives and premises. Many nursing theorists have incorporated or "borrowed" theories from other disciplines and then transmuted them to fit within the context of nursing so that their nursing theories comprise shared knowledge used in a distinctive way (Timpson, 1996).

A related issue is whether professional nurses should consistently use only one nursing model, or use various models and theories from nursing and other disciplines in their practice. Most professions, like nursing, have multiple theories that represent divergent and unique perspectives about the phenomena of concern to their practice. Within nursing, conceptual models and theories range from broad conceptual models, or grand theories,

to specific practice theories. There are advantages and disadvantages to using one or more theories in clinical practice. Depending on the nurse's knowledge and clinical practice area, some nursing models and theories may be more appropriate than others. However, some would argue that use of only one nursing theory limits the nurse's assessment to only those things addressed by the theory, and the nurse may be forced to "fit" the client situation to the theory.

Others believe that nurses should consider a variety of nursing theories and select the model or theory that best "fits" the client's health problems. The majority of early nursing theories were based on traditional scientific methods and reflect a reductionistic perspective of humans as passive beings, consisting of elementary parts that respond to external stimuli in a linear, causal, and predictive way (Benner & Wrubel, 1989). Nursing models based on this perspective ultimately dehumanize individuals into disparate parts and systems and lead to fragmented, nonholistic nursing care (Aggleton & Chalmers, 1986). More contemporary nursing models view humans as continuously changing during reciprocal interactions with their environment, thus individual reactions to nursing care are not predictable, nor can they be controlled. However, these newer nursing models are more abstract than earlier models and are less likely to offer specific guidelines for nursing actions. Professional nurses are expected to develop unique, creative nursing actions suitable for each client's health problem and lifestyle, and theories from other disciplines may be integrated to complement and strengthen some limitations in both early and contemporary nursing models.

Cody (1996) contends that eclecticism, or selecting the best theory from other sources, is not necessarily wrong, but constantly borrowing theories from other disciplines does not contribute to the science of nursing or differentiate nursing from other professions. He believes that nursing practice ought to reflect a coherent, nursing theoretical base to guide practice in specific ways and contribute to the quality of care.

Since professional nurses provide health care for a variety of clients, each of whom is unique yet may have similar health concerns, nurses must use a broad knowledge base from nursing and other disciplines to select and apply relevant models and/or theories that are congruent with the client's situation. Health care, based on appropriate nursing models and theories, that integrates appropriate family, behavioral, and developmental theories, is most likely to achieve desired client health outcomes.

Structure of Nursing Knowledge and Perspective Transformation

Advanced practice nurses must first understand the structure of nursing knowledge and the process of transforming nursing models and theories into useful perspectives prior to implementing theory-based practice. In her recent book, Fawcett (1995) described the structural hierarchy of nursing knowledge, or nursing science. Nursing's metaparadigm, which includes the major concepts of person, health, environment, and nursing, provides the foundation from which nursing philosophies, conceptual models, and theories are derived. Each nurse theorist developed unique definitions of her major concepts, based on her education, practice, and personal philosophy (values, beliefs, and assumptions) about humans, health, nursing, and environment. The theorist's philosophy also influenced her conceptual model, which describes how the concepts are linked: the model explains the relationships among client-health-nursing situations (Sorrentino, 1991). Conceptual nursing models are usually called "grand theories" because they are broad and abstract and may not provide specific directions for nursing actions. Some nurse theorists have developed midrange or practice theories from their models that describe specific relationships among the concepts and suggest hypotheses to be tested.

According to Rogers (1989), an individual's personal "meaning" perspective or conceptual model provides a frame of reference or lens that influences how one perceives, thinks, and behaves in the world, yet most people are not aware of how their perspective influences and affects their view of themselves, others, and their world because underlying beliefs are held in the unconscious mind. In practice, nurses' perceptions, thoughts, feelings, and actions are guided by their personal framework or perspective of nursing, which provides a cognitive structure based on their assumptions, beliefs, and values about nursing (Fawcett, 1995). Many nurses unconsciously use a medical or institutional model as their perspective for organizing care. The prevalent values of such models or perspectives are efficiency, standardized care, rules, and regulations, such as "critical care pathways" (Rogers, 1989). As nurses become aware of the differences between the present and potential possibilities of nursing practice, they experience a cognitive dissonance or discomfort from an awareness of "what is" versus "what could be" (Rogers, 1989). Thus, only when nurses experience cognitive dissonance in practice will they change their frame of reference and use nursing models and theories.

For professional nurses to apply conceptual nursing models and theories, a dramatic change, or "perspective transformation," must occur (Fawcett, 1995; Rogers, 1989). Perspective transformation is the process of moving from one frame of reference or perspective to another, when unresolved dilemmas arise and create dissonance in one's current perspective (Mezirow, 1979). It is a process of critical reflection and analysis of other explanations or perspectives that might resolve the dilemma and explain or guide one's understanding and actions. The process involves gradually acquiring a new perspective that leads to fundamental changes in the way nurses experience, interpret, and understand their world and their relationships with others (Fawcett, 1995).

Fawcett (1995) describes nine phases leading to "perspective transformation." Initially, the prevailing stability of the current nursing practice is disrupted when use of a nursing

conceptual model or theory-based practice is introduced. Dissonance occurs as nurses consider their own perspective for practice and the challenge of changing to a new conceptual model or theory. Some nurses identify discrepancies between their current practice and how the new model or theory could affect their practice. Confusion may follow as nurses struggle to learn about the model or theory and how to apply it in practice. Nurses often feel anxious, angry, and unable to think during these phases and may grieve the loss of familiar perspectives of nursing. Their former perspective no longer seems useful, yet they have not internalized the new model or theory well enough to use it effectively. While dwelling with uncertainty, nurses acknowledge that their confusion is not due to personal inadequacy, and as their anxiety diminishes, they begin to critically examine former practice methods and explore the possibilities of implementing a new model or theory (Fawcett, 1995; Rogers, 1989).

With the discovery that a new model or theory is coherent and meaningful, synthesis occurs. As ways to apply the new model become clearer, new insights assist nurses to understand the usefulness of the conceptual model or theory in nursing practice (Fawcett, 1995). Resolution occurs as nurses become comfortable using the new model; they may feel a sense of empowerment and view their practice differently. Gradually, nurses consciously change their practice during reconceptualization; they shift from their former patterns to new ways of thinking and acting within the new model or theory. The final phase, return to stability, occurs when nursing practice is clearly based on the new nursing model or theory. Acceptance of a new perspective or paradigm, along with the corresponding assumptions, values, and beliefs concludes the transformation process.

Models and theories from nursing and other disciplines provide the cognitive structures that guide professional nursing practice. This body of knowledge helps nurses explain "what they know" and the rationale for their nursing actions that facilitate the client's health (Fawcett, 1997). Theory-based nursing practice depends on the depth of nurses' knowledge of models and theories and their understanding about how to apply them in practice (Alligood, 1997a). Nursing models and theories represent ideal, logical, unique perspectives or "maps" of the person and health. They provide a structure and systematic approach to examine clients' situations, identify relevant information, interpret data for nursing diagnoses, and plan effective nursing care through critical thinking, reasoning, and decision making (Alligood, 1997a; Mayberry, 1991; Timpson, 1996).

Nurses must use critical thinking skills to apply models and theories to their clients' health concerns. Paul and Nosich's (1991) definition of critical thinking is a commonly accepted one:

> Critical thinking is the intellectually disciplined process of actively and skillfully conceptualizing, applying, analyzing, synthesizing, or evaluating information gathered from, or generated by, observation,

experience, reflection, reasoning, or communication, as a guide to belief and action. (p. 4)

According to Cradock (1996), it is not what they know that makes nurses advanced practitioners, but how they use what they know. They must make expert clinical decisions based on reflection, complex reasoning, and critical thinking to apply theoretically based knowledge to diverse client situations (Spiracino, 1991). Critical thinking incorporates ideas from both models or theories with clinical experience and provides the structure for unique, creative nursing practice with each client (Alligood, 1997a; Field, 1987; Mayberry, 1991; Sorrentino, 1991). Several nurse authors believe that nursing theories will become the stimuli for reflection and critical thinking, leading to realms for creative expressions in nursing practice (Chinn, 1997; Marks-Moran & Rose, 1997). Theory-based nursing and critical thinking are the foundations of advanced nursing practice (Mitchell, 1992). Specific critical thinking skills for each component of the nursing process are identified in **Table 28-1**.

Models and Theories Applicable in Advanced Nursing Practice

Theory-based nursing practice is the creative application of various models, theories, and principles from nursing, medical, behavioral, and humanistic sciences. Models and theories from relevant disciplines provide

Table 28-1   Application of Critical Thinking Skills to the Nursing Process

Components and Definitions	Critical Thinking Skills and Activities
Assessment An ongoing process of data collection to determine the client's strengths and health concerns	Collect relevant client data by observation, examination, interview and history, and reviewing the records Distinguish relevant data from irrelevant Distinguish important data from unimportant Validate data with others
Diagnosis The analysis/synthesis of data to identify patterns and compare with norms and models A clear, concise statement of the client's health status and concerns appropriate for nursing intervention	Organize and categorize data into patterns Identify data gaps Recognize patterns and relationships in data Compare patterns with norms and theories Examine own assumptions regarding client's situation Make inferences and judgments of client's health concerns Define the health concern and validate with the client and health team members Describe actual and potential concerns and the etiology of each diagnosis Propose alternative explanations of concerns
Planning Determination of how to assist the client in resolving concerns related to restoration, maintenance, or promotion of health	Identify priority of client's concerns Determine client's desired health outcomes Select appropriate nursing interventions by generalizing principles and theories Transfer knowledge from other sciences Design plan of care with scientific rationale
Implementation Carrying out the plan of care by the client and nurse	Apply knowledge to perform interventions Compare baseline data with changing status Test hypotheses of nursing interventions Update and revise the care plan Collaborate with health team members
Evaluation A systematic, continuous process of comparing the client's response with the desired health outcomes	Compare client's responses with desired health outcomes Use criterion-based tools to evaluate Determine the client's level of progress Revise the plan of care

the knowledge base to understand various aspects of the client's health concerns and guide appropriate nursing management. In advanced nursing practice, the client may be an individual, families or an aggregate, such as a community or special population. Knowledge of relevant models and theories from nursing and other disciplines enables the nurse to select those that "best fit" each client. This section provides a brief overview of some nursing, family, community, and other models and theories that may be relevant and useful to nurse practitioners.

Nursing Models and Theories

Numerous nursing models and theories have been reported in the literature since the 1950s. Some well-known nurse theorists' works are cited: readers are encouraged to seek other sources for more information about their models and theories. The early nurse theorists' conceptual models focused on individual clients and described nursing goals and activities. Peplau's "Interpersonal Model" described a goal-directed, nurse–client interpersonal process to promote the client's personality and living. Orlando's model explained a deliberative nursing approach to understand nurse–patient relationships and the communication process. Hall's "Core-care-cure Model" expanded and clarified nursing actions to promote clients' health. Levine's model identified four principles of human conservation to guide nursing activities.

More contemporary nursing theories have been published since 1970, when Rogers introduced her "Science of Unitary Man."

She described mutually evolving relationships between humans and their environment that are expressed as changing energy fields, patterns, and organization. Orem's "Self-care Model" identified requisites for an individual's self-care, and specific nursing systems to deliver care according to the client's self-care needs. King designed a systems model that included the individual, family, and society, then developed her "Theory of Goal Attainment," which described nurse–patient transactions to achieve the client's goals. Roy's "Adaptation Model" identified three types of stimuli that affect a patient's four modes of functioning. She described how the nurse identifies maladaptive behaviors and alters stimuli to enhance the client's adaptation. Paterson and Zderad developed a model of "Humanistic Nursing." Leininger's "Transcultural Nursing Model" explained differences between universal and cultural specific views of health and healing, and how nurses can provide culturally congruent health care. According to Watson, nursing is the art and science of human care: nurses engage in transpersonal caring transactions to assist persons achieve mind–body–soul harmony. Johnson's "Behavioral Systems Model" focused on nurturing, protecting, and stimulating the individual's seven subsystems to maintain balance and stability. Neuman designed a complex "Health Care Systems" model that identified different types of stressors and levels of defense: nursing actions were based on three levels of prevention. Parse developed a "Man–living–health Theory" in which nurses assist individuals to explore their past–present–future life experiences and illuminate possible life-style choices to enhance their health and lives. Newman's theory of "Health as expanding consciousness" considers disease as part of health, and explores time and rhythm pattern recognition with changes in life and health.

Family Models

Although most nursing models were originally designed to focus on individual clients, a few are applicable to families. King views the family as a social system or group of interacting individuals, and family health as dynamic life experiences. Roy views the family as part of the client's immediate social environment, whereas Neuman's concept of family is harmonious relationships among family members. These nurse theorists focused on the individual client with the family seen as context. If the family is viewed as the client, the nurse must decide what the model should focus on—family development, interactions and stress, family systems, structure and function, or a combination of these models, such as the Calgary Family Model.

Family development models are based on the premise that the life cycle of families follows a common sequence of events from marriage through childrearing, retirement, and bereavement. Most are based on the typical nuclear two-parent family and emphasize the stages and adult's responsibilities to accomplish desired goals. Duvall's (1977) model is well-known, and Stevenson (1977), a nurse theorist, also designed a family model.

Family interactional models view family members as a unit of interacting personalities within a dynamic life process. These models focus on how members' perceptions and interpretations of themselves and other family members determine their behaviors and actions. Also, these models consider how members' roles affect their interaction with others. Satir's "Family Interaction Model" is an example. Family stress and coping models, based on the work of Lazarus and Folkman, were developed by Moos and Billings (1982) to identify how the family appraised the situation, dealt with their problems, and handled the resulting emotions. McCubbin and McCubbin (1993) designed the "Double ABCX Model," which examines family life stressors and resources, along with changes that affect their adaptation to health problems, and ability to manage family crises. Curran's (1985) "Healthy Family Model" identified characteristics of healthy families and common stressors affecting families.

Family systems models view the whole family as greater than and different from the sum of its parts or members. These models focus on the family with a hierarchy of subsystems (mother–father, parent–child) and supersystems in the community (social, occupational, recreational, and religious networks) that interact with the family system. Olson, Russell, and Sprenkle's (1983) model identifies 16 types of family systems based on the premise that a balance must be maintained in family cohesion, so that members do not become too enmeshed or too distant, and adaptability, wherein too much change creates chaos and too little change leads to rigidity. Communication between family members is the third dimension. The "Beaver's System Model" (Beavers & Voeller,

1983) examines the structure, flexibility, and competence of a family and its members. Centripetal families enjoy close family relationships, while centrifugal families seek satisfaction outside the family.

Family structural–functional models view the family as a social system composed of nuclear and extended family members, and their social–communicative interactions to achieve family functions. According to Friedman (1992), the structural components include family composition, values, communication patterns, members' roles, and the power structure. Functional components of this model include physical necessities and care, economic, affective, and reproductive behaviors, socialization and placement of family members, and family coping abilities. The structural and functional components are interrelated, and each part is affected by changes in other parts.

A model that combines many of the above models is the Calgary Family Model, developed by Wright and Leahey (1994). The major components include the internal and external family structure, similar to Friedman's (1992) model, along with family context, such as race, ethnicity, social class, religion, and environment. Family functions are viewed as "instrumental" or daily living activities, and "expressive" activities, including communication (emotional, verbal, and behavioral), problem-solving, roles, influences, beliefs, and alliances or coalitions. Family developmental stages and tasks, similar to Duvall's (1977), are also part of this comprehensive model.

Any family model may be combined with and complement a nursing model because nursing practice may involve individual clients or families. Nurses with knowledge of various family models are more likely to select the most appropriate and relevant one to meet the family's health concerns.

Community Models

There are many community models that are useful to nurses, but they differ according to whether "community" is considered a target population or aggregate or a geographical area. McKay and Segall (1983) described an aggregate model, in which the focus is on a group of individuals who share common characteristics, but may not interact with each other. Shamansky and Pesznecker (1981) identified three interdependent factors that constitute a geographical community: (1) persons who reside in an area; (2) space and time, which includes the community's history and environmental features; and (3) purpose factors that explain functional processes such as government policies, educational services, and forms of communication. The "Community-as-Client Model," designed by Anderson, McFarlane, and Helton (1986) combines both the aggregate and geographical community. It addresses the following eight subsystems of the aggregate in the community: physical environment, education, safety and transportation, politics and government, health and social services, communication, economics, and recreation. A community nursing process model was developed by Goeppinger, Lassiter, and Wilcox (1982) that examines the following eight processes in a community: commitment of members, awareness of others' views, articulation of community needs, effective communication within and among members, conflict containment and accommodation, participation in organizations, management of relations with the larger society, and mechanisms to facilitate participant interactions and decision making. Knowledge of several community models facilitates selection of the most appropriate one.

Other Useful Models and Theories

Nurses, and theorists in other disciplines, have developed many relevant models and theories that are useful in advanced nursing practice. Some of these models include Maslow's Hierarchy of Needs, Erikson's "Stages of Development," Piaget's "Cognitive Development of Children," Pender's (1987) "Health Promotion/Disease Prevention" model, and Loveland-Cherry's (1989) "Family health promotion" model. In addition, there are numerous theories of stress, crises, coping, grief, bereavement, death, and dying developed in psychology and behavioral disciplines. Nurses have transformed some of these theories to encompass a health–illness context. Nurses who are cognizant of a variety of nursing, family, community, and behavioral models and theories are more likely to select the "best fitting" model for their clients.

Selection of Relevant Models and Theories

This section provides an overview of several nurse scholar's criteria and guidelines for selecting models and theories. Meleis (1997)

identified six criteria to guide selection of suitable models and theories for practice. McKenna (1997a) described seven selection criteria based on a review of the literature. Kim (1994) constructed a framework for practice theories with four dimensions to consider in selecting nursing models and theories. Fawcett and associates (1992) suggested that nurses consider three questions to determine the best "fit" between the client's health concerns and various models and theories. Relevant criteria from the above scholars' work were integrated with the author's prior work to delineate five guidelines for selecting appropriate models and theories (Christensen & Kenney, 1996).

Meleis (1997) wrote that selecting models and theories for nursing practice is both a subjective and objective process. She identified six criteria for nurses to consider in the selection process.

- Personal—the nurse's comfort with the theory and congruency with the nurse's own philosophical views of life
- Mentor—the model or theory learned from a nurse mentor or educator
- Theorist—their reputation in the discipline and degree of recognition
- Literature—support the amount of literature available about the theory and the theory's significance for one's specialty
- Sociopolitical congruency—the model or theory's acceptability within the nurse's workplace and whether major structural or practice changes are required

- Utility—the ease in which nurses can understand and apply the model or theory in practice settings

McKenna (1997a) reviewed the literature and identified the following seven criteria for selecting models and theories.

- The type of client—the client's needs should direct the choice because the theory provides guidelines to achieve the client's goals.
- Healthcare setting—the type of clinical setting and nursing practice are contextual factors that affect selection of theories.
- Parsimony/simplicity—simple and realistic theories are more likely to be understood and applied in practice.
- Understandability—nurses must understand a theory if they are expected to use it.
- Origins of the theory—the credibility, prior use, and testing of the theory should also be considered.
- Paradigms as a basis for choice—nurses must decide between the totality or simultaneity paradigm, as each provides a different view of clients and nursing actions.
- Personal values and beliefs—the theory must be congruent with the nurse's own views about humans, health, and nursing.

In her article on practice theories, Kim (1994) defined two dimensions of theories, which include four "sets of practice theories" relevant to selecting models and theories. One dimension is the "target," which addresses both the philosophy of care for the person and the philosophy of therapy for the client's problems. The other dimension is the "nurse–agent," which includes two phases, deliberation, and enactment. The four "sets of practice theories" serve to guide nurses in choosing theories that will (1) explain the patient's problems and ideas about therapy for the problems; (2) provide ideas about how the nurse should approach the patient, such as through communication, caring, or empowerment; (3) explain how to make decisions about appropriate nursing actions for the patient; and (4) explain what happens during enactment of nursing actions. Kim proposed that a science of nursing practice could be developed from this framework.

Fawcett and associates (1992) identified questions to guide nurses' selection of appropriate theories and models. The nurse must understand the differences among various models and theories in nursing and other disciplines to answer these questions. The following three questions will help the nurse identify the most appropriate model:

1. Does the theory or model address the client's problems and health concerns?
2. Are the nursing interventions suggested by the model consistent with the client's expectations for nursing care?
3. Are the goals of nursing actions, based on the model or theory, congruent with the client's desired health outcomes?

These questions help nurses decide which models and theories will assist them to organize the data into patterns, identify other health concerns, and determine congruency of the client's and nurse's view of nursing and health.

The first step toward theory-based nursing practice is the conscious decision to use theories in practice (Fawcett, 1997). The second step is recognizing that use of conceptual nursing models and theories requires a major change in how the nurse thinks about and interacts with clients to alleviate their health concerns. This change, referred to earlier as a "perspective transformation," occurs gradually as the nurse discards one framework of practice and learns another perspective. Adopting and applying new models and theories in practice depends on nurses having knowledge of various models and theories and understanding how these models and theories relate to each other (Alligood, 1997a).

Guidelines for Selecting Models and Theories for Nursing Practice

After deciding to implement theory-based nursing practice, the author believes that each nurse must engage in the five steps described here:

1. Consider your personal values and beliefs about nursing, clients, health, and environment. Each nurse has a personal frame of reference or perspective of nursing practice, based on his/her conscious or unconscious assumptions, beliefs, and values about nursing. One's perspective of nursing provides a cognitive structure that guides one's perceptions, thoughts, feelings, and nursing actions (Fawcett, 1995). Clarifying one's own values and beliefs about clients, health, and nursing practice is necessary before a "perspective transformation" can occur.

2. Examine the underlying assumptions, values, and beliefs of various nursing models, and how the major concepts are defined. After clarifying one's own values and beliefs, the nurse examines the definitions of major concepts in various models and theories to determine whether they are congruent with one's own beliefs (Alligood, 1997a). Nursing models and theories are based on different values and beliefs about the nature of the client's behaviors and abilities, what is health and environment, and what nursing actions facilitate clients' health. Each nursing model and theory provides a unique view for specific nursing practice. Some nursing models reflect a "totality" paradigm, and view humans as having separate biological, social, psychological, and spiritual parts that respond to environmental stimuli or change, and the nurse's role is to facilitate adaptation or equilibrium to maintain health. Other nursing models reflect a "simultaneity" paradigm, and believe humans are intelligent beings, capable of making informed decisions about their lives, and that they continuously engage in a dynamic, mutual interaction with their environment. In this paradigm, the nurse's role is to guide clients in choosing lifestyles and/or therapies that are acceptable

to them and facilitate their growth and life–health process.

3. Identify several models that are congruent with your own values and beliefs about nursing, clients, and health. Each nurse must consider whether the theorist's underlying values are congruent with one's own personal values and beliefs about clients, health, and nursing because the theorist's values guide the nurse's critical thinking and reasoning processes (Alligood, 1997a). Models and theories reflect the theorist's views about people and nursing. They directly effect how nurses approach their clients, what information they gather, how that information is processed, what nursing activities are appropriate, and, what client outcomes are expected based on the model. For example, some traditional nursing models define the person as a bio–psycho–social being who responds to environmental stimuli, and health results from nursing actions that lead to predictable changes. These models would be incongruent for contemporary nurses who believe that people are free agents, dynamically interacting with their environment as a whole, and capable of making rational decisions, and that the nurse's role is to assist clients to explore various options and choose ones that are acceptable with their values and lifestyle.

4. Identify the similarities and differences in client focus, nursing actions, and client outcomes of these models. Nursing models and theories consist of concepts with specific definitions, and statements that describe how the concepts are interrelated. Some propose specific nursing actions and expected client outcomes. The major concepts guide what data is collected during the assessment and how the data is organized to identify and interpret bio–behavioral patterns and determine nursing diagnoses. Nursing models also guide development of the nursing care plans and designate desired outcomes to evaluate. By comparing various models, nurses recognize which ones are congruent with their values and beliefs about nursing and offer the best "fit" with the client's health concerns.

5. Practice applying the models and theories to clients with different health concerns to determine which ones best "fit" specific situations and guide nursing actions that will achieve desired client outcomes. The nurse explores specific models in depth, and may analyze their usefulness before implementing them. By comparing several models and examining the attributes of the client, the focus of nursing actions, and the proposed outcomes, the nurse will acquire a more in-depth understanding of different models. Each nursing model describes different areas for assessment, unique nursing diagnoses, and specific nursing interventions to assist the client toward health. The nurse must decide which models and theories are most appropriate for each client. Which one offers the best "fit" for the client's health concerns? Selecting appropriate models and theories for each unique client health situation requires nurses to use their broad knowledge base from various disciplines, critical thinking skills, clinical expertise, and intuition to identify the best 'fit' between the client's health concerns and nursing models (Fawcett, et al., 1992).

Application of Theory-Based Nursing Practice

The choice of theories and models suitable to the client's health concerns occurs during the initial data assessment process. The initial data focus on the client's primary expressed concerns and how they are related to or affect the client's lifestyle and patterns of living. These data assist the nurse to identify and understand the client's common and unique patterns. The client's view of health, along with past and present "lived experiences," and future lifestyle and health concerns, are also considered. Using this information, the nurse considers various models and theories from nursing and other disciplines that are relevant to the client's unique health concerns, and congruent with the nurse's own beliefs. Then, the nurse selects those models and other theories that best "fit" the client's situation and health concerns and will systematically direct nursing practice.

The major concepts of the chosen models and theories guide each component of the nursing process, as shown in **Table 28-2.** The concepts serve as categories to guide additional data collection. They suggest, either directly or indirectly, what information is relevant and should be collected. The models and theories assist the nurse to organize, categorize, and interpret pertinent data that illustrate the client's bio–behavioral patterns and identify appropriate nursing diagnoses that are linked to relevant etiological factors.

Nursing and other models and theories guide development of a care plan by suggesting appropriate types of nursing interventions and specific nursing actions. Desired client outcomes are derived from the models and theories and define what changes in the client should be evaluated. For example, if Roy's model is chosen, data about the client's physiological needs, self-concept, role mastery, and interdependence, along with related stimuli would be collected, and used to identify adaptive and maladaptive behavioral patterns. The nurse who uses Orem's Self-Care Model would assess and judge clients' ability to meet their universal and developmental self-care requisites and whether they had any health deviations. From analysis of this data, the nurse would diagnose self-care deficits and determine appropriate nursing plans for partial, compensatory, or health education nursing care. Nursing care plans are based on the model and describe the client's desired outcomes, along with nursing actions to achieve the client's outcomes. Nurses who use Johnson's Behavioral Systems Model would consider ways to nurture, protect, or stimulate the client to facilitate health, whereas the Neuman's Health Care System's model assists the nurse to explore ways to reduce stressors within the three levels of disease prevention.

Some nurses believe that family models complement nursing models and provide a more holistic and comprehensive perspective of clients and their health concerns. Selection of a family model occurs after the nurse gathers preliminary data about the family and identifies its unique and common patterns. Then the nurse decides whether the "family as context" or "family as client" would

Table 28-2   Theory-Based Nursing Practice

Component	Nursing Process Use	Nursing Model Use
Assessment	Describes how to collect data	Guides what data to collect
Diagnosis	Describes how to process data	Guides organizing, categorizing, and interpreting data
	Provides format for nursing diagnosis	Provides concepts for nursing diagnosis
	Describes *how* to plan	Guides *what* to plan
	Facilitates development of care plan unique to client	Designates appropriate types of nursing interventions
Implementation	Describes phases of implementation	Directs model-specific nursing actions
Evaluation	Identifies *how* to evaluate	Guides *what* to evaluate
General	Requires accountability through use of systematic approach to nursing practice	Enhances accountability of theory-based practice
	Process enhances continuity of care	Provides a comprehensive, coherent approach to care of client

be more appropriate and best "fit" the client's situation. Also, the nurse's perception and definition of family and health guide the selection of a family model. For example, a pediatric nurse who works in an outpatient clinic may choose Orem's Self-Care Model to guide care of a nine-year-old child with an ear infection and the mother's treatment of the child. Friedman's Family System model may complement Orem's model and enhance understanding of the family's structure and functions. The nurse may also use Erikson's Developmental Framework to help the mother recognize and encourage her child's normal developmental behaviors. Pain management theories may also be applied to reduce the child's earache.

This example illustrates how nurses examine and judge the value of various models and theories and select those that are most congruent and useful and best "fit" the client's health concerns and the nurse's perspective of practice. Gradually, nurse practitioners develop an expertise in selecting theories and models that are appropriate and relevant to their client's health concerns and congruent with their own views of advanced practice.

Summary

This chapter described the importance and value of applying models and theories from nursing and other disciplines in advanced nursing practice. Issues related to the nursing theory-practice gap were discussed, along with concerns about using only one nursing model in practice and about integrating models and theories from other disciplines with nursing models and theories. The structure of nursing knowledge was explained and the need for a "perspective transformation" to occur prior to implementing theory-based nursing practice. Critical thinking, logical reasoning, and creatively applying nursing models and theories were emphasized. Different types of nursing, family, community, and other models and theories were discussed. Finally, the process of selecting and applying models and theories was thoroughly described.

In the last few decades, the emergence of nursing models and theories has illuminated several nursing paradigms and explicated their underlying assumptions, beliefs, and values that guide nursing practice. The science of nursing and empirical patterns of knowing is represented by these nursing models and their theories. Application of models and theories from nursing and other disciplines depends on nurses having a broad knowledge base and understanding how models and theories are interrelated. Empowerment of nurses through "perspective transformation" and the use of nursing models and theories is essential. They provide the framework for critical thinking within the context of nursing and guide the reasoning that professional nurses need to survive in an era of cost containment and evidence-based practice. Use of models and theories from nursing and related health disciplines

enables nurses to demonstrate accountability for their decisions and actions through scientific explanation and provides a coherent approach to theory-based nursing practice.

References

Aggleton, P. J., & Chalmers, H. (1986). Nursing models and the nursing process. Basingstoke: Macmillan.

Alligood, M. R. (1997a). Models and theories: Critical thinking structures. In M. R. Alligood and A. Marriner-Tomey. Nursing Theory: Utilization & Application, St. Louis: C. V. Mosby, pp. 31–45.

Alligood, M. R. (1997b). Models and theories in nursing practice. In M. R. Alligood and A. Marriner-Tomey. Nursing Theory: Utilization & Application, St. Louis: C. V. Mosby, pp. 15–30.

Anderson, E. T., McFarlane, J. M., & Helton, A. (1986). Community as client: A model for practice. Nursing Outlook, 3(5), 220.

Beavers, W. R., & Voeller, M. N. (1983). Family models: Comparing and contrasting the Olson circumplex models with the Beaver's systems model. Family Process, 22, 85–98.

Benner, P., & Wrubel, J. (1989). The primacy of caring. Menlo Park, CA: Addison-Wesley.

Chinn, P. L. (1997). Why middle-range theory? ANS, 19(3), viii.

Christensen, P. J., & Kenney, J. W. (1996). Nursing process: Application of conceptual models, 4th ed. St. Louis: C.V. Mosby.

Cody, W. K. (1996). Drowning in eclecticism. Nursing Science Quarterly, 9(3), 86–88.

Cradock, S. (1996). The expert nurse: Clinical specialist or advanced practitioner? In Gary Rolfe (Ed.). Closing the theory-practice gap: A new paradigm for nursing. Oxford, UK: Butterworth-Heinemann Ltd.

Curran, D. (1985). Stress and the healthy family. Minneapolis, MN: Winston Press.

Duvall, E. M. (1997). Marriage and family development, 5th ed. Philadelphia: Lippincott.

Fawcett, J. (1995). Implementing conceptual models in nursing practice. In J. Fawcett (Ed.). Analysis and evaluation of conceptual models of nursing, 3rd ed. Philadelphia: F. A. Davis.

Fawcett, J. (1997). Conceptual models of nursing, nursing theories, and nursing practice: Focus on the future. In M. R. Alligood and A. Marriner-Tomey (Eds.). Nursing Theory: Utilization & Application. St. Louis: C. V. Mosby, pp. 211–221.

Fawcett, J., Archer, C. L., Becker, D., et al. (1992). Guidelines for selecting a conceptual model of nursing: Focus on the individual client. Dimen Critical Care Nursing, 11(5), 268–277.

Field, P. A. (1987). The impact of nursing theory on the clinical decision making process. Journal of Advanced Nursing, 12, 563–571.

Firlet, S. I. (1985). Nursing theory and nursing practice: Separate or linked? In J. McCloskey & H. K. Grace (Eds.). Current issues in nursing. Boston: Blackwell Scientific Publications, pp. 6–19.

Friedman, M. M. (1992). Family nursing: Theory and practice, 3rd ed. New York: Appleton & Lange.

Goeppinger, J., Lassiter, P. G., & Wilcox, B. (1982). Community health is community competence. Nursing Outlook, 30(8), 464.

Kenney, J. W. (1996). Relevance of theory-based nursing practice. In P. J. Christensen & J. W. Kenney (Eds.). Nursing Process: Application of Conceptual Models, 4th ed. St. Louis: C. V. Mosby, pp. 1–23.

Kim, H. S. (1994). Practice theories in nursing and a science of nursing practice. Scholarly Inquiry for Nursing Practice: An International Journal, 8(2), 145–158.

Loveland-Cherry, C. J. (1989). Family health promotion and health protection. In P. Bomar (Ed.). Nurses and family health promotion: Concepts, assessment, and interventions. Baltimore, MD. Williams & Wilkins.

Marks-Moran, D., & Rose, P. (Eds.). (1997). Reconstructing nursing: Beyond art and science. Philadelphia: Bailliere Tindall.

Mayberry, A. (1991). Merging nursing theories, models, and nursing practice: More than an administrative challenge. ANS, 15, 44.

McCubbin, M. A., & McCubbin, H. I. (1993). Families coping with illness: The resiliency model of family stress, adjustment and adaptation. In C. B. Danielson, B. Hamel-Bissell, & P. Winstead-Fry (Eds.). Families, health and illness: Perspectives on coping and intervention. St. Louis: Mosby, pp. 21–65.

McKay, R., & Segall, M. (1983). Methods and models for the aggregate. Nursing Outlook, 31(6), 328.

McKenna, H. (1997a). Choosing a theory for practice. In Hugh McKenna (Ed.). Nursing theories and models. New York: Rutledge, pp. 127–157.

McKenna, H. (1997b). Applying theories in practice. In Hugh McKenna (Ed.). Nursing theories and models. New York: Rutledge, pp. 158–189.

Meleis, A. I. (1993). Nursing research and the Neuman model: Directions for the future. Panel discussion conducted at the Fourth Biennial International Neuman Systems Model Symposium, Rochester, NY.

Meleis, A. I. (1997). Theoretical nursing: Development and progress, 3rd ed. Philadelphia: Lippincott.

Mezirow, J. (1979). Perspective transformation. Adult Education, 28(3), 100–110.

Mitchell, G. (1992). Specifying the knowledge base of theory in practice. Nursing Science Quarterly, 5(1), 6–7.

Moos, R. H., & Billings, A. G. (1982). Conceptualizing and measuring coping resources and processes. In L. Goldberger & S. Breznitz (Eds.). Handbook of stress. New York: Free Press.

Olson, D. H., Russell, C. S., & Sprenkle, D. H. (1983). Circumplex models of marital and family systems: VI. Theoretical update. Family Processes, 22, 69–83.

Paul, R. W., & Nosich, G. M. (1991). Proposal for the national assessment of higher-order thinking (revised version). The United States Department of Education Office of Educational Research and Improvement, National Center for Education Statistics.

Pender, N. J. (1987). Health promotion in nursing practice. New York: Doubleday.

Rogers, M. E. (1989). Creating a climate for the implementation of a nursing conceptual framework. Journal of Continuing Education in Nursing, 20(3), 112–116.

Shamansky, S. L., & Pesznecker, B. (1981). A community is. . . . Nursing Outlook, 29(3), 182–185.

Smith, M. C. (1994). Beyond the threshold: Nursing practice in the next millennium. Nursing Science Quarterly, 7(1), 6–7.

Sorrentino, E. A. (1991). Making theories work for you. Nursing Administration Quarterly, 15(3), 54–59.

Spiracino, P. (1991). The reciprocal relationship between practice and theory. Clinical Nurse Specialist, 5(3), 138.

Stevenson, J. (1977). Issues and crises during middlescence. New York: Appleton-Century-Crofts.

Timpson, J. (1996). Nursing theory: Everything the artist spits is art? Journal of Advanced Nursing, 23, 1030–1036.

Wright, L. M., & Leahey, M. (1994). Nurses and families: A guide to family assessment and intervention, 2nd ed. Philadelphia: F. A. Davis.

CHAPTER 29

What Will Count as Evidence in the Year 2050?

Francelyn M. Reeder, RN, PhD

In scientific discussions *what counts as evidence* is an eternal question that disserves attention whenever we face another era in pursuit of knowledge in any field. However, this is particularly important when integrated, complex systems are the focus of concern, involving human beings in the context of the environment, the world, and the universe. I propose that the answer for the year 2050 calls for a comparable kind of evidence, identifiable as *cosmic patterns of change in the life world*. Identifying which approach is fitting and adequate to pursue evidence of this kind, without breaking down the integral nature of the human–environment relationship, could be achieved through the process of *pattern recognition of change in life-world relationships*. I identify the kind of evidence to be pursued by addressing questions of what, why, when, how, and by whom.

What and Why Now?

Current realities taken to the global level carry a sense of urgency to ask new questions, suggesting a shifting of priorities. For example, Al Gore's (2006) explorations and concerns about global warming provide substantive issues that need answers about the effect of global warming on all forms of life on the planet and the atmosphere, given the suggestion that human beings play a large part in its formation by the way we live. In his book, *An Inconvenient Truth*, Gore's claims were substantiated with research on environment and cultural influences, suggesting that the way human beings make choices to live more and more by consumption of earth resources, such as fossil fuels, influences substantially the life world of the planet and universe, leaving an imbalance between human

Source: Reeder, F.M., Nursing Science Quarterly, Vol. 30, no. 3, pp. 208-211, copyright © 2007 by SAGE Publications. Reprinted by Permission of SAGE Publications.

and environmental fields. Concomitantly, an urgent call to seek ways to stabilize the climate has been made by environmentalist groups based on the research evidence from scientists in atmospheric and oceanic science (Deutch & Moniz, 2007; Pope, 2007). Coal is the economic fuel of choice for new electricity-generating power plants at today's fuel prices. Deutch and Moniz (2007) asked, so what is the problem? The environmental impact? The recognition that global warming is related to choices human beings make and the way we live our lives on earth and in the universe is a clarion call to moral responsibility to the planet and the universe. The evidence is building not only in popular awareness by environmentalists, but by serious scientists and moral leaders from all nations, and particularly from the economically most privileged populations.

Knowledge is not static but open-ended; insights take us forward to another *standpoint* and *viewpoint*. New vistas empower us to see more clearly; new standpoints give new grounds out of which to base knowledge rooted in contemporary reality to answer questions relevant to the times. Perspective is important in making the choice to pursue the question of what shall count as evidence in 2050. Where in the world and context does the question of evidence reside? Perspectives?

Philosopher of science, Karl Popper (Bartley, 1976; Popper, 1978) described three worlds in which we live: (1) the world of nature, (2) the world of human beings,

and (3) the constructed world made by human beings, that is, our cultures, religions, civilizations, architecture, museums, libraries, schools, cities, farms, ranches, technologies to save and use energy, and communities. All are designed to meet our social, cultural, technological, business, and educational needs as well as needs for health, relaxation, travel, and comfort. They use resources of the earth and the universe on a daily basis. Using the stuff of the earth and sky and accumulated bodies of knowledge will continue to require our best intellect, will, spirit, soul, and judgment to address the human story/ predicaments of our times.

It is important to dwell with the question, how will the nature of evidence be enlarged enough to grasp the current realities recognized in our thirst to know? Currently, the view of evidence receiving the greatest attention remains on what is known as *the prevailing view*. It focuses on isolated, five-sense perceptible things obtained through microscopic and macroscopic views of the physical world and universe. As recently as March 2007 this view of evidence has been the *gold standard* for scientific approaches, particularly to support or deny the value of allopathic medicine practices, while having less association with complementary and alternative medicine (CAM) practices. Calhoun (2007) raised the question, because most CAM practices are complex and focus on healing rather than curing, are evidence-based medicine principles sufficient for making clinical decisions about CAM?

Contributions from Human Sciences and from the Discipline of Nursing

A larger view of evidence circa 2050, supported by authors who grasp the nature of human beings in the environment and the universe, is necessary. Even so, human science disciplines that separate human productions and activities from the environment will still not provide an adequate source of evidence to answer our questions about life processes in the world and universe. It seems the evidence called for in 2050 is of the scope and integrity that reflects the relationships between inhabitants of the earth and heavens as a civilization, one that respects the life world and provides the basis for making choices as to how we shall live together.

Inquiry into the experience of human beings in the environment has been conducted from these two paradigms of science. From positivist science, inquiry is conducted from the third person point of view, through study of the microscopic and macroscopic, five-sense perceptible entities of the physical world isolated from the lived world context. This is comparable with the first world domain Popper (1978) identified as made up of earth and given material of the universe as the focus of interest in the prevailing view of evidence.

The phenomenological point of view, or integral view of evidence, described by phenomenologist Husserl (1948/1979), acknowledges the necessity of being in the world as the knower and knowing the world of nature, the world of living human experience, and the constructed, created world. All are necessary for knowledge of all things possible. The principle of intentionality contains Husserl's theory of knowledge recommended in this column to enlarge the notion of evidence adequate to the year 2050 and beyond.

Further, the integral world view accesses evidence through study of the life world from a first-person point of view. Most importantly, as known intentionally *by someone* in that world through a sensorium including not only five senses but also feelings, intuitions of the world in the present and of the past through memory (retention), and the future, through imagination and sense of the possible, all of which together is the foundation of knowing anything and everything at all. Groopman (2007) wrote about a current problem in medicine. Physicians, he reported, diagnose diseases based on what is called *pattern recognition*; to form patterns in our minds, we use shortcuts in thinking, so-called *heuristics*. Usually, a doctor generates one or two hypotheses about what is wrong within the first minutes of seeing the patient and listening to his or her story. Groopman (2007) stated that often, "we are correct in these rapid judgments, but too often we can be wrong. . . . Physicians are rarely taught about 'pitfalls in cognition'" (p. C3). "Often in today's world where there is intense pressure to see as many patients as possible, the quick judgment is often rewarded! Unfortunately, working in haste is a setup for errors in thinking" (Groopman, 2007, p. C1). *Anchoring* or attaching firmly to one possibility so tightly not considering other possibilities is called *premature closure*. Discounting discrepant or contradictory data is called *confirmation bias*. The mind cherry-picks the available information to confirm the anchored assumption, rather than revising the working diagnosis. Later, when a blood test reveals a serious problem, a misdiagnosis is sadly recognized as having been made (Groopman, 2007).

Now and in 2050 evidence that counts must consider the principle of intentionality (Reeder, 1984) that builds on Husserl's (1948/1979) phenomenological view of evidence from all modes of awareness and possible points of view for the basis of knowing anything at all. Pattern seeing recommended by nurse theorists of the unitary paradigm presents an alternative approach to evidence that is essential in this discussion. Cowling (2006) and Butcher (2005) took the discussion further toward pattern recognition and approaches to processing and building a basis for knowledge (for practice and life in general). This is consistent with Reeder's (1984) phenomenological integral world view in the development of comprehensive knowledge avoiding the pitfalls of premature closure before all evidence is in, considering all data available, before naming or closing the exploration.

Integral evidence necessary for 2050 as presented is congruent with the study of healing relationships or teaching relationships of sentient, thinking, feeling beings in the world. Further, first being in the world so that a presentation of the life world sustains the relationship between the knower and the known, where objects are not separated from the observer in an effort to examine them, but in relationship between the earth as walked upon and the *other* is related to and intentionally known. Thus, the knowledge gained from both the prevailing view and integral view on evidence with these methods of inquiry provide a different access and exploration of the world, the lived world, comprised of all three worlds of Popper (for example, the first world, or the given world of earth and sky; the second world, or that of human beings; and the third world, the constructed world). In the context of the lived world of 2050 it is expedient and necessary to consider why a more comprehensive view would require evidence that ultimately represents the life world as it unfolds and represents all inhabitants on the earth and in the universe, and why it is important to not accept views of evidence isolated out of site or forgetful of the whole life-world as adequate evidence for 2050.

Another question to be considered is who will provide possible directions in the decision as to what kind of evidence is large enough for the task of encompassing the human–environment relationship envisioned for 2050? The standpoint, or ground out of which we can think about future views of evidence, has roots within the discipline of nursing beginning with Florence Nightingale, with the promise of extending into the future, through the works of nurse theorists. This is specifically for nurse theorists whose works have focused on the mutual relationship of human beings and the environment and knowing participation in the world.

Rogers (1990), Newman (1997), Barrett (1990), and Parse (1995) addressed the relationship of human beings with the environment, with world views large enough to sustain knowledge development foundational to the discipline and practice of nursing. The work of Davidson and Ray (1991) on complexity science and the science of unitary human beings revealed patterns of knowing participation in the environment, illuminating the nature of choice, about how we can knowingly participate in change through a mutual process of human beings in the evolving world and universe. Barrett's development of the theory of power as knowing participation in change is central to this discussion and substantially suggests the moral relationship of humans as inhabitants on the earth and in the universe to the discussion of what shall count as evidence in 2050.

The disciplinary work of Watson (2003, 2005) on human caring science provides a view from international nurse scholars on the question of what counts as evidence in the sacred science of human caring. Her writings on Levinas' (1969) idea of belonging before we have our being have implications for how we should live in relation to all beings on the earth. In particular, it illuminates the moral relationship of humans with other inhabitants who share the earth and sky.

The concept of knowing participation in change by humans in mutual process with the environment (Barrett, 1990) is central to this chapter and is intentionally extended by this author to include all conscious beings who belong to this world sharing in the life world with all earthly creatures. Choice is truly manifest in their life patterns of migration, foraging, building shelters, expressing choices for survival, depending on the fruits of the earth and the air we breathe, and are considered contributors to the present discussion about what counts as evidence for 2050.

Davidson and Ray (1991) highlighted *choice* in the results of their dissertation investigating the science of unitary human beings to frame a study on the unitary relationship of humans in their environments as described by office workers, as they make choices to pattern their environment to enhance their performance, and also their sense of well-being in the workplace. Phenomenologists, beginning with the writings of Husserl (1948/1979), provided perspectives on knowing that require examining the world by first being in it so that a presentation of the life world sustains the relationship between the knower and the known. Objects are not separated or isolated from the natural environment, as in the circle depicted on the left, or from the observer in an effort to know them, but in the relationship between the earth as observed, as walked upon, not separated for inner and outer elements and processes or separated, but held as making up the resources of the environment. From the integral point of view, the life world of both human and the earth, or created world, can be understood. Life choices, if based on our knowledge of all three worlds of Popper's (1978) emphasis on earth and universe as given, human, and the created/constructed environmental world, can lead to choices for the future that will create a sustainable world for all inhabitants. Taking seriously the ability to knowingly participate in the environment and universe and attributing knowing participation to *all* inhabitants of the earth should be the basis for choice in the use of the environment for a viable future.

Also, if belonging before being is an enduring, persistent point of view, as proposed by Levinas (1969), and a reoccurring theme in human consciousness and now in theoretical writings, it is a truth to be included in viewpoints and standpoints about what shall count as evidence for the future survival, not only of the human race but also of all living beings. Then, belongingness of all creatures on earth and in the universe is an essential moral stance to be included in the kind of evidence that must count in the year 2050. All voices and life patterns of expression must be heard and counted!

References

Barrett, E. A. M. (1990). Health patterning with clients in a private practice environment. In E. A. M. Barrett (Ed.), *Visions of Rogers' science-based nursing* (pp. 105–115). New York: National League for Nursing.

Bartley, W. W. (1976). The philosophy of Karl Popper: Part 1. Biology and evolutionary epistemology. *Philosophia, 6,* 463–494.

Butcher, H. K. (2005). The unitary field pattern portrait research method: Facets, processes, and findings. *Nursing Science Quarterly, 18,* 293–300.

Calhoun, C. (2007). Are EBM principles sufficient for making clinical decisions about CAM? *Integrative Cancer Therapies, 6,* 217–218.

Cowling, W. R. (2006). A unitary healing praxis model for women in despair. *Nursing Science Quarterly, 19,* 123–132.

Davidson, A. W., & Ray, M. A. (1991). Synthesis in nursing knowledge: An analysis of two approaches. *Journal of Advanced Nursing, 21,* 870–974.

Deutch, J., & Moniz, E. (2007, March 15). The future of fossil fuel. *The Wall Street Journal,* p. A17.

Gore, A. (2006). *An inconvenient truth.* Emmas, PA: Rodale.

Groopman, J. (2007, March 19). Cognitive pitfalls too often lead to mistaken diagnosis. *The Boston Globe,* pp. C1–C3.

Husserl, E. (1979). *Experience and judgment* (L. Landgrebe, Ed.; J. S. Churchill & K. Ameriks, Trans.). Evanston, IL: Northwestern University. [Original work published 1948.]

Levinas, E. (1969). *Totality and infinity.* Pittsburgh, PA: Duquesne.

Newman, M. (1997). Evolution of the theory of health as expanding consciousness. *Nursing Science Quarterly, 10,* 22–25.

Parse, R. R. (Ed.). (1995). *Illuminations: The human becoming theory in practice and research.* New York: National League for Nursing.

Pope, C. (2007). Ways and means—Prevent, prepare, repair. *The Sierra Magazine, 92*(2), 6.

Popper, K. (1978, April). The Tanner lectures on human values: Three worlds. Paper presented at the University of Michigan, Ann Arbor, MI.

Reeder, F. (1984). Philosophical issues in the Rogerian science of unitary human beings. *Advances in Nursing Science, 6*(2), 14–23.

Rogers, M. E. (1990). Nursing science of unitary, irreducible human beings: Update 1990. In E. A. M. Barrett (Ed.), *Visions of Rogers' science-based nursing* (pp. 5–11). New York: National League for Nursing.

Watson, J. (2003). Caring science: Ethics of face and hand—an invitation to return to the heart and soul of nursing and our deep humanity. *Nursing Administration Quarterly, 27,* 197–202.

Watson, J. (2005). Love and caring: Belonging before being as ethical cosmology. *Nursing Science Quarterly, 18,* 304–305.

CHAPTER 30

An Ontological View of Advanced Practice Nursing

Cynthia Arslanian-Engoren, RN, PhD

Frank D. Hicks, RN, PhD

Ann L. Whall, RN, PhD, FAAN, FGSA

Donna L. Algase, RN, PhD, FAAN, FGSA

Identifying, developing, and incorporating nursing's unique ontological and epistemological perspective into advanced practice nursing practice places priority on delivering care based on research-derived knowledge. Without a clear distinction of our meta-theoretical space, we risk blindly adopting the practice values of other disciplines, which may not necessarily reflect those of nursing. A lack of focus may lead current advanced practice nursing curricula and emerging doctorate of nursing practice programs to mirror the logical positivist paradigm and perspective of medicine. This chapter presents an ontological perspective for advanced practice nursing education, practice, and research.

Key words: *advanced practice nursing, epistemology, graduate nursing education, nursing knowledge, ontology.*

The profession and discipline of nursing has struggled for decades to define and refine its disciplinary focus and unique contributions to health care. Although multiple theoretical perspectives exist to assist in guiding practitioners and scientists in their respective work, we continue to be hindered in fostering a unifying framework that is helpful to all of nursing's varied practitioners. Across the globe nurses are pursuing advanced education to keep up with the demands of an ever-expanding knowledge base and the omnipresent need for effective healthcare services. Graduate nursing education has been prevalent in the United States for more than 50 years. Yet, trends in nursing education in the United States may not necessarily be headed toward an advancement of nursing knowledge or nursing practice if these programs are based on a medical model that has as its main goal the transmission of medical knowledge. With the multiplicity of

Source: Used with permission of Springer Publishing Company, from Research and Theory for Nursing Practice, Volume 19, Number 4, 2005 , pp. 315-322(8)

educational entrees to nursing at the graduate level, it is more crucial than ever to define the unique perspective of nursing and its relation to health care. The purpose of this chapter is therefore to explicate an ontological view of nursing that may be helpful to advanced practice nurses (APNs) and nurse scientists. Advances in developing nursing knowledge are synthesized into a coherent framework, and suggestions presented for nurses to incorporate into clinical practice.

Case for a Disciplinary Focus

Identifying, developing, and incorporating nursing's unique ontological and epistemological perspective into APN practice places priority on delivering care based on knowledge derived from the disciplinary perspective of nursing. Moreover, practicing from a strong nursing perspective that is theoretically grounded and steeped in specialized knowledge assists our efforts to gain recognition and respect as a profession and an academic discipline. Without such grounding the very future of the profession and discipline is at stake. It is imperative that APNs be able to delineate their unique contribution and perspective to healthcare delivery. For without a clear distinction of our meta-theoretical space, we risk blindly adopting the practices, views, and values of other disciplines (Whall, 2005), which may not necessarily reflect those of nursing. A lack of disciplinary focus may lead current APN curricula and emerging doctor of nursing practice (DNP) programs in the United States

to mirror the logical positivist, reductionistic paradigm and perspective of medicine.

Equally disturbing are national certifications that may embrace a medical focus, thus neglecting the nursing focus that should be inherent in APN programs. The question that must then be asked is as follows: Does the current system of educating APNs mirror the focus of medicine (i.e., laboratory data interpretation, medication management, and medical diagnoses) or nursing? A review of such educational content should include an emphasis on nursing diagnoses, questions that address the meta-paradigm of nursing, and inquiries that address holistic, patient-centered care. If national examinations for advanced practice nursing are limited in scope to medical phenomena of interest, these examinations will not reflect the essence or values of nursing. Failing to differentiate the practice of APNs compared with physicians and physician assistant colleagues further blurs the essential nursing core of disciplinary knowledge that should be inherent in any advanced nursing degree program. Although diagnostic reasoning processes are essential to all healthcare professions, the questions, data, and clinical labels applied in these processes are specific to each profession and reflect knowledge generated through related research in the discipline.

Advanced Practice Nurses and Knowledge Development

By virtue of their education and experience and the emphasis on holistic care and health promotion, APNs are in a prime position to provide affordable, expert, and efficient health care to diverse populations. Moreover, as clinical experts, APNs have a unique and significant part to play in advancing the development of nursing knowledge. Often believed to be the sole responsibility of academicians, clinical practice in essence is *the field* for knowledge development, because it is in the practice arena that nursing's phenomena of interest are encountered. Indeed, there is a largely untapped source of nursing knowledge embedded within nurses' daily practice (Benner, 1984; Benner, Tanner, & Chesla, 1996). By virtue of their exposure and participation in clinical nursing, APNs are in a prime position to add to and shape the body of nursing knowledge from a nursing perspective.

Knowledge development from a unique nursing perspective defines the boundaries of nursing and delineates the nature and application of nursing knowledge that explicates nurses' unique contribution to the healthcare team. Without this, nurses merely interpret what other disciplines have come to know. Without a unique and clearly articulated body of knowledge, nursing will never truly achieve the independence and stature of a profession. Thus, nursing practice will depend on others to legitimate and guide it.

If knowledge is power, then nursing knowledge is the power base of the profession and its development is the responsibility of both practicing and academic nurses. Many nurses are daunted by the prospect of developing knowledge and often feel ill-prepared to assume this charge and actualize

this process. Such feelings are understandable if one considers there may be a lack of attention paid to nursing knowledge and its development in today's APN nursing education programs. Given the emphasis on medical care and the medical approach taken in many graduate nursing curricula, it may be unlikely that the nursing knowledge embedded in clinical practice can ever be realized by today's APN.

Developing a World View: Philosophy, Science, and Nursing Science

A philosophy of science is the umbrella under which all science emerges. Its importance is especially noted in the formation of a world view that influences the work of scientists and, ultimately, nursing clinicians. A world view seeks to answer two types of philosophical questions fundamental to knowledge development. The first, the ontological question, seeks to answer the nature of phenomena (i.e., What is this thing?). The second, the epistemological question, seeks to answer how the phenomena are known (i.e., How do we come to understand this thing?). As a means of looking at the world and interpreting its experiences, a world view contains both explicit and implicit assumptions, beliefs, and values about the world and how one goes about gaining an understanding of it. Moreover, a world view identifies phenomena worthy of attention and investigation, ultimately affecting the focus of nursing practice, education, and research (Whall & Hicks, 2002).

Nursing philosophers and scientists who have articulated their ontological and epistemological views include Rogers (1970, 1990), Parse (1981, 1998), and Watson (1985, 1995). Each has a unique way of viewing the world and nursing's place in it. These views have had a significant influence on the way nurses investigate phenomena and practice their profession and have even influenced the ways in which some nurses have been educated. Over the last 50 years common themes have emerged that form the basis of nursing's disciplinary identity. These themes, sometimes known as the "meta-paradigm," common to all nursing theory, and extremely important in today's education, include person, environment, health, and nursing. The way these themes are explicated, however, varies greatly among theorists. For example, Neuman (2002), Parse (1981, 1998), and Rogers (1990) view humans as unitary beings that cannot be divided into parts, whereas Roy (1995) and Orem (1991) view them as holistic beings comprised of several facets of human experience (e.g., psychosocial, physiological). For Rogers (1970, 1990) the environment and person are in constant mutuality, whereas Nightingale (1860/1969) viewed the person and environment as separate entities that influence one another. Health is sometimes viewed as an objectified phenomenon by some theorists, whereas Rogers (1990) viewed health as a culturally defined and socially enforced concept, and Neuman (2002) conceptualized it as a state of consciousness. Although individual theorists have added or interpreted concepts from

their world view (King, 1971, 1995; Orem, 1991; Roy, 1995; Watson, 1985, 1995), their resulting theories and frameworks clearly reflect nursing's historic meta-paradigm concepts and our holistic view. Therefore, it is especially important that existing APN programs and emerging DNP programs align themselves with the historic paradigmatic approach of nursing to deliver theory-based, culturally relevant, holistic care. To ignore nursing's scholarship is to deprive an emerging generation of practitioners and scientists of nursing's foundational knowledge and to impair the further building of knowledge that is so crucial to professional discipline and its related science.

Diversity in ontological approaches, although positive and exemplary of our scholarship, has led to divisions among nurse scientists and clinicians, resulting in a multiplicity of perspectives within the discipline that further confuse nursing's purpose and place in the world. A common complaint among graduate nursing students is that these multiple views make it impossible to understand and articulate the common nature of nursing. There is, however, an ontological perspective that synthesizes and unites these various views.

A New View: Nursing Processes

According to Reed (1997), the nature and substance of nursing derives from the fact that *nursing is* the substantive perspective of our discipline. That is, nursing is concerned with the human processes of well-being that are inherent among all human systems, whether individual, family, or community. However, that is not to dismiss the existence of sickness or pathology. Rather, we integrate knowledge of pathology into a view of and interaction with the person who, as a whole, is striving for well-being. On the other hand, medicine often tends to *disease-ify* normal health processes, such as birth or sleep. Nurses strive to help people to *health-ify* themselves, including overcoming disease or adapting to or integrating the limits imposed by irreversible pathologies.

Nursing processes emanate from persons, groups, and communities and are by their nature relational, contextual, and transformative. These processes are known by the intersection of complexity, integration, and well-being and are manifested by changes in complexity and integration that generate well-being. Our quest as nurses is to "understand the nature of and to facilitate nursing processes in diverse contexts of health experiences" (Reed, 1997, p. 77).

Within this ontological perspective individuals are open, living systems, intrinsically active, innovative, and capable of self-organizing. Self refers to the entire system, generating qualitative change out of ongoing events of life processes and the context (environment) in which they are situated. Complexity occurs when human systems experience or express variables (e.g., life events, physiological events) as parts, separated from the whole, rather than as patterns of the whole. Complexity provides diversity, specialization, and depth of experiences. Increasing complexity brings quantitative, not qualitative, change. Integration is the

system's ability to synthesize and organize experiences or phenomena that results in a change in form and depends on a certain level of complexity. Integration is transformative and involves qualitative change, providing organization, coherence, and breadth.

Well-being arises out of the intersection of complexity and integration, which are rhythmical in creating change. According to Reed (1997), well-being occurs when the particulars of a life experience are brought together and synthesized in a coherent way. Without this synthesis people feel *dis*-integrated, *dis*-associated, and *dis*-organized, in other words, *dis*-eased. Promoting well-being through a perspective of inherent processes of complexity and integration is distinctly nursing. If nursing is viewed as inherent human–environment processes that lead to well-being vis-à-vis complexity and integration, then it follows that the focus of nursing science should be on understanding those processes, whereas nursing practice assists those processes. Thus, instead of seeing nursing as something exterior to the patient/client/system, nursing is viewed as intrinsically inherent to the patient/client/system, something to be developed and nurtured in human systems. Within this ontological view the approach to understanding nursing processes is achieved with sensitivity to the contextual and holistic nature of the human system. Thus, nurses need to strive to understand and teach the complexities involved in human life processes as they influence and are influenced by well-being. The unique role of the nurse, then, becomes one that assists the human system in integrating the dynamic complexities that evolve from human–environment interactions and is thusly important in clinical practice.

Reed's (1997) view of nursing not only provides a unique perspective, but it also raises interesting philosophical and scientific questions, and presents a novel approach to nursing practice. The exciting ideas contained within this ontology hold promise for unifying and articulating the age-old questions of what is nursing and what do nurses do?

Application to Advanced Practice Nursing

Nursing's philosophic views and beliefs have led to a unique perspective that distinguishes APNs from other healthcare providers. The importance of this understanding cannot be underestimated. Grounding practice within this perspective, nurses will find it easy to understand their own contribution to health care as well as to articulate this to other members of an interdisciplinary team. A lack of understanding of the essence of nursing will threaten the existence of nursing as is now known and understood by society. The social contract between nursing and the public will be jeopardized, and it will be difficult to ascertain the role of nurses as compared with other healthcare providers. Nursing has a service to offer that has been historically understood by society. Not recognizing this unique nursing perspective and philosophic view will jeopardize nursing existence. This perspective should underpin APN education, practice, and research.

APN Education

As specialty curricula are developed and implemented for the education of APNs and nurses with DNP degrees, ontological and epistemological perspectives necessary to actualize these roles must be carefully considered. Although not negating the importance of natural, biological, organizational, and social science knowledge (e.g., pathophysiology, statistics, and psychology) commonly found within APN curricula, these alone do not provide the student with the advanced skills and knowledge necessary to deliver high-quality, advanced practice nursing. Indeed, many theoretical foundations shared with the medical discipline are used to prepare expert clinical practitioners. However, what distinguishes APNs from medical healthcare providers is the unique contribution of nursing's ways of knowing and holistic approach to the delivery of patient care. The clinical care provided by APNs focuses on the whole of a person's health and illness experiences (American Association of Colleges of Nursing, 1996). APN education, therefore, must focus on educating nurses to understand the essential nursing processes inherent in the human conditions and teach students to analyze the relationship of complexity, integration, and well-being. The mission of advanced practice nursing, "to provide expert, quality, and comprehensive nursing care to clients" (American Nurses Association, 1996, p. 1), must be grounded in the ontological and epistemological perspectives of the nursing discipline and reflected in professional competencies unique to nursing's pattern of knowing (Vinson, 2000).

APN Practice

The clinical practice of APNs must actualize the values and beliefs inherent within the discipline of nursing. Therefore, it is imperative that APNs who address the healthcare needs of patients do so from an advanced nursing perspective. APNs must not limit the focus of their care to just the differential medical diagnoses and prescribed pharmacological therapy. Instead, APNs must be mindful to include the integration of the family, the environment, and the human response to health and illness in the provision of health care, because this is what sets APNs apart from other healthcare professionals.

APNs must begin to reconceptualize their practice and endeavor to examine the multiplicity of patterns that evolve from the intersection of complexity, integration, and well-being. As such, the discernment of human health patterns may be able to capitalize on the existing nursing diagnosis taxonomy. Delineating and incorporating relevant nursing diagnoses into the plan of care illuminates the nursing component of APN practice. Firmly rooted in the epistemological and ontological values of the discipline, nursing diagnoses represent the essence of nursing—its focus, function, and future at an advanced practice level.

APN Research

Another available means to accentuate the nursing perspective within APN practice is through the utilization and generation of nursing research. Conceptual and philosophical consistency is obtained when scientists work under an overarching ontological world view. If nurse scientists and APNs both operated from this ontological world view, incorporating empirical knowledge with diverse ways of knowing, it would facilitate a richer and more holistic approach to patient care. Moreover, the application of nursing research to APN clinical practice anchors the delivery of care within a nursing perspective and communicates the value and importance of nursing investigations to clients, families, communities, and other healthcare professionals. The generation of nursing knowledge through scientific research advances the science of nursing from which APNs practice.

Conclusion

As the discipline of nursing continues to develop, the direction will be set by the philosophy and theories selected and the values espoused. To truly practice professional nursing at an advanced practice level requires a vast repertoire of skills coupled with a mastery of conceptual, empirical, and clinical knowledge of nursing. Embracing a paradigmatic perspective that unifies the values of the discipline of nursing will advance the profession, direct clinical practice, and enhance our understanding. Ignoring the complexity of nursing phenomena will lead to an incomplete nursing science (Whall & Hicks, 2002) that fails to serve its members or the public's healthcare needs.

References

American Association of Colleges of Nursing. (1996). *The essentials of master's education for advanced practice nursing.* Washington, DC: Author.

American Nurses Association. (1996). *Scope and standards of advanced practice registered nursing.* Washington, DC: Author.

Benner, P. A. (1984). *From novice to expert: Excellence and power in clinical nursing practice.* Menlo Park, CA: Addison-Wesley.

Benner, P. A., Tanner, C. A., & Chesla, C. A. (1996). *Expertise in nursing practice: Caring, clinical judgment and ethics.* New York: Springer Publishing Company.

King, I. M. (1971). *Toward a theory for nursing.* New York: Wiley.

King, I. M. (1995). The theory of goal attainment. In M. A. Frey & C. L. Seiloff (Eds.), *Advancing King's systems framework and theory of nursing* (pp. 23–33). Thousand Oaks, CA: Sage.

Neuman, B. (2002). *The Neuman systems model* (4th ed.). Upper Saddle River, NJ: Prentice Hall.

Nightingale, F. (1969). *Notes on nursing: What it is and what it is not.* New York: Dover Publications. [Original work published 1860.]

Orem, D. E. (1991). *Nursing: Concepts of practice* (4th ed.). St. Louis, MO: Mosby Year Book.

Parse, R. R. (1981). *Man-living-health: A theory of nursing.* New York: Wiley.

Parse, R. R. (1998). *The human becoming school of thought: A perspective for nurses and other health professionals.* Thousand Oaks, CA: Sage.

Reed, P. G. (1997). Nursing: The ontology of the discipline. *Nursing Science Quarterly,* *10*(2), 76–79.

Rogers, M. E. (1970). *An introduction to the theoretical basis of nursing.* Philadelphia: F. A. Davis.

Rogers, M. E. (1990). Nursing: Science of unitary, irreducible human beings. Update 1990. In E. A. M. Barrett (Ed.), *Visions of Rogers' science-based nursing* (pp. 5–11). New York: National League for Nursing.

Roy, C. L. (1995). Developing nursing knowledge: Practice issues raised from four philosophical perspectives. *Nursing Science Quarterly,* *8*(2), 79–85.

Vinson, J. A. (2000). Nursing's epistemology revisited in relation to professional educational competencies. *Journal of Professional Nursing,* *16*(1), 39–46.

Watson, J. (1985). *Nursing: Human science and human care.* Norwalk, CT: Appleton-Century-Crofts.

Watson, J. (1995). Postmodernism and knowledge development in nursing. *Nursing Science Quarterly,* *8*(2), 60–64.

Whall, A. L. (2005). "Lest we forget": An issue concerning the doctorate in nursing practice (DNP). *Nursing Outlook,* *53*, 1.

Whall, A., & Hicks, F. D. (2002). The unrecognized paradigm shift within nursing: Implications, problems, and possibilities. *Nursing Outlook,* *50,* 72–76.

CHAPTER 31

The Nurse Scholar of the 21st Century

Sandra Schimdt Bunkers, RN, PhD, FAAN

The professional nurse of the 21st century is called to be a nurse scholar. Webster's Ninth New Collegiate Dictionary (1990) defines scholar as '1. One who attends school or studies under a teacher; 2. a: one who has done advanced study in a special field; b: a learned person' (p. 1051). The professional nurse of the 21st century must be learned, must be mentored by wise and knowledgeable teachers, and must have the academic foundation for advancing the scholarship of service to humankind.

Nursing: A Call to Scholarship

Professional nursing today is a call to scholarship. Suggesting that the 21st century nurse be a nurse scholar implies that the discipline has a unique knowledge base from which one can draw on in the service of humankind. Nursing's history denotes a productive evolutionary journey of such knowledge development. Nursing began as a human service called into being by society. The knowledge base of our discipline was built as nurses, beginning with Florence Nightingale, carefully collected data on how to solve human health problems. Nurse scholar Marilyn Rawnsley (1999) points this out in writing the following:

It is the profession of nursing legitimized as a responsive human service that engendered the science of nursing. Nursing research, perhaps beginning with Nightingale's systematic data collection, was launched to solve problems encountered in practice. Nursing science as a legitimate academic endeavor, with theories aimed at understanding and explaining phenomena central to the discipline, evolved almost a century later. (p. 316)

It is true that nursing science has evolved. We are now at the point as a scientific discipline of having developed nursing theories encompassing more that one paradigm (or world-view to guide nurses in understanding the human health process). Nurse theorist Rosemarie Rizzo Parse identifies two competing worldviews in nursing, which she names the totality paradigm and the simultaneity paradigm. Parse (1996b) writes

> The discipline of nursing encompasses the knowledge in the extant frameworks and theories that are embedded in the totality and simultaneity paradigms. These theories and frameworks explicate the nature of nursing's major phenomenon of concern, the human–universe– health process. (p. 275)

Nurse scholars of the 21st century must be accountable for understanding these nursing theories and conceptual frameworks and utilizing them in guiding practice, research, education, and regulation. It is our challenge as nurse leaders today to merge the professional practice science (the problem solving for human health issues)

and the academic science (the creation of theories and conceptual frameworks) of our discipline. This merging of professional science and academic science is brought about in the formation of nursing theory–based education, practice, and regulation models. Examples of such models include The Health Action Model for Partnership in Community (Bunkers, Nelson, Leuning, Crane, & Josephson, 1999), an education-practice model originating in the Department of Nursing at Augustana College in Sioux Falls, South Dakota; a human becoming nursing theory-based parish nursing model created at First Presbyterian Church in Sioux Falls (Bunkers & Putnam, 1995); the nursing theory-based South Dakota Board of Nursing Regulatory Decisioning Model (Damgaard & Bunkers, 1998); and a model for teaching-learning based on the theory of human becoming (Bunkers, 1999b). These models are prototypes for nursing, providing a blueprint for creating nursing theory-guided practice, education, research, and regulation.

The demand to educate responsive, ethical, and intelligent knowledge-guided nurses has been echoed through time. Constance Schuyler (1992) writes in a commentary on Florence Nightingale the following:

> Nightingale believed that nursing education should develop both the intellect and the character of the nurse. Accordingly, she gave her students a solid background in the sciences to enable them to understand the theory behind their care. To develop character, she

assigned readings in the humanities to increase their understanding of human ethics and morals. She believed that nurses should never stop learning. She wrote to her student, 'To nurse is a field of which one may safely say: there is no end in what we may be learning every day.' (p. 11)

Nightingale was known to be brilliant. However, intellectual pursuits were not enough. She had a drive for action and this coupled with her brilliance spurred her on 'to be one of the greatest reformers of the 19th century' (Schuyler, 1992, p. 16). In addressing human suffering, Nightingale writes in 1859:

> No mockery in the world is so hollow as the advice showered upon the sick. It is of no use for the sick to say anything, for what the adviser wants is, not to know the truth about the state of the patient, but to turn whatever the sick may say to the support of his own argument, set forth, it must be repeated, without any inquiry whatever into the patient's real condition. . . . How little the real sufferings of illness are known or understood. (p. 57)

The scene is now around 1992. Nurse theorist Martha Rogers (1992) writes concerning the development of nursing knowledge:

> Over-emphasis on technology tends to over-shadow therapeutic modalities that can have real significance. Nurses must recognize that they do not create change in people, rather they participate in the process of change to the extent that they bring knowledge to the situation and recognize that the healing process has the potential for healing beyond that which we tend to recognize today. The answer to health will not be found in more drugs, more technology, or more hospitals. (p. 61)

In 1992, nurse theorist Callista Roy (1992) writes addressing her focus for nursing:

> I can amass in a week more evidence of human pain and suffering than Nightingale perceived in her lifetime. . . . Nightingale would be sure to respond in her characteristic way, noting that she need not wait until she fully understood the phenomena, nor definitively prove that a given approach could relieve such suffering, but rather she would use everything at her disposal, and all that she could garner from others, to relieve such suffering and find ways to prevent it. She would organize and teach nurses to work with people around the world to create life-giving environments, to free human bodies and spirits from all that hinders full life potential. (p. 69)

The date is 1997. Discussing the evolution of nursing science and in particular the human becoming theory's focus on quality of life from the person's perspective, nurse theorist Rosemarie Rizzo Parse (1997a) writes

> The journey of the evolution of the human becoming theory has not been simply an easy movement from one port to another, but, like all journeys, it has been an ebb and flow of intense and quiet moments, pleasures and challenges all at once. The journey is one of forging new paths for the discipline of nursing and other health-related disciplines and living with opportunities that arise when daring to question the prevailing paradigm. The author is open to the new, the mysteries of the yet-to-be discovered possibles in the quest for preserving the uniqueness of nursing in its contributions to the quality of life for humankind. (p. 36)

These nurse theorists are among many that are actively engaged in the continual scientific endeavor of knowledge development for the discipline of nursing. However, nursing needs to frame this nursing knowledge within an umbrella of values and beliefs.

Framing Nursing Knowledge

The knowledge base of nursing science, with an emphasis on the betterment of humankind, is composed of ideas concerning the person, health, the environment, the universe, and the focus of nursing. 'The core substance of nursing, like all other disciplines, resides in its theories and frameworks, historically created and developed by nurses' (Parse, 1995, p. 51). Along with this unique nursing knowledge, the discipline draws on the natural sciences, human sciences, arts, and humanities to understand phenomena. Although specific knowledge in these areas needs to be known so as to be a competent practitioner of nursing knowledge content changes. Knowledge is in a variety of settings, as time and society evolves, constantly being created and is an interchange between the knower and the known (Palmer, 1993).

Parker Palmer in To Know as We Are Known (1993) suggests three sources of knowledge:

> History suggests two primary sources for our knowledge. . . . One is curiosity; the other is control. The one corresponds to pure, speculative knowledge, to knowledge as an end in itself. The other corresponds to applied science, to knowledge as a means to practical ends. (p. 7)

Palmer (1993) goes on to identify one other source of knowledge: 'This is a knowledge that originates not in curiosity or control but in compassion, or love—a source celebrated not in our intellectual tradition but in our spiritual heritage' (p. 8). He suggests that the goal of knowledge arising from love 'is the reunification and reconstruction of broken selves and worlds' (p. 8).

All three sources of knowledge identified by Palmer are relevant to nurse scholars. All three sources of knowledge are sources of truth. Palmer (1993) suggests that truth is personal and truth is communal: it exists in relationship. He writes

> Truth is neither 'out there' nor 'in here,' but both. Truth is between us, in relationship, to be found in the dialogue of knowers and knowns who are understood as independent but accountable selves. (p. 56)

As independent and accountable selves, nurses must identify foundational values or tenets to guide the teaching–learning processes that will engage nursing's quest for truth in the 21st century. And, teaching-learning in the discipline is the responsibility of all nurse leaders.

Foundational Tenets in Guiding the Framing of Nursing Knowledge

In educating nurse scholars, this author suggests 16 foundational tenets that can frame nursing curriculum and guide nursing education, practice, and research in the 21st century. These 16 tenets need to be grounded in the theories and conceptual frameworks of nursing (see **Table 31-1**).

Honoring Human Freedom and Choice

The nurse scholar of the 21st century must seek to understand the interconnection between health and human freedom. This tenet implies that the nurse be a student of philosophy as well as a student of science. Jean-Paul Sartre (1956) writes in Being and Nothingness, 'Human freedom precedes

essence in man and makes it possible; the essence of the human being is suspended in her/his freedom. What we call freedom is impossible to distinguish from the being of human reality' (p. 60). Sartre's existential position is that humans are free to choose in situations. Parse's (1998) theory of human becoming posits that humans are open beings, freely choosing meaning in situations and bearing responsibility for these choices. 'The human is responsible for all outcomes of reflective–prereflective choices, even though many are unknown when making decisions' (Parse, 1998, p. 21). Nurse scholars must acknowledge and understand the role human freedom and choice play in persons cocreating patterns of health.

Cultivating an Attitude of Openness to Uncertainty and Difference

Nurse scholars need to cultivate an attitude of openness, openness to new ideas, changes in worldviews and to the unexpected. Jacob Bronowski in his book The Origins of Knowledge and Imagination (1978) writes

> Science is essentially a self-correcting activity. But more important, scientists are people who correct the picture of the moment with another one, as a natural evolution towards a 'true' picture of the world. We have spoken enough about truth to know that we are not going to get a final picture of the world. Nobody is going to find the truth one fine day, as I say, like a hat or an umbrella. . . . The creative personality is always one that looks on the world as fit for

---

Table 31-1   Tenets for Framing Nursing Knowledge

---

1. Honoring human freedom and choice

2. Cultivating an attitude of openness to uncertainty and difference

3. Appreciating the meaning of lived experiences of health

4. Understanding the nature of suffering

5. Committing to social justice

6. Believing in the imagination as a source of knowledge

7. Recognizing the significance of language in structuring mean and reality

8. Understanding health as a process

9. Understanding community as a process

10. Believing in the power of personal presence

11. Participating in scientific inquiry

12. Asserting the ethics of individual and communal responsibility

13. Emphasizing living in the present moment

14. Respecting life and nature

15. Acknowledging mystery

16. Focusing on quality of life

---

change and on herself/himself as an instrument for change. Otherwise, what are you creating for? If the world is perfectly all right the way it is, you have no place in it. The creative personality thinks of the world as a canvas for change and of herself/himself as a divine agent of change. (pp. 122–123)

Parse (1998) suggests that 'the human aspires and reaches beyond to that which is not-yet' (p. 46). The nurse scholar of the 21st century must look at differing views and differing lifestyles as an invitation to discover opportunities for new knowledge and creative growth for the self and the larger community. With such an attitude of openness to uncertainty and difference, unique possibilities will emerge in health care for the betterment of humankind.

Appreciating the Meaning of Lived Experiences of Health

Victor Frankl in his classic work Man's Search for Meaning (1984) suggests that the essence of human existence is to find meaning in life. This meaning of life 'always changes but never ceases to be' (Frankl, 1984, p. 115). According to Frankl, we can discover meaning in life 'in three different ways: (1) by creating a work or doing a deed; (2) by experiencing something or encountering someone; and (3) by the attitude we take toward unavoidable suffering' (p. 117). Nurse theorist Rosemarie Parse's human becoming theory and practice and research methodologies focus on understanding the meaning of lived experiences of health. 'Each human's reality is the meaning of the situation' (Parse, 1996b, p. 56).

For the nurse scholar of the 21st century, understanding the meaning the individual or community gives to their health experiences will make it possible for the nurse to work with others' reality. 'Understanding the meaning of the lived experience of another is the essence of coming to know another and valuing the other as a unique human being' (Bunkers, 1998, p. 62). Understanding is the basis for reflective, knowledgeable action.

Understanding the Nature of Suffering

Suffering, in most health literature, is connected with loss, pain, disfigurement, defeat, or harmful events (Daly, 1995). Philosopher Thich Nhat Hanh (1998) identifies suffering in such 'problems of the world like hunger, war, oppression, and social injustice' (p. 31). Hanh also connects suffering with lack of communication or using words that are untruthful or words of hatred or division. Perhaps the most important understanding of suffering is that suffering is unique to each

person. Mitchell (1991) views suffering 'as a lived experience which is multidimensional and which can be understood only from the perspective of the individual living it' (p. 101). Newman (1994a) suggests that 'suffering offers us the opportunity to transcend a particular situation' (p. 142). She suggests, 'The need is to let go, embrace our experience, and allow the expansion of consciousness to unfold' (Newman, 1994a, p. 142). Parse (1996a) suggests concerning suffering that 'joy–sorrow is a paradoxical rhythm lived by all human beings' (p. 80). In a study on joy–sorrow, Parse (1997b) found that participants talked about adversities, but also there were 'always pleasures, either remembered or in the immediate moment' (p. 85).

The nurse scholar of the 21st century must attend carefully to others' suffering and be aware of the meaning of the joy–sorrow rhythm in people's lives. By bearing witness to suffering and being with others in moments of joy and moments of pain and sorrow, the nurse will discover new ways of providing comfort and quality of life.

Committing to Social Justice

The commitment to social justice runs throughout the history of knowledge development in nursing. Starting with Florence Nightingale, considered one of the leading reformers of the 19th century, this history includes Margaret Sanger, Lillian Wald, and Livina Dock (Chinn, 1991). Margaret Sanger developed knowledge of birth control and fought against great resistance to distribute birth control to women desperate for it. Her attempts to develop support for family planning remains with us today in the development of theoretical constructs informing women's health. Lillian Wald was concerned for the extremely poor immigrants crowded in housing in New York City. She developed the House on Henry Street from which emerged concepts of community health nursing. Livina Dock, who was an active organizer in the House on Henry Street, worked for over 20 years to give women the right to vote (Chinn, 1991). Newman (1994b) suggests, 'It is necessary to connect all parts of the system, to integrate the similar and the dissimilar, unleashing the power of creativity' (p. 45). Such creative activity involves the human becoming concept of originating (Parse, 1998), which 'is inventing new ways of conforming—not conforming in the certainty–uncertainty of living' (p. 49).

The nurse scholar of the 21st century must be aware of the social and political forces of uncertainty influencing healthcare and quality of life. The nurse scholar must develop the ability to work with individuals, families, governmental systems and countries, not conforming to what has been but, instead, creating new ways for addressing human health challenges.

Believing in the Imagination as a Source of Knowledge

To imagine is to think of what can be. It is the process of imagining that generates new ideas and new ways of being in the world. Goleman, Kaufman, and Ray in The Creative Spirit (1992) suggest creativity is akin to leadership: 'A successful leader is someone who can persuade people to change their ideas or behavior. A successful creator is someone who gives other people a different way of looking at a world' (p. 26). These authors go on to suggest the art of creativity involves the capability to sift important information, selectively combine relevant information, and draw comparisons and analogies. 'The ability to see things in a fresh way is vital to the creative process, and that ability rests on the willingness to question any and all assumptions' (Goleman et al., 1992, p. 36). Parse (1998) suggests that through the process of imaging, reality is constructed: 'The human is a questioning being, however, and all that is imaged explicitly–tacitly is an answer to a question, and the questioning is a searching for certainty in knowing' (p. 36).

The nurse scholar of the 21st century must be prepared to question everything and use imaging as a means of addressing the known and the unknown, of creating what is yet to be. Daring to be different and inventing new ways of viewing the familiar holds the potential for transforming nursing knowledge.

Recognizing the Significance of Language in Structuring Meaning and Reality

Edward Murray in Imaginative Thinking and Human Existence (1986) writes, 'Without words, no thing may be; with words, much may be. . . . It will be remembered that language operates within the horizon sketched out or drawn by the human imagination' (p. 83). Human language exists both in speaking–being silent and moving–being still (Parse, 1995). Gemma Fiumara (1990) in The Other Side of Language: A Philosophy of Listening calls for a society that 'pays heed' to each other through active listening. Such listening Fiumara (1990) refers to as 'life-enhancing' (p. 17). Newman (1999) cites the importance of listening and silence in relating with the pattern of others: 'If we want to get in touch with this pattern, we need to listen to the silence, to listen with our hearts, as we attune ourselves to the rhythm of the other person' (p. 227). Parse (1998) suggests

> Languaging is not just the content of what a person says with words, but how the whole message is uncovered in the context of the situation. It is the rhythmical moments of silence, the choice of words of syntax, the intonation, the facial expressions, the gestures, the posture, and that which is not said and movements that are not made that constitute the symbolic expression characteristic of languaging as a concept of structuring meaning multidimensionally. (p. 40)

The nurse scholar of the 21st century must learn to use the languaging of speaking—being silent and moving—being still carefully and constructively. This scholar needs to develop the skill of listening multidemensionality to what is said and what is left unsaid in the human interconnectedness with others and the universe. The careful and deliberate use of language is vital in expanding understanding of human health experiences.

Understanding Health as a Process

Nursing and other disciplines have come to explore health as much more than the absence of disease. Ferguson (1980) describes health as an attitude that reflects accepting responsibility for self in developing purpose in life. Dossey (1982) describes health as a shared phenomenon created by the person with the environment. Newman (1994a) describes health as a process of expanding consciousness, which is the ability of the individual to interact with the environment. Parse defines health as a process of personal becoming; it is a living of value choices (Parse, 1990). These encompassing definitions of health as process reflect the complexity of human life and the opportunity nurses have to work with people in a variety of settings to address changing patterns of health.

The nurse scholar of the 21st century must understand health as the way one chooses to live and be attuned to the choices involved in living one's patterns of health. The nurse scholar will need to continue to seek ways of working with individuals and groups as they choose ways of living with complex health issues.

Understanding Community as a Process

Community is much more than a place. Community is a process of 'living in relationship' (Bunkers et al., 1999, p. 92). Such community interconnectedness involves the interrelationship of ideas, people, places, events, and personal histories (Parse, 1999a). Newman (1994a) suggests 'that the focus of our discipline is the unitary field that combines person–family– community all at once' (p. xix). Parse (1996a) posits that community, in its most abstract sense, is viewed as 'the universe, the galaxy of human connect-edness' (p. 4). Parse (1999a) suggests that 'no engagement with another is without commu-nity. The individual is community, the family is community, the group is community, the world is community' (p. 120).

The nurse scholar of the 21st century must understand the connections–discon-nections occurring in human relationships in community. For example, nursing practice must respond to 'the relational connection–disconnection issues of those underserved by health and human resources' (Bunkers et al., 1999, p. 93). The nurse scholar needs to be prepared to work with the complexity of community, knowing that it is not a place one goes to, but is a unitary process of rela-tionship that one engages in.

Believing in the Power of Personal Presence

The power of the personal presence of the nurse is cornerstone for nursing prac-tice in the 21st century. Philosopher Kabir Helminski (1992) writes

> Presence signifies the quality of consciously being here. It is the activation of a higher level of awareness that allows all our other human functions—such as thought, feeling, and action—to be known, developed, and harmonized. Pre-sence is the way in which we occupy space, as well as how we flow and move. (p. viii)

Scholars of nursing have long written about and developed theoretical constructs concerning the importance of presence in nursing. Peplau (1952/1991) in her land-mark book The Nurse– Patient Relationship detailed clearly for the first time the healing quality of the nurse's presence with those struggling with emotional issues. Watson (1997) writes about the 'transpersonal car-ing relationship' as core to nursing. Newman (1994a) identifies authentic presence as key in working with others and states,

> The new paradigm of health, essential to nursing, embraces a unitary pat-tern of changing relationships. . . . The task is not to try to change another person's pattern but to recognize it as information that depicts the whole and relate to it as it unfolds. (p. 13)

Parse posits that the nurse–person pro-cess is the core of nursing and is lived in true presence. True presence is an intentional, reflective way of being with others in bear-ing witness to their changing health patterns. Parse (1997a) writes,

> The nurse in true presence joins the reality of the person at all realms of the universe and is open to him or her without judging or labeling. The person at all realms of his or her universe experiences the intent of the nurse, which is to bear witness to changing health patterns. The intent of the nurse is languaged in his or her whole being, in all realms of the universe, so words the subtle knowing the messages given and

taken at are not necessary to live true presence in the nurse–person process. (p. 35)

These examples of the importance of the nurse's presence indicate that it is the quality of the relationship between the nurse and other, not the quantity nor the task conducted, that is of central importance. Quality of presence implies competence in the tasks/skills needed in the setting in which a nurse has selected to practice. However, even more than this, it implies competence in the nurse–person process. It is critical that the nurse scholar of the 21st century be exposed to beliefs and values that elevate the power of the nurse's personal presence.

Participating in Scientific Inquiry

Scientific inquiry in nursing is critical to the ongoing development of the discipline. Nurse scholar Judy Norris (1999) states, 'Inquiry can be thought of as a transformative act accomplished by intentionally expending cognitive effort in activities such as discourse, reflection, reading, writing, or analysis' (p. 197). And, the goal of the discipline of nursing is 'to expand knowledge about human experiences through creative conceptualization and research' (Parse, 1999b, p. 275). It must also be remembered that the practice of science is both an individual and a social activity, for even great minds cannot work in isolation (Bronowski, 1978).

The nurse scholar of the 21st century must be mentored within a community of scholars. This community of scholars needs to focus on developing scientific inquiry that will continue to advance nursing science. The nurse scholar will need skills in creatively conceptualizing, dialoguing, utilizing research findings, and conducting either basic or applied research. The challenge of generating new knowledge for the discipline will be an ongoing one.

Asserting the Ethics of Individual and Communal Responsibility

The development of nursing knowledge and the role of the nurse scholar must be grounded in integrity and honesty. Bronowski (1978) points out,

Knowledge cannot be gained unless you behave in certain ways. . . . Once you regard truth (truth in detail) as the cement of the scientific community, then it follows at once that people have got to behave so that the truth shall be apparent. (pp. 129–130)

Bronowski (1978) goes on to identify personal values necessary for science to be carried out: individual values of sensitivity, tolerance, and respect, and the community values of honesty, integrity, dignity, and authenticity—'which bind the scientific community together' (Bronowski, 1978, p. 132).

The nurse scholar of the 21st century must provide leadership in advancing the knowledge base of the discipline. Values reflecting individual and communal responsibility for knowledge development must be reflected in the education and practice of nurses. Fawcett (1999) suggests that it is the discipline of nursing's responsibility to see that 'nurse scholars will actively engage in integrated research-practice activities, using nursing methodologies to test and apply conceptual models of nursing and nursing theories in the provision of nursing services to people' (p. 313).

Emphasizing Living in the Present Moment

Philosopher Thich Nhat Hanh (1998) writes concerning life being available only in the present moment. He posits that living fully in the moment requires mindfulness:

> The Chinese character for mindfulness has two components: heart, or mind, and present moment. To be mindful means to be fully present in the moment—not one part of you washing the dishes while another part is wondering when the work will be finished. . . . Conscious breathing is the vehicle that brings us back to the present moment and keeps us here. . . . Mindfulness leads to concentration and wisdom. . . . Mindfulness makes life real, deep, and worth living. It helps us be in the here and now where true life can be encountered. It helps us get in touch with refreshing and healing elements within and around us. (pp. 37–38)

The nurse scholar of the 21st century will need to understand the power of attending to what is happening here and now. Focusing on the now bids us to not hold on to what was or try to force what will be. Newman (1994a, p. 68) suggests, 'There is not basis

for rejecting any experience as irrelevant. The important factor is to be fully present in the moment.' Parse (1998) writes about focusing on the moment in true presence as 'a special way of 'being with' in which the nurse is attentive to moment-to-moment changes in meaning as she or he bears witness to the person's or group's own living of value priorities' (p. 71). The nurse scholar must be prepared to practice a mindfulness that cultivates sensitive encounters with others in the present moment and cultivates the development of wisdom.

Respecting Life and Nature

The unitary interconnectedness of all that is summons nursing to be concerned with and attend to the health of the universe. Sylvia Earle in the book Sea Change: A Message of the Oceans (1995) conveys an urgent call to action to do something about the damage being done to our global environment and the universe. Earle writes passionately about her concern for oceanic life:

> There's plenty of water in the universe without life, but nowhere is there life without water. . . . The living ocean provides the cornerstone of the life-support system for all creatures on our planet, from deep-sea starfish to desert sagebrush. That's why the ocean matters. If the sea is sick, we'll feel it. If it dies, we die. Our future and the state of the oceans are one. (p. xii)

The nurse scholar of the 21st century must be concerned with the treatment and care of nature. This scholar must study the interrelationship of life on this planet with the universe. Parse (1998) posits that the human–universe–health process is a mutual process and that 'quality of life is the meaning one gives to one's life at the moment in cocreation with the universe' (Parse, 1994b, p. 18). Respect for life and nature must coexist with respect for the advances of modern science and civilization.

Acknowledging Mystery

It is important for nurse scholars of the 21st century to know that there is much we do not know or understand. 'Acknowledging mystery involves recognizing that there is a power greater than ourselves present in the universe' (Bunkers, 1999a, p. 29). Nursing in the 21st century must work with the mystery of not knowing and acknowledge 'that not knowing is simply the first step toward truth' (Palmer, 1993, p. 72). Parse (1998) suggests that fundamental to understanding humans is 'the notion of the human as mystery—an appreciation of the unexplainable in human becoming' (p. 43). Acknowledging mystery and the unexplainable provides the nurse scholar of the 21st century with the foundation for developing questions for advancing nursing science.

Focusing on Quality of Life

The meaning individuals give experiences constitutes their quality of life (Parse, 1994a). Frankl (1984) suggests that meaning 'boils down to becoming aware of a possibility against the background of reality or . . . to becoming aware of what can be done about

a given situation' (p. 145). Gioiella (1994) writes about quality of life from an international perspective. She suggests quality of life is seen as a universal human goal: 'Nursing has a commitment internationally to work to achieve this goal' (p. 1). Theory development in nursing demonstrates various definitions of quality of life. Peplau (1994) suggests, 'Human relationships are a major determinant of quality of life' (p. 10). Leininger (1994) suggests that quality of life 'is culturally constituted and patterned' (p. 22). Parse (1994a) posits that quality of life 'is what the person there living the lie says that it is' (p. 17); 'the unitary perspective is essential to capture the meaning of quality of life now and in the next millennium' (p. 20).

The nurse scholar of the 21st century must be prepared to understand the meanings persons give to life experience, thus being in concert with their quality of life issues. As Florence Nightingale addressed the challenges to quality of life posed to her by the meanings she gave experiences in the Crimean War, so too will the nurse scholar of the 21st century be challenged to respond to quality of life issues for the betterment of humankind.

Conclusion

The development of the nurse as scholar is a journey, a journey that began over a century ago. Parse (1994b) identifies three crucial processes involved in scholarship: 'perpetual curiosity, a focused commitment, and a willingness to risk challenge' (p. 143). On this journey of scholarship, perpetual curiosity must be fostered in those who will question and who wish to discover the new. A focused commitment must be modeled by mentors of the discipline and lived in their day-to-day practice of both the art and science of nursing. A willingness to risk challenge calls for courage to push forward with nursing theory and model development in expanding nursing science. Are we, the nursing community of today ready for this challenge of scholarship? Florence Nightingale (1859) wrote in Notes on Nursing, 'For it may safely be said, not that the habit of ready and correct observation will by itself make us useful nurses, but that without it we shall be useless with all our devotion' (p. 63). A habit of ready and correct observation, a habit of continual scholarship, is the call for nursing in the 21st century.

References

Bronowski, J. (1978). The origins of knowledge and imagination. London: Yale University Press.

Bunkers, S. S. (1998). Considering tomorrow: Parse's theory-guided research. Nursing Science Quarterly, 11, 56–63.

Bunkers, S. S. (1999a). Emerging discoveries and possibilities in nursing. Nursing Science Quarterly, 12, 26–29.

Bunkers, S. S. (1999b). The teaching-learning process and the theory of human becoming. Nursing Science Quarterly, 12, 227–232.

Bunkers, S. S., Nelson, M., Leuning, C., Crane, J., & Josephson, D. (1999). In E. Cohen & V. De Back (Eds.), The outcomes mandate: Case management in health care today (pp. 92–100). St. Louis: Mosby.

Bunkers, S. S., & Putnam, V. (1995). A nursing based model of health ministry: Living Parse's theory of human becoming in parish nursing. In Ninth Annual Westberg Parish Nurse Symposium: Parish nursing: Ministering through the arts (pp. 197–212). Northbrook, IL: Advocate Health Care.

Chinn, P. (1991). Theory and nursing: A systemic approach. St. Louis: Mosby.

Daly, J. (1995). The view of suffering within the human becoming theory. In R. R. Parse (Ed.), Illuminations: The human becoming theory in practice and research (pp. 45–59). New York: National League for Nursing Press.

Damgaard, G., & Bunkers, S. S. (1998). Nursing science-guided practice and education: A state board of nursing perspective. Nursing Science Quarterly, 11, 142–144.

Dossey, L. (1982). Space, time and medicine. Boulder, CO: Shambhala.

Earle, S. (1995). Sea change: A message of the oceans. New York: Fawcett Columbine.

Fawcett, J. (1999). The state of nursing science: Hallmarks of the 20th and 21st centuries. Nursing Science Quarterly, 12, 311–315.

Ferguson, M. (1980). The Aquarian conspiracy: Personal and social transformation in the 1980s. Los Angeles: J. P. Tarcher.

Fiumara, G. C. (1990). The other side of language: A philosophy of listening. New York: Routledge.

Frankl, V. (1984). Man's search for meaning. New York: Simon & Schuster.

Gioiella, E. C. (1994). Quality of life: An international commitment. Nursing Science Quarterly, 7, 1.

Goleman, D., Kaufman, P., & Ray, M. (1992). The creative spirit. New York: Dutton.

Hanh, T. N. (1998). Interbeing. Berkeley, CA: Parallax Press.

Helminski, K. E. (1992). Living presence. New York: Putnam.

Leininger, M. (1994). Quality of life from a transcultural nursing perspective. Nursing Science Quarterly, 7, 22–28.

Mitchell, G. (1991). Nursing diagnosis: An ethical analysis. Image: Journal of Nursing Scholarship, 23, 99–103.

Murray, E. (1986). Imaginative thinking and human existence. Pittsburgh: Duquesne University Press.

Newman, M. (1994a). Health as expanding consciousness (2nd ed.). New York: National League for Nursing Press.

Newman, M. (1994b). Into the 21st century. Nursing Science Quarterly, 7, 44–46.

Newman, M. (1999). The rhythm of relating in a paradigm of wholeness. Image: Journal of Nursing Scholarship, 31(3), 227–229.

Nightingale, F. (1859). Notes on nursing. London: Harrison.

Norris, J. R. (1999). The Internet: Extending our capacity for scholarly inquiry in nursing. Nursing Science Quarterly, 12, 197–201.

Palmer, P. (1993). To know as we are known. San Francisco: Harper-Collins.

Parse, R. R. (1990). Health: A personal commitment. Nursing Science Quarterly, 3, 136–140.

Parse, R. R. (1994a). Quality of life: Sciencing and living the art of human becoming. Nursing Science Quarterly, 10, 16–21.

Parse, R. R. (1994b). Scholarship: Three essential processes. Nursing Science Quarterly, 7, 143.

Parse, R. R. (1995). Building the realm of nursing knowledge. Nursing Science Quarterly, 8, 51.

Parse, R. R. (1996a). Community: A human becoming perspective. Illuminations: The Newsletter of the International Consortium of Parse Scholars, 5(1), 1–4.

Parse, R. R. (1996b). The human becoming theory: Challenges in practice and research. Nursing Science Quarterly, 9, 55–60.

Parse, R. R. (1997a). The human becoming theory: The was, is, and will be. Nursing Science Quarterly, 10, 32–38.

Parse, R. R. (1997b). Joy-sorrow: A study using the Parse research method. Nursing Science Quarterly, 10, 80–87.

Parse, R. R. (1998). The human becoming school of thought. Thousand Oaks, CA: Sage.

Parse, R. R. (1999a). Community: An alternative view. Nursing Science Quarterly, 12, 119–121.

Parse, R. R. (1999b). Nursing: The discipline and the profession. Nursing Science Quarterly, 12, 275–276.

Peplau, H. E. (1991). Interpersonal relations in nursing. New York: Springer Publishing Company. (Original work published 1952.)

Peplau, H. E. (1994). Quality of life: An interpersonal perspective. Nursing Science Quarterly, 7, 10–15.

Rawnsley, M. (1999). Response to Fawcett's 'The state of nursing science.' Nursing Science Quarterly, 12, 315–318.

Rogers, M. (1992). Nightingale's notes on nursing: Prelude to the 21st century. In D. Carroll (Ed.), Notes on Nursing by Florence Nightingale (Commemorative edition) (pp. 58–62). Philadelphia: J. B. Lippincott Company.

Roy, C. (1992). Vigor, variables, and vision: Commentary of Florence Nightingale. In D. Carroll (Ed.), Notes on Nursing by Florence Nightingale (Commemorative edition) (pp. 63–71). Philadelphia: J. B. Lippincott Company.

Sartre, J. P. (1956). Being and nothingness. New York: Philosophical Library, Inc.

Schuyler, C. (1992). Florence Nightingale. In D. Carroll (Ed.), Notes on Nursing by Florence Nightingale (Commemorative edition) (pp. 3–17). Philadelphia: J. B. Lippincott Company.

Watson, J. (1997). The theory of human caring: Retrospective and prospective. Nursing Science Quarterly, 10, 49–52.

Webster's ninth new collegiate dictionary. (1990). Springfield, MA: Merriam-Webster.

Index